Mothers, Babies, and Cocaine:
The Role of Toxins in Development

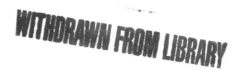

Mothers, Babies, and Cocaine:
The Role of Toxins in Development

Edited by

Michael Lewis
Margaret Bendersky
Robert Wood Johnson Medical School

LEA LAWRENCE ERLBAUM ASSOCIATES, PUBLISHERS
1995 Hillsdale, New Jersey   Hove, UK

Copyright © 1995 by Lawrence Erlbaum Associates, Inc.
 All rights reserved. No part of the book may be reproduced in
 any form, by photostat, microform, retrieval system, or any other
 means, without the prior written permission of the publisher.

Lawrence Erlbaum Associates, Inc., Publishers
365 Broadway
Hillsdale, New Jersey 07642

Library of Congress Cataloging-in-Publication Data

Mothers, babies, and cocaine : the role of toxins in development /
 edited by Michael Lewis, Margaret Bendersky.
     p.   cm.
   Includes bibliographical references and index.
   ISBN 0-8058-1583-X. — ISBN 0-8058-1584-8 (pbk.)
   1. Cocaine habit.   2. Drug abuse in pregnancy.   3. Fetus—Effect
of drugs on.   4. Children of prenatal subtance abuse—Development.
I. Lewis, Michael, 1937 Jan. 10–   . II. Bendersky, Margaret.
RG580.D76M68   1995
618.3′268—dc20   94-42935
                                                      CIP

Books published by Lawrence Erlbaum Associates are printed on acid-free
paper, and their bindings are chosen for strength and durability.

Printed in the United States of America
10 9 8 7 6 5 4 3 2

Contents

Foreword   ix
Coryl LaRue Jones

Preface   xi

PART I: MODELS

1   Developmental Toxicity of Cocaine: Mechanisms
of Action   5
Diana L. Dow-Edwards

2   Prenatal Cocaine Exposure and Child Outcome:
What Do We Really Know?   19
Barry M. Lester, Kiti Freier, and Lyn LaGasse

3   Incipient Hazards of Cocaine: Lessons
from Environmental Toxicology?   41
Bernard Weiss

4   Methadone During Pregnancy: A Brief Review
of Clinical Outcome and a New Animal Model   57
Donald E. Hutchings and Ann C. Zmitrovich

PART II: METHODS

5   A Review of Developmental Exposure Models
    for CNS Stimulants: Cocaine   71
    Charles V. Vorhees

6   The Problem of Confounding in Research on Prenatal
    Cocaine Effects on Behavior and Development   95
    Daniel R. Neuspiel

7   Strategies for Detecting the Effects of Prenatal Drug
    Exposure: Lessons from Research on Alcohol   111
    Joseph L. Jacobson and Sandra W. Jacobson

8   A Cohort Study of Prenatal Cocaine Exposure:
    Addressing Methodological Concerns   129
    Heather Carmichael Olson, Therese M. Grant,
    Joan C. Martin, and Ann P. Streissguth

9   Measuring the Effects of Prenatal Cocaine Exposure   163
    Margaret Bendersky, Steven M. Alessandri,
    Margaret Wolan Sullivan, and Michael Lewis

10 Meconium Drug Analysis   179
    Enrique M. Ostrea, Jr.

PART III: OUTCOMES

11 Alterations in Cognitive Function Following Prenatal
    Cocaine Exposure: Studies in an Animal Model   207
    Linda Patia Spear

12 Neurophysiological Effects of Prenatal Cocaine
    Exposure: Comparison of Human and Animal
    Investigations   229
    Robert Needlman, Deborah A. Frank, Marilyn Augustyn,
    and Barry S. Zuckerman

13 Developmental Dilemmas for Cocaine-Abusing
    Parents and Their Children   251
    Linda C. Mayes and Marc H. Bornstein

14 Temperament in Cocaine-Exposed Infants   273
       Steven M. Alessandri, Margaret Wolan Sullivan,
       Margaret Bendersky, and Michael Lewis

15 Attentional and Social Functioning of Preschool-Age
       Children Exposed to PCP and Cocaine in Utero   287
       Leila Beckwith, Senobia Crawford, Jacqueline A. Moore,
       and Judy Howard

16 Cocaine Use Among Pregnant Women: Socioeconomic,
       Obstetrical, and Psychological Issues   305
       Nanci Stewart Woods, Marylou Behnke, Fonda Davis Eyler,
       Michael Conlon, and Kathleen Wobie

PART IV: INTERVENTION

17 Effective Early Intervention for Children Prenatally
       Exposed to Cocaine in an Inner-City Context   335
       Abigail Baxter, Linda S. Butler, Richard P. Brinker,
       Wynetta A. Frazier, and Delores M. Wedgeworth

18 Cocaine Exposure and Intervention
       in Early Development   355
       Tiffany Field

       Author Index   369

       Subject Index   393

Foreword

Coryl LaRue Jones
National Institute on Drug Abuse

The material represented in this volume on the effects of maternal cocaine use during pregnancy and the role of toxins in human development could not have been conceptualized a mere 10 years ago when cocaine began to become a drug of choice among drug-using women of childbearing age. In 1986, when the Public Health Service convened its expert panel to examine the scientific basis for the content of prenatal care, tobacco and alcohol use during pregnancy were identified as major problems, but drug abuse was presented as an undifferentiated problem of a special population of addicted women who could be treated with methadone. The panel and the public had to be made aware of the differences among the different types of illicit drugs, of the fact that methadone was a pharmaceutical intervention for opiate addiction—not other drugs and not cocaine—and that knowledge of drug use needed to become a mainstream concern because of its impact on health care, child development, and society. The point had to be made that "crack babies" do not exist, they are babies exposed to cocaine among many other things, including tobacco, alcohol, marijuana, heroin, and lead, and subjected to malnutrition and other ramifications of maternal lifestyle, biology, and genetic vulnerability.

In the mid-1980s technologies needed to be developed to assess the presence/absence of a range of drugs, contaminants, and their metabolites. Urine screening was and is useful in determining compliance in drug treatment, but was not and is not adequate for studies of cocaine exposure. Meconium assays and hair analysis were just entering the scene. Postnatal passive exposures needed to be assessed. Models needed to be developed of direct and indirect pharmacologic and behavioral effects. The behavior of the neonate and young child needed to be considered as an interactive contributing factor to adult behaviors toward the child. The ways in which drug use affected maternal behaviors needed to be considered. Identifying primary care providers and their characteristics would influence how a child might behave in assessment situations involving attachment or the accuracy of maternal reports. Child environments and cultural attributes also needed to be factored into the models. Child abuse, neglect, and violence in the home and immediate environment pervaded such research, and political battles raged about criminalizing drug use by pregnant women. Reporting requirements regarding maternal drug use as child abuse varied by jurisdiction and could determine child custody. Investigators had to assume responsibility for reporting child abuse and neglect and inform potential subjects that they might be reported if they participated in such studies. Such factors burdened progress but sharpened awareness of factors which confounded research on human development and drug abuse. HIV infection was an exclusion factor unless the study focused on pediatric AIDS.

The National Institute on Drug Abuse (NIDA) had supported treatment research for pregnant and parenting women as far back as NIDA's own conception in 1974, but the baby was not the identified subject; the mother was. Determining biologic paternal links was (and remains) a legal quagmire in human studies. The heroin-addicted mother usually kept her baby as they moved into their troubled future. Cocaine use by pregnant women changed this.

Whereas opiates are sedative, and the user "comes down" slowly after heroin use, cocaine is a fast-acting stimulant with a quick rush and a rapid descent in which depression and suicidal ideation are known risks. Cocaine users began to use heroin and other drugs to cope with the rapid decline from a cocaine episode. The baby exposed to cocaine became a child of a polydrug-abusing mother. The prenatal cocaine pharmacologic model fell short, and the complex drug-involved model became a state-of-the-science necessity.

A time factor may also exist. A close look at studies of the short- and long-term effects of marijuana exposure and barbiturate exposure indicates that significant effects identified postnatally abate to trends or disappear during childhood—or are overwhelmed by environmental factors, as in the heroin and methadone studies—but emerge again in early adolescence when memory, concentration, and cumulative small effects interfere with learning and performance. This scientific need to develop complex longitudinal models that incorporate pharmacologic, genetic, familial, and environmental factors in the dynamics of human development research has increased demands for an integrated link between basic research with animal models and clinical research in natural environments.

Major steps have occurred in drug abuse research. A first step was bringing the best minds in child development research into the drug abuse research field. Another step was the closer link between basic and clinical research. This volume is a testament to the significant contributions made by these joint ventures.

Preface

An alarming number of women use substances of abuse during pregnancy. The nationwide prevalence has been estimated to be as high as 20%, exposing nearly half a million fetuses to potentially damaging substances every year. But what are the effects of such prenatal exposure on the developing fetus? Cocaine, particularly in the form of crack, is one of the drugs of choice of many users, including women of childbearing age. Will children whose mothers smoked crack or used other substances of abuse during pregnancy be the tremendous burden on our medical and education resources that some have predicted? The answers to these questions are far from clear, but it is important that answers be found. Research efforts are underway in many laboratories around the country. Scientists have gone beyond the early models of simple cause and effect. We are at an exciting juncture in thinking about long-term sequelae of prenatal drug and toxin exposure.

Research on this topic is of both theoretical and practical importance. The theoretical importance rests in the need to test both general and specific models of development. For example, what are the interactive effects of drug exposure and environment on children's development? Is it the cocaine exposure in utero that causes infant patho-development and, if so, what are its specific effects? As we shall see, using cocaine when pregnant may itself be a marker for environments that cause patho-development. In the chapters that follow, these and other questions are raised from both animal and human studies.

This volume is both timely and unique. It grows out of a conference sponsored by the Center for Human Development and Developmental Disabilities, an interdisciplinary effort of the Department of Pediatrics, Robert Wood Johnson

Medical School—University of Medicine and Dentistry of New Jersey. In addition to the participants represented in the chapters, Barbara Ostfeld, Mujahid Anwar, David Mandelbaum, and Karol Kaltenbach also attended and contributed to the volume through discussions. This volume is the first in a series that aims to address topics pertaining to developmental disabilities and retardation. This collection of chapters addresses the critical question of the effects of prenatal exposure to cocaine and related toxins on the developing central nervous system. It looks at the consequences for early neurodevelopmental function as well as more complex outcomes, which include learning ability, responses to stress, and emotional development; areas with profound implications for long-term functioning. The volume presents integrated theories deriving from a multiple risk model of development. Unlike previously published works, this perspective emphasizes the interrelated effects of a variety of developmental forces, both organismic and environmental, that contribute to long-term outcome. The chapters cover a wide range of topics, from models of the mechanism of effects of cocaine and other toxins to methodological issues involved in doing human research in an area fraught with difficulties. Results from animal as well as human research add to the breadth of information on the topic of toxins and development.

The volume is divided into four parts. In the first, models involved in the study of toxins and development are presented. Part II presents the various methodological issues encountered in the study of toxins. Outcomes as a consequence of exposure is the content of the third part, and Part IV deals with issues related to intervention.

We hope that this volume will appeal to researchers and clinicians from a variety of disciplines, including toxicology, pharmacology, neuroscience, behavioral medicine, developmental psychology, medical practice, social service providers, and education. In order to address this diverse set, we have tried to present complex information with much of the technical terminology fully explained or reduced. It is our hope that this volume will underscore the importance of this problem both in terms of popular interest as well as scientific study.

Finally, we would like to express appreciation to David Carver, Chairman of the Department of Pediatrics, for supporting this conference series. In addition, we wish to thank Barbara Britten, Vice President; Linda Dite, Director of Maternal–Child Health Nursing; and Patricia Gilbert, Director of the High-Risk Infant Follow-up Clinic, at Mercer Medical Center, and Sonya Imaizumi, Neonatologist at the Medical College of Pennsylvania, without whose support our work in the area of prenatal substance abuse would not be possible.

Michael Lewis
Margaret Bendersky

I

▼▼▼▼▼▼▼▼▼

MODELS

Research in a new area of inquiry typically advances according to a standard pattern. A theory is generated that is subject to empirical inquiry. Based on the findings, the theory may be refined and again tested by appropriately designed studies. This cycling of theory and empirical test continues until a detailed valid theory evolves, which explains all of the observed data, and on which accurate predictions can be based. The four chapters in this section present the current state of theoretical and empirically based conceptualizations of the effects of cocaine. The authors present potential mechanisms of effects of cocaine from the direct pharmacological action on developing fetal cells, to the effects on early neurobehavior, and the long-term, indirect functional consequences through complex organism and environment interactions over time. The section also provides suggestions for appropriate research models to advance our understanding further.

Dow-Edwards reviews what is known of the specific pharmacologic effects of cocaine on a developing organism. Cocaine inhibits reuptake of three major neurotransmitters—dopamine, serotonin, and norepinephrine; acts as a potent local anesthetic that has the potential to disrupt the normal development of excitable tissues; and is a powerful vasoconstrictor that could reduce the flow of oxygen-rich blood to a fetus. The challenge is not only to study cocaine's mechanisms of action on the developing brain further, but to elaborate a model of how these direct effects translate into functional impact on an organism.

Lester, Freier, and LaGasse take up this challenge: "What do we really know?" They offer a multiple risk systems model that accounts for both the short-term acute and longer term developmental effects of prenatal cocaine exposure. This model has not only been informed by early research on the effects of cocaine exposure, but also by lessons learned over the last three decades of research on the development of other high-risk populations, in particular preterm infants. In this model, the direct and indirect actions of cocaine affect neuroregulatory mechanisms that may result in early behavioral disorders of attention, arousal, affect, and action. There is then an interaction between these short-term neurobehavioral effects and environmental factors that can exaggerate the child's vulnerability, resulting in longer term problems, or help the child to regulate his or her behavior with few long-term problems as a consequence. The authors powerfully convey the complexities of a developmental model with a multiplicity of environmental variables and range of potential behavioral effects.

The remaining chapters in this section propose models for approaching the study of cocaine's impact that have been field tested in other areas of behavioral teratology and hazard risk assessment. Weiss recommends a model for approaching the question of effects of prenatal exposure derived from the process of risk assessment used to identify environmental chemical pollutants. He describes four stages of risk assessment: hazard identification, dose–response assessment, exposure assessment, and risk characterization. Weiss contends that cocaine has been identified as a developmental neurotoxicant; however, the succeeding risk assessment steps have not been taken. Not only is the dose-response curve ill defined, but exposure assessment is lacking, particularly the cumulative or low-level exposure risk. Without this information, the actual risk of prenatal cocaine exposure cannot be adequately characterized. Weiss reminds us that a broad perspective of the potential effects of cocaine exposure is in order at this stage of our knowledge. He presents examples of long latency onset diseases such as cancers, Parkinson's disease, and amyotrophic lateral sclerosis, and well-studied environmental chemicals including lead and mercury, which he feels provide valuable lessons to the cocaine researcher.

In the final chapter of this section, Hutchings and Zmitrovich review some of the methodological and interpretive issues encountered in prenatal methadone exposure research and offer a new animal model. Of particular concern to these authors is the comparability of animal dosing regimens to human patterns of use. The authors also describe disruptions in the rest–activity cycle and acoustic startle of the 3- to 4-week-old rat, which they suggest are useful indicators of a compound's potential to produce neonatal abstinence effects. These lessons in pharmacological teratology can be applied to the design of animal research into effects of prenatal cocaine exposure.

All of the authors agree that there is still much to learn at all levels of the question of effects of prenatal cocaine exposure. They suggest that through the application of lessons from previous research with other high-risk populations, and the generation of hypotheses based on models of cocaine's specific effects, the field can take a giant step toward a complete answer to this pressing question.

1

▼▼▼▼▼▼▼

Developmental Toxicity of Cocaine: Mechanisms of Action

Diana L. Dow-Edwards
State University of New York
Health Sciences Center at Brooklyn

Since the mid-1980s, much attention has been paid to the effects of cocaine on human development. Several excellent reviews have been published (e.g., Neuspiel & Hamel, 1991). In general, the consensus among clinicians is that cocaine use during pregnancy is associated with several adverse outcomes. However, the evidence for long-term neurobehavioral sequelae in exposed children is more difficult to obtain due to a myriad of confounding factors such as maternal polydrug and alcohol consumption, smoking, and several lifestyle factors that all contribute to adverse outcomes of exposed children. Cocaine alone probably does not produce structural defects (with the possible exception of hydronephrosis) but does appear to produce some neurobehavioral alterations that vary according to the population under study (see Hutchings, 1993). Due to the inherent problems in doing clinical research in this area, researchers have relied on studies of animals, particularly the rat, to determine whether cocaine exposure during development produces a consistent pattern of biological effects. Fortunately, the effects of cocaine on the nervous system of the rat are similar, in many ways, to those on the nervous system of humans, and because we know much more about developmental neurochemistry in the rat than in humans, we can address questions about the mechanisms of action only in the animal model (Dow-Edwards, 1991).

The purpose of this chapter, then, is to review the evidence that cocaine produces its neurobehavioral effects in exposed neonates through specific pharmacologic effects. Cocaine has a complex pharmacology. First, it acts as an inhibitor of reuptake of three major neurotransmitters: dopamine, serotonin, and norepinephrine (thus potentiating their actions). Cocaine also is a potent local anesthetic, a property that could potentially alter the developmental course of all excitable tissues. Lastly, cocaine is a potent vasoconstrictor that could reduce blood supply to and oxygenation of the fetus—factors that are known to produce adverse postnatal outcomes. Other effects of cocaine, such as binding to the muscarinic cholinergic receptor, have not been adequately investigated and therefore are not discussed.

HYPOXIA

Evidence abounds that chronic or intermittent hypoxia during gestation produces permanent neurobehavioral alterations (Longo & Hermans, 1992; Mactutus & Fechter, 1986). The work of Woods, Plessinger, and Clark (1987) and others (Moore, Sorg, Miller, Key, & Resnik, 1986) has shown that cocaine reduces uteroplacental perfusion in sheep in a dose-dependent manner. That is, the degree of vasoconstriction and hypoxia produced by maternal intravenous (IV) cocaine administration closely parallels the maternal plasma cocaine levels (Woods, Plessinger, Scott, & Miller, 1989). Fetal oxygen pressures fall significantly and remain low for approximately 15 min following the highest dose of cocaine given (Woods et al., 1987). Because the sheep is an excellent model for the human cardiovascular system, these studies provide strong evidence that the vasoconstrictive effects of cocaine must be considered as important mechanisms of action in producing developmental toxicity in humans. The work in sheep, however, cannot, a priori, be extrapolated to the rat due to differences between rodents and sheep in the responses to cocaine. The early studies on the effects of cocaine on the cardiovascular system in rodents were sparse and contradictory. In some vascular beds in certain experimental models, cocaine actually could be considered a vasodilator. Systemic blood pressure, for example, decreases between 40% and 45% following 5 mg/kg cocaine IV in a pentobarbital anesthetized rat (Pitts, Udom, & Marwah, 1987). The pressure returns to control levels within 5 min. However, if the rat is alert, the pressure initially rises and then returns to baseline within 1 min after the cocaine is administered.

Only recently the effects of pregnancy on the cardiovascular responses to cocaine administration have been examined in the rat. Hohmann, Keve, Osol, and McLaughlin (1990) reported that in mesenteric veins, the potentiation of the response to transmural stimulation by cocaine was greater in the pregnant than nonpregnant rat. In mesenteric arteries, Crandall, Keve, and McLaughlin (1990) found that although pregnancy decreased the response to norepinephrine, it increased the response to cocaine. Together, these studies indicate that pregnancy increases the vasoconstrictive actions of cocaine in the mesentary but that the effects of natural catecholamines can be reduced by pregnancy. Therefore, in order to attribute a portion of the neurobehavioral effects of cocaine exposure during rodent development to the vasoactive effects of the drug, these effects need to be determined empirically.

We recently completed a study where cocaine was administered at 60 mg/kg intragastric (IG) to 22-day pregnant, nonanesthetized rats (1 day prior to parturition) and then uteroplacental blood flow was determined using [^{14}C]iodoantipyrine just after the time of the peak plasma cocaine concentration. If cocaine produced vasoconstriction in the rat that paralleled the plasma cocaine levels as Woods et al. (1989) showed for the sheep, then, at 17 min postintubation, we should have seen the maximal cardiovascular effect because, at 15 min, the plasma levels are maximal in the rat (Dow-Edwards, 1990). The effects of cocaine on physiologic variables important to the blood flow determination are shown in Table 1.1. Although cocaine had no effect on maternal blood gases and pH, hematocrit, or systolic and diastolic blood pressure, it did significantly reduce heart rate compared to precocaine levels. There were also no significant effects of cocaine on fetal blood gases and pH with the exception that fetal pO$_2$ was reduced compared to those whose mothers received saline. Rates of blood flow were decreased by 27% and

TABLE 1.1
Physiological Variables Collected Prior to Iodoantipyrine Infusion

	Control (n = 7)		Cocaine (60 mg/kg) (n = 7)	
Maternal Data				
Body weight	418 ± 8		422 ± 11	
Rectal temperature	37.0 ± .1		37.2 ± .1	
B.P. mean (mmHg)	102 ± 2		98 ± 5	
Hematocrit %	.35 ± .02		.36 ± .03	
pH	7.373 ± .016		7.392 ± .030	
pCO$_2$ (mmHg)	28.5 ± 1.2		26.0 ± 1.6	
pO$_2$ (mmHg)	101.7 ± 7.4		109.3 ± 5.8	
HCO$_3$	16.5 ± 0.9		15.6 ± 0.9	
	Before	*After*	*Before*	*After*
Systolic	123 ± 3	122 ± 3	121 ± 3	115 ± 4***
Diastolic	93 ± 6	88 ± 2	100 ± 5	95 ± 4***
Heart Rate	443 ± 10	446 ± 22	488 ± 12	425 ± 12**
Fetal Data[a]				
pH	7.061 ± .022		7.042 ± .065	
pCO$_2$ (mmHg)	73.7 ± 7.7		63.1 ± 7.7	
pO$_2$ (mmHg)	6.1 ± 1.1		2.7 ± 0.8*	
HCO$_3$	19.7 ± 1.6		17.1 ± 1.7	

[a]Data from sample with lowest pO$_2$.
*Significantly different from control value ($p < .05$ t test).
**Significantly different from predrug value ($p = .006$, paired t test).
***Different from predrug value ($p = .06$, paired t test).

30% in the uterus and placenta, respectively, following cocaine administration (Dow-Edwards, Grose, Freed-Malen, & Hughes, 1993).

Morishima, Cooper, Hara, and Miller (1992) recently examined the effects of cocaine administered IV to pregnant rats and found that cocaine decreased heart rate, cardiac output, and cerebral, myocardial, and utero placental blood flow in pregnant rats compared to precocaine baselines. Systemic blood pressure was significantly increased. In nonpregnant rats, cocaine only decreased cerebral blood flow. Therefore, although they did not quantify fetal blood gas or pH concentrations, their study and our study can generally be taken as evidence that cocaine reduces uteroplacental perfusion in the pregnant rat. Hypoxia should, therefore, be considered as a possible mechanism whereby cocaine produces neurobehavioral alterations in the offspring of rats as it most certainly does in humans.

A few studies have appeared that provide indirect evidence for the importance of hypoxia in producing cocaine's developmental toxicity. For example, prenatal cocaine administration increases ornithine decarboxylase activity in much the same way as hypoxia alone does (Bondy, Nakla, Ali, & Ahmad, 1990; Longo & Hermans, 1992; Seidler & Slotkin, 1993). Webster, Brown-Woodman, Lipson, and Ritchie (1991) provided evidence that ip cocaine produced structural changes in the brain that closely resemble those produced by clamping a uterine artery. However, to date, the hypoxic profile of the fetus, either human or rodent, produced by maternal cocaine administration has not been adequately documented and reproduced to demonstrate that the neurobehavioral effects of prenatal cocaine exposure are the result of the hypoxia produced by the drug. Therefore, further work is needed in this area.

LOCAL ANESTHETIC EFFECTS

Cocaine is a potent local anesthetic and, in fact, its only clinical use today is as such. In this regard, cocaine blocks Na channels and, therefore, would attenuate action potentials in excitable cells (Matthews & Collins, 1983). The effects of exposure to local anesthetics during development have not been adequately studied. Numerous studies have appeared that document the effects of local anesthetics used peripartum and some have examined the teratology and toxicology of lidocaine (Fujinaga & Mazze, 1986; Ramazzotto, Curro, Paterson, Tanner, & Coleman, 1985). Smith, Warton, Kurtz, Mattran, and Hollenbeck (1986) and Teiling et al. (1987) examined the neurobehavioral effects on offspring of a single maternal injection of lidocaine, and are not in agreement about the effects, but none has examined the neurobehavioral consequences of long-term administration during pregnancy. One can, however, predict that cocaine would have long-term functional consequences based on other studies that show that the propagation of action potentials is critical for normal synaptic formation and neuronal function (Wiesel, 1982, in the visual system and van der Loos & Woolsey, 1973, in the somatosensory system). In addition, there is evidence that nerves from young rabbits are more sensitive to local anesthetics than nerves in adult rabbits (Benzon et al., 1988). Therefore, lidocaine or other local anesthetics can be administered to developing animals to mimic the local anesthetic effects of cocaine. This approach should enable an assessment of the importance of these effects on the overall developmental toxicity of cocaine. Recently, two papers have compared the effects of lidocaine to those of cocaine in the neonatal rat (Anderson-Brown, Slotkin, & Seidler, 1990; Koegler, Seidler, Spencer, & Slotkin, 1991). In both cases, the effects of lidocaine did not resemble the effects of cocaine. That is, cocaine alone inhibited DNA synthesis and decreased ornithine decarboxylase, whereas lidocaine at equivalent doses did not. On the other hand, Stewart and colleagues (W. Slikker, personal communication, July, 1993) examined the effects of lidocaine (40 mg/kg/day) administered during the last 2 weeks of pregnancy in the rat and found that lidocaine-exposed pups exhibited an amount of stereotypy (following quinpirole, a D-2 agonist, challenge) that was equal to that seen in the pups exposed to an equal dose of cocaine prenatally and challenged with the same quinpirole doses.

Our laboratory examined the effects of lidocaine in comparison to cocaine on cerebral blood flow in the 10-day-old rat pup. At this age, the rat brain is still developing and blood flow can be used as an indicator of overall cerebral functional activity. Although we have not completed the analysis, preliminary examination of the results indicates that cocaine and lidocaine do produce similar effects on brain function but that these effects are quite subtle. Therefore, until a full analysis of the acute effects of lidocaine on the developing brain and several experiments documenting the consequences of chronic lidocaine exposure on neurobehavioral development have been completed, the contribution of the local anesthetic effects of cocaine to its overall toxicity will not be known.

REUPTAKE INHIBITION: DOPAMINE

Certainly the actions of cocaine on the dopamine system have received the greatest amount of interest in recent times. This is perhaps because it is fairly well accepted that the reinforcing effects of cocaine are due to its ability to inhibit dopamine reuptake (e.g., Koob & Bloom, 1988; Ritz, Lamb, Goldberg, & Kuhar, 1987). Briefly, cocaine binds to and inhibits the dopamine carrier in the presynaptic terminal, thus increasing the amount of dopamine in the synapse, that is, potentiating the effect of dopamine. The dopamine carrier has been functionally identified in the rat brain as early as 16 days of gestation (Fiszman, Zuddas, Masana, Barker, & di Porzio, 1991; Hanbauer & Grilli, 1992; Yotsumoto & Nomura, 1981) and, in the adult, is located in several important neuronal structures, including the caudate nucleus, the accumbens, the olfactory tubercle, subthalamus, ventral tegmental area, substantia nigra, and anterior olfactory nucleus

(Javitch, Strittmatter, & Snyder, 1985). In the adult, acute cocaine administration results in an increase in dopamine concentration in the caudate (Church, Justice, & Byrd, 1987). Because one cannot a priori assume that drug effects in the fetus are the same as those seen in the adult and because alterations in neurochemical measures in the fetus following maternal drug administration could be secondary to changes in maternal physiology in addition to direct actions of the drug, the effects of cocaine on the dopamine system must be examined in the developing brain before this mechanism can be established as that producing the developmental toxicity. It is clear, however, that a growing body of evidence indicates that cocaine has effects on the development of the dopamine system. For example, changes in dopamine receptors (Dow-Edwards, Freed, & Fico, 1990; Henderson, McConnaughey, & McMillian, 1991; Scalzo, Ali, Frambes, & Spear, 1990), neurotransmitter content, metabolism in dopamine-rich regions of brain (Dow-Edwards et al., 1990), response to dopamine challenge drugs (Meyer, Sherlock, & Macdonald, 1992; Peris, Coleman-Hardee, & Millard, 1992; W. Slikker, personal communication, July, 1993), and changes in spontaneous action potentials of dopamine neurons (Minabe, Ashby, Heyser, Spear, & Wang, 1992) have all been described following prenatal cocaine administration. Therefore, the potential for cocaine to produce its developmental toxicity through its effects on the dopamine system is certainly there. To date, however, the empirical evidence is just evolving.

The use of newly synthesized compounds that mimic specific actions of cocaine has enabled investigators to begin to tease out cocaine's complicated effects. One such compound, GBR 12909 (Anderson, 1989) is a potent inhibitor of the dopamine carrier, but it differs from cocaine in that it slowly dissociates from the carrier compared to cocaine and it does not increase extracellular dopamine as much as cocaine does (Rothman et al., 1991). Therefore, although both compounds may bind to the same carrier and therefore have the same topographic distribution of effects within the developing nervous system, they do not produce identical neurochemical responses in terms of extracellular dopamine levels. In spite of this difference, the use of GBR 12909 in developmental studies should help us to determine whether inhibition of dopamine reuptake alone could produce long-term neurobehavioral alterations. One such study (W. Slikker, personal communication, July, 1993) shows that GBR 12909 (10 mg/kg/day) administered during the last 2 weeks of pregnancy in the rat resulted in offspring that were similar to those produced by cocaine at 40 mg/kg regarding stereotypic responses to the D-2 agonist quinpirole. The problem with this study as well as others is that drugs were administered to the mother and effects on offspring were examined without quantifying the amount of drug that reaches the fetal brain (or plasma). We have examined the effects of cocaine in comparison with GBR 12909 on function in the developing brain following chronic exposure (Frick, Grose, Hughes, Freed, & Dow-Edwards, 1993). In this study postnatal rat pups between 11 and 20 days of age received either cocaine, GBR 12909, or vehicle and then on Day 21 were administered their final dose of drug or vehicle and examined 20 min later for brain functional activity using the deoxyglucose method (Sokoloff et al., 1977). Preliminary analysis of the data indicates that cocaine stimulates metabolism in 36 of 56 brain regions and that in all cases, there are no statistically significant differences between the cocaine and the GBR 12909 exposed groups. A study to evaluate the effects of cocaine compared to GBR 12909 on behavioral responses to D1 and D2 agonists is currently underway in our lab. However, at this point, it is safe to say that the bulk of evidence does indicate that cocaine's effect on the developing dopamine system appear to be very important to its long-term neurobehavioral toxicity.

EFFECTS ON THE SEROTONIN SYSTEM

Cocaine is a potent inhibitor of serotonin (5-HT) reuptake in adult brain (Ross & Renyi, 1969) as well as the uptake of the 5-HT precursor tryptophan and the activity of the 5-HT synthetic enzyme tryptophan hydroxylase (Knapp & Mandell, 1972). The importance of serotonin in brain development has been examined by a number of investigators. Serotonin appears early in development and is involved in the regulation of morphogenetic events such as cell migration, axonal outgrowth, and synaptogenesis (Lauder, 1988). Serotonin uptake has been identified as early as 16 days of gestation in the rabbit and therefore presumably the carrier would be available to be bound by cocaine at that time. Fetal 5-HT synthesis can be manipulated by altering tryptophan availability (Arevalo, Alfonso, Castro, & Rodriguez, 1991). Therefore, blocking tryptophan uptake by cocaine can also be expected to produce long-term alterations in serotonergic function. However, the effects of cocaine on the 5-HT system have been characterized in the mature brain only. Therefore, the ontogeny of cocaine's effects on the 5-HT system needs to be fully characterized. In adult brain, serotonin reuptake sites can be labeled with ^3H paroxetine and are localized in such important structures as the cerebral cortex, the hippocampus, the hypothalamus, the basolateral amygdala, the dorsal and medial raphe, the substantia nigra, and the interpeduncular nucleus, in addition to traditionally dopaminergic structures such as the caudate and globus pallidus (Hrdina, Foy, Hepner, & Summers, 1990). Alterations in the development of the serotonin system have been shown to result from administering blocking agents and neurotoxins (e.g., 5,7 DHT; Pranzatelli & Martens, 1992; Sikich, Hickok, & Todd, 1990). Akbari, Kramer, Whitaker-Azmitia, Spear, and Azmitia (1992) found that prenatal cocaine decreases paroxetine binding, an indicator of 5-HT terminals, at 1 day and 1 week postnatal.

We have examined the effects of fluoxetine, a drug that inhibits serotonin reuptake in much the same way as cocaine does, on brain function in the developing rat (Frick, Hughes, Grose, Freed, & Dow-Edwards, 1992). In this study, cocaine, fluoxetine, or vehicle (at 25 mg/kg) were administered during postnatal Days 11–20. On Day 21, the pups received their last dose of drug 20 min prior to the deoxyglucose study. These data indicate that, as before, cocaine stimulated metabolism in several brain regions but that in most brain regions, fluoxetine produced rates of metabolism that were similar to the controls. In addition, littermates were examined for behavioral responses to serotonergic challenge drugs and showed that cocaine effects were very different from fluoxetine effects. That is, whereas developmental exposure to cocaine enhanced the acoustic startle response to 8 OH-DPAT, a $5HT_{1a}$ agonist, and MCPP, a $5HT_3$ agonist, fluoxetine exposure during development altered the baseline startle responsivity and thus appeared to attenuate the 8 OH-DPAT response and increase the MCPP response (Hughes, Grose, & Dow-Edwards, 1992). In another behavioral measure, developmental exposure to cocaine enhanced the behavioral depression seen in males following quipazine, a nonspecific 5-HT agonist, and attenuated it in females. Fluoxetine-exposed males showed no statistically significant response to quipazine challenge and fluoxetine-exposed females resembled cocaine-exposed females in their responses (Hughes, Grose, & Dow-Edwards, 1993). Therefore, our laboratory has completed three independent studies comparing developmental exposure to equal doses of fluoxetine or cocaine and found that, on the whole, the two drugs produce qualitatively different responses to 5-HT specific drugs in both developing as well as mature rats. Others have examined a group of pups exposed to fluoxetine (12.5 mg/kg/day) prenatally and found that the stereotypic and locomotor responses to quinpirole, a D-2 agonist, were not similar to those produced in the prenatal cocaine-exposed pups (W. Slikker, personal communication, July, 1993). Of course, all of these studies are limited by the fact that the neurochemical responses to these drugs are not thoroughly characterized in developing animals and although both inhibit reuptake of 5-HT, cocaine's effects on the serotonin system are considerably more complex than fluoxetine's. An in vivo and in vitro comparison of the neurochemical response to cocaine and fluoxetine should be completed in the developing brain before drawing any conclusions based on fluoxetine's effects about the importance of cocaine's effects on the serotonin system in the production of cocaine's developmental toxicity.

REUPTAKE INHIBITION: NOREPINEPHRINE

The third neurotransmitter that cocaine inhibits the reuptake of is norepinephrine (NE; Carmichael & Israel, 1973). Uptake of norepinephrine can be identified in the brain at 18 days of gestation (Coyle & Axelrod, 1971). The noradrenergic cells in the locus coeruleus extend their processes rostrally to innervate the frontal cortex first and then arch caudally to innervate the lateral cortex, parietal cortex, and then occipital cortex by the time the rat is born (Levitt & Moore, 1979). Uptake processes are mature by 9 days of age. ^3H desmethylimipramine, which labels noradrenergic uptake sites is densest in the locus coeruleus, anterior-ventral thalamus, bed nucleus of stria terminalis, and paraventricular and dorsal nuclei of hypothalamus. The cortex exhibits moderate levels of binding except in the cingulate cortex (Biegon & Rainbow, 1983). Disruption of these systems in adults produces a wide range of behavioral alterations from hyperactivity to catelepsy (Moore & Bloom, 1979). Therefore, alterations in these systems produced by cocaine certainly have the potential to produce long-term alterations in behavior. Prenatal cocaine exposure has been shown to alter noradrenergic endpoints. For example, increased beta adrenergic receptors at 30 days of age (Henderson et al., 1991), increased tyrosine hydroxylase immunoreactive fibers in hippocampus at 28 days of age (Akbari & Azmitia, 1992), and persistent noradrenergic hyperactivity (Seidler & Slotkin, 1992) have been described. Unfortunately little experimental evidence has been published that would demonstrate that these changes in the noradrenergic system are due to cocaine's effects on norepinephrine uptake specifically. However, in one study (W. Slikker, personal communication, July, 1993), desipramine, an inhibitor of norepinephrine uptake, was administered at 10 mg/kg/day to pregnant rats and the authors found that the pups were different from cocaine-exposed pups following challenge with a D-2 agonist, quinpirole. Of course, this is a single study and limited by the variability of delivery of the two drugs to the fetal tissues, the selection of a single dose of a relatively nonspecific NE reuptake inhibitor for comparison, and the selection of a dopamine challenge drug rather than an NE challenge drug. Therefore, further examination of cocaine as a norepinephrine reuptake inhibitor is needed before any conclusion can be drawn regarding the importance of cocaine's noradrenergic effects on its developmental toxicity.

SUMMARY

Although a great deal is known about cocaine's effects in the adult brain, we are still learning what cocaine does to the developing brain. The five major actions of the drug must first be analyzed individually by using pharmacologic agents that mimic specific effects of cocaine (e.g., the GBR 12909 compound for the dopamine effects or lidocaine for the local anesthetic effects). Then, when each action is well characterized, the combined effects can be examined. It is particularly important to determine whether the hypoxia produced in the fetus following maternal cocaine administration interacts with the effects on specific neurotransmitter systems. At this point, cocaine's effects on the dopaminergic system and the cardiovascular effects appear to be the most significant. However, because none of cocaine's mechanisms of action has been adequately investigated, it is premature to draw any firm conclusions at this time.

We do know that developmental exposure to cocaine alters several neurochemical measures related to the dopamine system. Our studies of brain metabolism have shown that dopaminergic regions as well as nondopaminergic regions exhibit long-term alterations in function following developmental cocaine exposure (Dow-Edwards, Freed, & Milhorat, 1988; Dow-Edwards et al., 1990; Dow-Edwards, Freed-Malen, & Hughes, 1993). However, because no neurochemical system operates independently, it is expected that effects on one neurotransmitter would induce alterations in other neurotransmitters within a given circuit. Our studies have also shown that cocaine effects are gender specific. For example, prenatal cocaine alters metabolism in male rats, whereas female rats appear to exhibit most of the behavioral abnormalities. Postnatal cocaine exposure affects brain metabolism in female rats, whereas both genders show behavioral alterations. Interestingly, fluoxetine's effects resemble cocaine's effects in females but not in males (Frick et al., 1992; Hughes et al., 1992). Therefore, until investigators examine both genders (with the females in a single phase of oestrus), utilize probes that mimic specific pharmacologic actions of cocaine, and study both prenatal and postnatal development in the rodent, it will not be possible to fully understand what cocaine is doing to the developing nervous system.

REFERENCES

Akbari, H. M., & Azmitia, E. C. (1992). Increased tyrosine hydroxylase immunoreactivity in the rat cortex following prenatal cocaine exposure. *Developmental Brain Research, 66*, 277–281.

Akbari, H. M., Kramer, H. K., Whitaker-Azmitia, P. M., Spear, L. P., & Azmitia, E. C. (1992). Prenatal cocaine exposure disrupts the development of the serotonergic system. *Brain Research, 572*, 57–63.

Anderson, P. H. (1989). The dopamine uptake inhibitor GBR 12909: Selectivity and molecular mechanisms of action. *European Journal of Pharmacology, 166*, 493–504.

Anderson-Brown, T., Slotkin, T. A., & Seidler, F. J. (1990). Cocaine acutely inhibits DNA synthesis in developing rat brain regions: Evidence for direct actions. *Brain Research, 537*, 197–202.

Arevalo, R., Alfonso, D., Castro, R., & Rodriguez, M. (1991). Fetal brain serotonin synthesis and catabolism is under control by mother intake of tryptophan. *Life Sciences, 49*, 53–66.

Benzon, H. T., Strichartz, G. R., Gissen, A. J., Shanks, C. A., Covino, B. G., & Datta, S. (1988). Developmental neurophysiology of mammalian peripheral nerves and age-related differential sensitivity to local anesthetic. *British Journal of Anesthesiology, 61*, 754–760.

Biegon, A., & Rainbow, T. C. (1983). Localization and characterization of [³H]desmethylimipramine binding sites in rat brain by quantitative autoradiography. *Journal of Neuroscience, 3*, 1069–1076.

Bondy, S. C., Nakla, M., Ali, S. F., & Ahmad, G. (1990). Cerebral ornithine decarboxylase levels following gestational exposure to cocaine. *International Journal of Developmental Neuroscience, 8*, 337–341.

Carmichael, F. J., & Israel, Y. (1973). In vitro inhibitory effects of narcotic analgesics and other psychotropic drugs on the active uptake of norepinephrine in mouse brain tissue. *Journal of Pharmacology and Experimental Therapeutics, 186*, 253–260.

Church, W. H., Justice, J. B., & Byrd, L. D. (1987). Extracellular dopamine in rat striatum following uptake inhibition by cocaine, nomifensine and benztropine. *European Journal of Pharmacology, 139*, 345–348.

Coyle, J. T., & Axelrod, J. (1971). Development of the uptake and storage of l-[³H]norepinephrine in the rat brain. *Journal of Neurochemistry, 18*, 2061–2075.

Crandall, M. E., Keve, T. M., & McLaughlin, M. K. (1990). Characterization of norepinephrine sensitivity in the maternal splanchnic circulation during pregnancy. *American Journal of Obstetrics and Gynecology, 162*, 1296–1301.

Dow-Edwards, D. L. (1990). Fetal and maternal cocaine levels peak rapidly following intragastric administration in the rat. *Journal of Substance Abuse, 2*, 427–437.

Dow-Edwards, D. L. (1991). Cocaine effects on fetal development: A comparison of clinical and animal research findings. *Neurotoxicology and Teratology, 13*, 347–352.

Dow-Edwards, D. L., Freed, L. A., & Fico, T. A. (1990). Structural and functional effects of prenatal cocaine exposure in adult rat brain. *Developmental Brain Research, 57*, 263–268.

Dow-Edwards, D. L., Freed, L. A., & Milhorat, T. H. (1988). Stimulation of brain metabolism by perinatal cocaine exposure. *Developmental Brain Research, 42*, 137–141.

Dow-Edwards, D. L., Freed-Malen, L. A., & Hughes, H. E. (1993). Long-term alterations in brain function following cocaine administration during the preweanling period. *Developmental Brain Research, 72*, 309–313.

Dow-Edwards, D. L., Grose, E. A., Freed-Malen, L. A., & Hughes, H. E. (1993). Alterations in uteroplacental blood flow and fetal physiology following maternal cocaine administration in the rat. *Teratology, 47*, NBTS 21.

Fiszman, M. L., Zuddas, A., Masana, M. I., Barker, J. L., & di Porzio, U. (1991). Dopamine synthesis preceded dopamine uptake in embryonic rat mesencephalic neurons. *Journal of Neurochemistry, 56*, 392–399.

Frick, G. S., Grose, E. A., Hughes, H. E., Freed, L. A., & Dow-Edwards, D. L. (1993). The role of dopaminergic reuptake blockade in producing cocaine's effects on cerebral function in periweanling rats. *Society of Neuroscience Abstracts, 19*, 757.13.

Frick, G. S., Hughes, H. E., Grose, E. A., Freed, L. A., & Dow-Edwards, D. L. (1992). The role of serotonergic reuptake blockade in producing cocaine's effects on cerebral function in periweanling rats. *Society of Neuroscience Abstracts, 18*, 619.8.

Fujinaga, M., & Mazze, R. I. (1986). Reproductive and teratogenic effects of lidocaine in Sprague-Dawley rats. *Anesthesiology, 65*, 626–632.

Hanbauer, I., & Grilli, M. (1992). Molecular mechanisms involving transport and release of dopamine in primary cultures of mesencephalic neurons. *Neurochemistry International, 20*(Suppl.), 101S–105S.

Henderson, M. G., McConnaughey, M. M., & McMillen, B. A. (1991). Long-term consequences of prenatal exposure to cocaine or related drugs: Effects on rat brain monoaminergic receptors. *Brain Research Bulletin, 26*, 941–945.

Hohmann, M., Keve, T. M., Osol, G., & McLaughlin, M. K. (1990). Norepinephrine sensitivity of mesenteric veins in pregnant rats. *American Journal of Physiology, 259*, R753–759.

Hrdina, P. D., Foy, B., Hepner, A., & Summers, R. J. (1990). Antidepressant binding sites in brain: Autoradiographic comparison of [^{3}H] imipramine localization and relationship to serotonin transporter. *Journal of Pharmacology and Experimental Therapeutics, 252*, 410–418.

Hughes, H. E., Grose, E. A., & Dow-Edwards, D. L. (1992). Perinatal exposure to cocaine or fluoxetine interacts with gender in predicting the acoustic startle response following 8OHDPAT and MCPP injection in adult rats. *Society of Neuroscience Abstracts, 18*, 155.3.

Hughes, H. E., Grose, E. A., & Dow-Edwards, D. L. (1993). Perinatal exposure to cocaine or fluoxetine interacts with gender in predicting motor activity following quipazine injection in adult rats. *Teratology, 47*, NBTS 22.

Hutchings, D. E. (1993). The puzzle of cocaine's effects following maternal use during pregnancy: Are there reconsilable differences? *Neurotoxicology and Teratology, 15*, 281–312.

Javitch, J. A., Strittmatter, S. M., & Snyder, S. H. (1985). Differential visualization of dopamine and norepinephrine uptake sites in rat brain using [^{3}H]mazindol autoradiography. *Journal of Neuroscience, 5*, 1513–1521.

Knapp, S., & Mandell, A. J. (1972). Narcotic drugs: Effects on 5HT biosynthetic enzymes. *Science, 177*, 1209–1211.

Koegler, S. M., Seidler, F. J., Spencer, J. R., & Slotkin, T. A. (1991). Ischemia contributes to adverse effects of cocaine on brain development: Suppression of ornithine decarboxylase activity in neonatal rat. *Brain Research Bulletin, 27*, 829–834.

Koob, G. F., & Bloom, F. E. (1988). Cellular and molecular mechanisms of drug dependence. *Science, 242*, 715–723.

Lauder, J. M. (1988). Neurotransmitters as morphogens. *Progress in Brain Research, 73*, 365–387.

Levitt, P., & Moore, R. Y. (1979). Development of the noradrenergic innervation of neocortex. *Brain Research, 162*, 243–259.

Longo, L. D., & Hermans, R. H. M. (1992). Behavioral and neurochemical sequelae in young rats of antenatal hypoxia. *Early Human Development, 29*, 83–90.

Mactutus, C. F., & Fechter, L. D. (1986). Perinatal hypoxia: Implications for mammalian development. In E. P. Riley & C. V. Vorhees (Eds.), *Handbook of behavioral teratology* (pp. 427–470). New York: Plenum.

Matthews, J. C., & Collins, A. (1983). Interaction of cocaine and cocaine congeners with sodium channels. *Biochemical Pharmacology, 32*, 455–460.

Meyer, J. S., Sherlock, J. D., & Macdonald, N. R. (1992). Effects of prenatal cocaine on behavioral responses to a cocaine challenge on postnatal day 11. *Neurotoxicology and Teratology, 14*, 183–189.

Minabe, Y., Ashby, C. R., Heyser, C., Spear, L. P., & Wang, R. Y. (1992). The effects of prenatal cocaine exposure on spontaneously active midbrain dopamine neurons in adult male offspring: An electrophysiological study. *Brain Research, 586*, 152–156.

Moore, R. Y., & Bloom, F. E. (1979). Central catecholamine neuronal system: Anatomy and physiology of the norepinephrine and epinephrine system. *Annual Review of Neuroscience, 2*, 113–168.

Moore, T. R., Sorg, J., Miller, L., Key, T. C., & Resnik, R. (1986). Hemodynamic effects of intravenous cocaine on the pregnant ewe and fetus. *American Journal of Obstetrics and Gynecology, 155*, 883–888.

Morishima, H. O., Cooper, T. B., Hara, T., & Miller, E. D. (1992). Pregnancy alters the hemodynamic responses to cocaine in the rat. *Developmental Pharmacology and Therapeutics, 19*, 69–79.

Neuspiel, D. R., & Hamel, S. C. (1991). Cocaine and infant behavior. *Developmental and Behavioral Pediatrics, 12*, 55–64.

Peris, J., Coleman-Hardee, M., & Millard, W. J. (1992). Cocaine in utero enhances the behavioral response to cocaine in adult rats. *Pharmacology, Biochemistry and Behavior, 42*, 509–515.

Pitts, D. K., Udom, C. E., & Marwah, J. (1987). Cardiovascular effects of cocaine in anesthetized and conscious rats. *Life Sciences, 40*, 1099–1111.

Pranzatelli, M. R., & Martens, J. M. (1992). Plasticity and ontogeny of the central 5-HT transporter: Effect of neonatal 5,7-dihydroxytryptamine lesions in the rat. *Developmental Brain Research, 70*, 191–195.

Ramazzotto, L. J., Curro, F. A., Paterson, J. A., Tanner, P., & Coleman, M. (1985). Toxicological assessment of lidocaine in the pregnant rat. *Journal of Dental Research, 64*, 1214–1217.

Ritz, M. C., Lamb, R. J., Goldberg, S. R., & Kuhar, M. J. (1987). Cocaine receptors on dopamine transporters are related to self-administration of cocaine. *Science, 237*, 1219–1223.

Ross, S. B., & Renyi, A. L. (1969). Inhibition of uptake of tritiated 5-hydroxytryptamine in brain tissue. *European Journal of Pharmacology, 7*, 270–277.

Rothman, R. B., Mele, A., Reid, A. A., Akunne, H. C., Greig, N., Thurkauf, A., deCosta, B., Rice, K. C., & Pert, A. (1991). GBR12909 antagonizes the ability of cocaine to elevate extracellular levels of dopamine. *Pharmacology, Biochemistry and Behavior, 40*, 387–397.

Scalzo, F. M., Ali, S. F., Frambes, N. A., & Spear, L. P. (1990). Weanling rats exposed prenatally to cocaine exhibit an increase in striatal D2 dopamine binding associated with an increase in ligand affinity. *Pharmacology, Biochemistry and Behavior, 37*, 371–373.

Seidler, F. J., & Slotkin, T. A. (1992). Fetal cocaine exposure causes persistent noradrenergic hyperactivity in rat brain regions: Effects on neurotransmitter turnover and receptors. *Journal of Pharmacology and Experimental Therapeutics, 263*, 413–421.

Seidler, F. J., & Slotkin, T. A. (1993). Prenatal cocaine and cell development in rat brain regions: Effects on ornithine decarboxylase and macromolecules. *Brain Research Bulletin, 30*, 91–99.

Sikich, L., Hickok, J. M., & Todd, R. D. (1990). 5-HT$_{1A}$ receptors control neurite branching during development. *Developmental Brain Research, 56,* 269–274.

Smith, R. F., Wharton, G. G., Kurtz, S. L., Mattran, K. M., & Hollenbeck, A. R. (1986). Behavioral effects of mid-pregnancy administration of lidocaine and mepivacaine in the rat. *Neurobehavioral Toxicology and Teratology, 8,* 61–68.

Sokoloff, L., Reivich, M., Kennedy, C., Des Rosiers, M. H., Patlak, C. S., Pettigrew, K. D., Sakurada, O., & Shinohara, M. (1977). The [^{14}C]Deoxyglucose method for the measurement of local cerebral glucose utilization: Theory, procedure, and normal values in the conscious and anesthetized albino rat. *Journal of Neurochemistry, 28,* 897–916.

Teiling, A. K. Y., Mohammed, A. K., Minor, B. G., Jarbe, T. U. C., Hiltunen, A. J., & Archer, T. (1987). Lack of effects of prenatal exposure to lidocaine on development of behavior in rats. *Anesthesia and Analgesia, 66,* 533–541.

van der Loos, H., & Woolsey, T. A. (1973). Somatosensory cortex: Structural alterations following early injury to sense organs. *Science, 179,* 395–398.

Webster, W. S., Brown-Woodman, P. D. C., Lipson, A. H., & Ritchie, H. E. (1991). Fetal brain damage in the rat following prenatal exposure to cocaine. *Neurotoxicology and Teratology, 13,* 621–626.

Wiesel, T. N. (1982). Postnatal development of the visual cortex and the influence of environment. *Nature, 299,* 583–591.

Woods, J. R., Plessinger, M. A., & Clark, K. E. (1987). Effect of cocaine on uterine blood flow and fetal oxygenation. *Journal of the American Medical Association, 257,* 957–961.

Woods, J. R., Plessinger, M. A., Scott, K., & Miller, R. K. (1989). Prenatal cocaine exposure to the fetus: A sheep model for cardiovascular evaluation. *Annals of the New York Academy of Science, 562,* 267–279.

Yotsumoto, I., & Nomura, Y. (1981). Ontogenesis of the dopamine uptake into P2 fractions and slices of the rat brain. *Japanese Journal of Pharmacology, 31,* 298–300.

2

▼▼▼▼▼▼▼

Prenatal Cocaine Exposure and Child Outcome: What Do We Really Know?

Barry M. Lester
Kiti Freier
Lyn LaGasse
Brown University School of Medicine

Science progresses in stages or what Kuhn (1962) described as revolutions. Sometimes the progress of science is affected, either negatively or positively, by factors outside of the scientific domain. Most often these factors are social and political. The "cocaine" story is one that is affected in this manner. Even as this chapter goes to press there is a strong societal reaction, a re-evaluation of that reaction, and now we are starting to witness a backlash—denial that a problem exists.

No doubt the cocaine problem took our society by surprise. Unprepared, the academic, health-care, political, and legal communities floundered and quickly called cocaine an "epidemic." Based on scant evidence and in some cases methodologically poor studies, a "rush to judgment" (Mayes, Granger, Bornstein, & Zuckerman, 1992) was rendered that cocaine use during pregnancy resulted in serious obstetrical and perinatal problems with adverse child outcome. It did not take long for our society to believe that cocaine use during pregnancy caused irreparable brain damage; that these children were doomed, destined to become retarded, antisocial, and a burden on society. The fact is, if we take away the sensationalism and the hype and take a serious look at our knowledge base in this area it is still pretty scant, which is not to say that we have not learned a lot: We have. Primarily, we have learned to ask the right questions. Although we have a much better understanding of the problem than we had when research findings first appeared in press, in the mid-1980s, we still know very little about the effects of cocaine on child outcome.

EPIDEMIOLOGY

What do we know about the incidence and prevalence of cocaine use by pregnant women, and even more important, how do we know it? There are two ways to know if a woman used illegal drugs during pregnancy: self-report or toxicology analysis.

The 1992 National Institute on Drug Abuse (NIDA) Household Survey showed that although the prevalence of crack and cocaine has declined overall, in some groups the drug continues to be used at high or increasing rates. Not surprisingly it is inner-city minority groups that are most affected. In addition, women of childbearing age seem to be particularly susceptible. Prevalence rates range from 3% to almost 50% with the highest rates among centers that serve poor areas and inner-city mothers. There are two problems with these data. First, they are based on self-report, which is known to be especially unreliable when illegal activities are involved. Second, the report is based on individuals living in households; that is, you have to live in a household to be in the survey. Such criteria may exclude large numbers of the drug-using population.

DRUG TOXICOLOGY

The validity of epidemiological statistics improves as better toxicology assays become available. Urine screens have been the standard, however, they only reflect use over the preceding 72 hrs. The meconium assay is a more recent development and has the advantage of recording drug use through the second half of pregnancy. Hair analysis is a third technique that has the potential to provide an even longer record of drug use, although there are methodological problems with the assay and difficulties in obtaining informed consent in some cases that have limited the use of this technique so far.

Epidemiological information is also affected by the populations that are screened. Pregnant women are typically screened when they have a prior history of drug use or when there are clinical reasons to suspect drug use. There are no official criteria for clinical suspicion; each hospital determines its own policy. In general, criteria include obstetrical events such as lack of prenatal care, premature labor, and placental abruption. Because these conditions are more often associated with poverty, the poor and minorities are screened more often. Therefore, most of what we know about drug use comes from pregnant women living in poverty.

It is possible to do anonymous screens in which the patient is not identified. One such study was done with pregnant women in Florida and the surprising finding was that the incidence of illegal drug use in general, and not specifically cocaine, was comparable between lower-class and middle-class patients. If replicated, these findings would change the way society thinks about illegal drug use during pregnancy. It would also provide the methodological opportunity to study drug-exposed children growing up in more enriched environmental conditions.

Another problem with toxicology assays is how to separate drugs used for treatment from drugs of abuse. Treatment drugs may include prescription medication taken during pregnancy or obstetrical medication used during labor and delivery. Opiates, for example, used for pain medication can result in a positive toxicology screen but may not indicate illegal drug use. On the other hand, some mothers abuse prescription medication such as codeine. Therefore, even if a positive toxicology screen is challenged because the mother had taken prescription medication, she may, in fact, have been abusing prescription medication or taking illegal drugs as well. These questions cannot be answered by a toxicology analysis alone and in some cases the drug use history may never be known.

Epidemiological information is even more suspect when it comes to alcohol use during pregnancy. Alcohol is the most common "other" substance of abuse that is used with cocaine, yet there is no toxicology assay to determine if alcohol was used during pregnancy. The only method available is self-report. Although one might argue that because alcohol is legal, mothers are more likely to report, mounting societal pressure has made mothers reticent to report alcohol use. We know this from clinical studies in which mothers report substantially more alcohol use to a case manager or counselor after they have established a trusting relationship than they reported on initial intake. In addition, some questionnaire and clinical interview methods for determining level of alcohol use are more sensitive than others and when more sensitive methods are used the amount of alcohol reported is much higher than in the more traditional screening procedures.

PHARMACOLOGY

Most of the studies on in utero cocaine exposure and child outcome have been descriptive of the behavioral characteristics of the children but have not been driven by theoretical models based on our understanding of how cocaine affects the nervous system. Although description is appropriate in the early stages of science, we are now at a juncture in this field where we need to begin to generate hypotheses about drug use and behavior based on what we know about the pharmacology and neurobiology of cocaine.

Data on the pharmacological effects of cocaine come from animal studies and typically the rat model is used. There is certainly question about the validity of animal findings when applied to the human and whether or not the rat model is even appropriate. With these caveats in mind, we start by noting that cocaine is a central nervous system (CNS) stimulant that affects the monoaminergic transmitters in the CNS; dopamine, norepinephrine, and serotonin. Cocaine blocks the reuptake of these neurotransmitters (Gawin & Kleber, 1988). The reuptake process is primarily responsible for terminating the actions of both adrenergic impulses and circulating catecholamines. When the process is blocked, more circulating catecholamines are available centrally and peripherally. These effects are likely to lead to neurophysiologic, autonomic, and behavioral arousal. For example, the euphoria and increased motor activity produced by cocaine are mediated by enhanced neurotransmission in the brain (Spitz & Rosecan, 1987). The physiological effects of tachycardia and vasoconstriction with hypertension seen with cocaine use are mediated by increased amounts of circulating catecholamines in the periphery (Moore, Sorg, Miller, Key, & Clark, 1986; Richie & Greene, 1985).

EFFECTS ON THE FETUS

Cocaine easily crosses the placenta and the blood brain barrier. As discussed by Mayes (1994) there is a continuum of biologic vulnerability for the developing fetal brain and how cocaine is likely to affect brain development depending on the timing of the exposure. Three phases of brain development have been described by Volpe (1992): (a) proliferation for neurons in the first 2 to 4 months and for glial cells from 5 months to 1 year postnatally, (b) neuronal migration in the third to fifth month, and (c) organization from the sixth month to several years postnatally. Exposure to cocaine during the first half of gestation would be expected to affect processes of cytogenesis and histogenesis, whereas exposure during the second half of pregnancy would affect processes of differentiation, specification, and the growth of specific brain areas (Mayes, 1994).

The monoamine system affects synaptogenesis, neural growth, and cell proliferation (Lauder, 1988), suggesting one set of mechanisms by which cocaine may affect behavior. There has been some attempt to try and understand the effects of cocaine on development through the study of neurotransmitters and behavior. Monoaminergic neurotransmitters play an important role in the central control of basic processes including autonomic function, state regulation, and responses to sensory stimuli (Jacobs, 1985). The effects of cocaine on autonomic system activity mediated by monoaminergic transmitters is suggested by findings that elevated circulating norepinephrine levels and heart rates were found in prenatally exposed infants at 2 months of age (Doberczak, Shanzer, Senie, & Kandall, 1988; Salamy, Eldredge, Anderson, & Bull, 1990). A preliminary study showed some evidence that higher levels of norepinephrine were related to poorer responsiveness on the Brazelton scale (Mirochnick, Meyer, Cole, Herren, & Zuckerman, 1991).

Cocaine use during pregnancy may affect neuroregulatory mechanisms that result in disorders of behavioral regulation. The monoaminergic system affects would lead to disturbances associated with limbic, hypothalamic, and extrapyramidal function (Volpe, 1992). Lester and Tronick (1994) proposed a model of the effects of cocaine on behavior shown in Fig. 2.1. This model is based on a theory

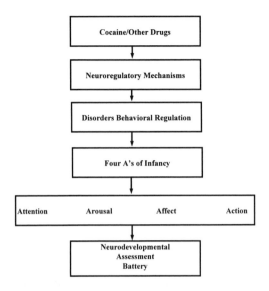

FIG. 2.1.   Theoretical model of the effects of prenatal cocaine exposure on child behavior.

of mutual regulation (Tronick, 1989) in which the infant's and young child's normal development is dependent on the regulatory capacities to control homeostatic, attentional, affective, and behavioral states. The regulatory systems include physiological systems, coping behaviors, cognitive processes, emotional social processes, and linguistic-speech capacities. When these regulatory processes are operating effectively, the infant can actively engage the world of people and their environment (world of objects). If regulatory capacities fail to generate well-organized states, this requires supplementary regulatory input from the environment.

The model in Fig. 2.1 suggests that cocaine affects neuroregulatory mechanisms, which in turn result in disorders of behavioral regulation. These disorders of behavioral regulation are manifest as the "Four A's of Infancy": *attention, arousal, affect,* and *action.* These four areas seem to be most affected by prenatal drug exposure. As explained later in this chapter, the ability of the drug-exposed infant to recover from disorders in behavioral regulation will require regulatory input from the caregiving environment.

Attention refers to visual and auditory abilities that relate to the intake and processing of information from the environment. *Arousal* includes control and modulation of behavioral states from sleep to waking to crying, and the ability to display the entire range of states, from excitation to inhibition to incoming stimuli. *Affect* relates to the development of sociability and emotion, the mutual regulatory processes of social interaction and social relationships. *Action* indicates perceptual-motor function, the development of fine and gross motor skills, and the acquisition of knowledge and social exchange through motor patterns.

Direct and Indirect Effects

In addition, cocaine has both direct and indirect effects on the fetus and infant (Jones & Lopez, 1988). We know from preclinical studies that the teratogenic effects of a drug can be produced by an action on the maternal animal, directly on the fetus, or by alteration of normal maternal–fetal metabolic pathways (Inglass, Curley, & Prindle, 1952). Direct effects include the action of cocaine on the fetus consequent to transfer of the drug through the placenta. These systemic effects of cocaine on the nervous system are probably mediated by the changes in synaptic transmission resulting in an excess of neurotransmitter at the receptor sites (Richie & Greene, 1985). This mechanism affects the sympathetic nervous system and produces vasoconstriction, an acute rise in arterial blood pressure, tachycardia, and a predisposition to ventricular arrhythmia and seizures (Cregler & Mark, 1986; Tarr & Macklin, 1987).

Indirect effects can be attributable to changes in the fetal environment and effects on the mother's CNS that place the infant at risk. During pregnancy, uterine blood vessels supplying oxygen and nutrients to the developing fetus are maximally dilated, but they vasoconstrict in the presence of catecholamines. Cocaine blocks the reuptake of catecholamines (Richie & Greene, 1985), thereby increasing their concentration, resulting in vasoconstriction of the uterine arteries and impaired oxygen delivery to the fetus.

In pregnant cocaine-using women, vasoconstriction, sudden hypertension, or cardiac arrhythmias may interrupt blood supply to the placenta and reduce profusion to various fetal tissues in early gestation, causing deformation or disruption of morphogenesis in late gestation (Bingol, Fuchs, Diaz, Stone, & Gromisch, 1987). Vasoconstriction, tachycardia, and increased blood pressure caused by cocaine all increase the chance for intermittent intrauterine hypoxia, preterm labor, precipitous labor, and abruptio placenta followed by hemorrhage, shock, and anemia (Tarr & Macklin, 1987). Vasoconstriction at the uterocomplex coupled with anorexic effects of cocaine might explain the growth retardation that occurs in approximately 25% of the offspring of cocaine-using mothers (Fulroth, Phillips, & Durand, 1989; Hadeed & Siegel, 1989; Yoon, Kim, Mac Hee, Checola, & Noble, 1989). Hypoxia by means of vasoconstriction has been shown to reduce fetal weight in animal studies (Mahalik, Gautieri, & Mann, 1984).

In summary, cocaine has a specific direct effect on brain function and an indirect effect through the influence of fetal nutritional status and it is possible that these direct and indirect effects have different influences on neurobehavioral functioning.

Figure 2.2 is taken from a study in which direct and indirect effects of cocaine were studied using acoustic cry analysis as the neurobehavioral outcome (Lester et al., 1991). Two neurobehavioral syndromes were identified consistent with direct versus indirect effects of cocaine. Excitable cry characteristics (e.g., higher

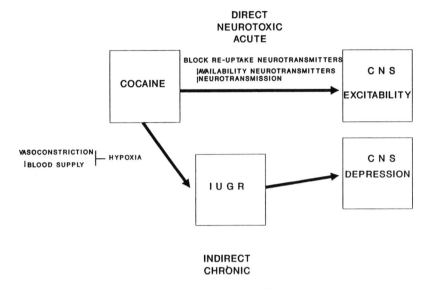

FIG. 2.2. Model of neurobehavioral effects of cocaine.

pitch, more variability, and longer cries) were related to the direct effects of cocaine. The action of cocaine on mesolimbic systems (Wise, 1984) trigger the cry, which is activated by the hypothalamic-limbic system and controlled by midbrain and brain stem regions (Lester & Boukydis, 1991). The effects of cocaine on the tegmentum and on the raphe nuclei (Wise, 1984) could directly affect midbrain and brain stem control.

Depressed cry characteristics (longer latency to cry onset, fewer cries, and lower amplitude cries) were related to indirect effects because this cry profile was associated with cocaine exposure, low birth weight, or intrauterine growth retardation (IUGR). Placental vasoconstriction can decrease the nutrient supply to the fetus, causing hypoxia and IUGR. Depressed catecholamine responses have been found in IUGR rat pups (Shaul, Cha, & Oh, 1989) and depressed behavior in IUGR human infants has been reported in other cry studies (Lester & Zeskind, 1978), feeding behavior (Mullen, Garcia-Coll, Vohr, & Oh, 1988), and the Brazelton scale (Lester, Garcia-Coll, Valcarcel, Hoffman, & Brazelton, 1986).

The notion of excitable and depressed neurobehavioral syndromes in cocaine-exposed infants is supported in several studies. For example, in studies using a narcotic withdrawal index, some findings suggest heightened responsivity, increased motor tone, and irritability consistent with excitability, whereas in other studies the infants are described as underaroused and lethargic. In our clinical experience with the Brazelton scale we have also observed these dual patterns. In addition, there appears to be a third or "mixed" pattern in which the exposed infant initially appears as underaroused, hard to wake up, and difficult to bring to a quiet alert state. They then become highly excitable, irritable, hypertonic, and remain in an insulated cry state. These infants appear to be unable to modulate their level of arousal once awake. They are primarily in lower (sleep) states or higher (cry) states and are unable to maintain a state of quiet alertness, although some can with massive consolability maneuvers by the examiner.

Appendix A shows a system for scoring the Brazelton scale on the excitable and depressed dimensions. This system is currently being used in several studies. In a study by Tronick, Frank, Cabral, and Zuckerman (1994) a dose–response relationship was reported between prenatal cocaine use and the excitability cluster at 2 weeks of age. A higher level of exposure was related to increased excitability supporting the direct cocaine effect. The depression cluster was not related to level of exposure and the correlation between the excitability and depressed clusters was low, suggesting that these two clusters represent different behavioral patterns.

There are several important qualifiers to these attempts to relate cocaine neurobiology and pharmacology to behavior. We already mentioned the potential limitation of the rat model. But, in addition, both animal and human studies are based on an "insult" model, that is, how a teratogen could alter normal developmental pathways. We have neither theory nor empirical work on compensation or "recovery" models, that is, how might the brain adjust, reorganize, or compensate for cocaine exposure; would "recovery" be affected by the timing of the insult given what we know about the stages of brain growth (Volpe, 1992)? It is far from clear whether the compensation capacities of the rat brain compare with the compensation capacities of the human brain. The insult model also does not determine how an insult translates to behavior. It is already one level of speculation to suggest how, for example, the monoaminergic system relates to behavior; it is yet another level to suggest how alterations in the monoaminergic system may affect behavior. Finally, the pharmacological models have not addressed the issue of polydrug use. We know that cocaine is rarely used alone (see following), and a variety of other substances are often used in conjunction with cocaine. Little is known about the pharmacology of how cocaine interacts with other drugs, let alone how polydrug use would affect behavior.

NEURODEVELOPMENTAL ASSESSMENT

Traditional tests of developmental outcome such as the Bayley Scales provide global estimates of neurobehavioral function and have the advantages of being standardized, widely known, accepted, and relatively easy to administer and score. However, these measures may not be suitable to detect the subtle and specific effects of cocaine. Thus, it is possible that current findings showing no significant differences or contradictory results may reflect inappropriate testing and not the status of neurobehavioral function. Lester and Tronick (1994) developed a neurodevelopmental battery for drug-exposed infants based on the Four A's of Infancy as part of a large multisite longitudinal study of prenatal drug exposure and child outcome for the National Institutes of Health (NIH). It includes state-of-the-art assessments that we believe will be sensitive to even subtle effects of cocaine. The battery should also help identify behavioral patterns such as the neurobehavioral excitable and depressed syndromes described earlier. The ability to describe these patterns of individual differences will enable us to identify specific mechanisms by which cocaine affects behavior, as well as to develop clinical programs that deal with the specific behavioral domains affected.

SURVEY OF NEUROBEHAVIORAL OUTCOME

Our knowledge base of the neurodevelopmental outcome of cocaine-exposed infants is relatively small and quite varied. Keep in mind, however, that this is a young field; although the first behavioral study appeared in 1985, most of the literature has been published since 1989. We have conducted a survey of the published literature of neurobehavioral studies on cocaine-exposed infants and summarized the findings of those studies that met methodologically acceptable criteria.

The criteria we used were borrowed from the meta-analysis conducted by Lutiger, Graham, Einarson, and Koren (1991), who were interested in the reported obstetrical and perinatal problems linked to cocaine use during pregnancy likely to adversely affect child outcome. The following list shows a partial list of deleterious outcomes that were initially attributed to cocaine.

- Pregnancy loss, including spontaneous abortion and stillbirth
- Abruptio placentae
- Precipitous labor
- Prematurity
- Low birth weight
- Short birth length
- Small head circumference
- IUGR
- Congenital malformations
- Apnea
- Abnormal pneumogram
- Sudden Infant Death Syndrome (SIDS)
- Perinatal cerebral infarction
- IVH
- Seizures
- Periventricular leukomalacia
- Low Apgar

However, findings from these studies were limited by serious methodological problems, including use of case reports, no control groups, inadequate control of confounding variables, and unreliability of methods to identify users and nonusers. In the Lutiger et al. (1991) meta-analysis, published articles between 1975 and 1989 that met the following criteria were included: cocaine use in pregnancy, assessment of pregnancy or fetal outcome, a cohort or case-control design, a control group, human subjects, original work, and published in English. Of 45 articles reviewed, only 20 met the inclusion criteria. When cocaine users were compared with polydrug users not using cocaine the few reproductive effects associated with cocaine were increased genitourinary malformations and shorter gestational age. When the control groups consisted of nondrug users, cocaine was associated with a higher risk for spontaneous abortion, shorter gestational age, smaller head circumference, shorter birth length, and lower birth weight.

In our review of neurobehavioral studies, the criteria we used were: neurodevelopmental outcome measure, cocaine use during pregnancy, human subjects, original research, inclusion of a comparison or control group, peer review publication, and use of statistical analysis. We initially identified 60 neurodevelopmental studies on the effects of cocaine. Of these, 10 were eliminated because they did not meet one or more of the methodological criteria cited. Of the 50 studies, only 7 (14%) were conducted with infants up to 4 months of age; two studies have been reported with infants older than 2 years old. Only the cohort studied by Chasnoff, Griffith, Freier, and Murray (1992) was followed to age 3 and this group was a convenience sample of mothers in a drug treatment program. Therefore, most of what we know about the neurobehavioral effects of cocaine is based on early infancy and what little follow-up is available is from a sample that may not be representative of the population of drug-using mothers.

Table 2.1 shows a list of the neurobehavioral outcomes that were used in the studies that met our criteria. In addition, we report the number of studies in which each assessment was used and the number of times a statistically significant effect (at least $p < .05$) was reported. Of the 16 different measures reported, only 3 have been used in four or more studies; 2 were withdrawal measures based on the narcotic addiction literature and one was the Brazelton scale suggesting limited replication in our database. A withdrawal syndrome has not been identified in cocaine-exposed infants and it is not clear in studies that did show effects of withdrawal if withdrawal effects may have been due to the presence of drugs other than cocaine. Eight studies have been reported using the Brazelton scale and seven studies have shown cocaine effects. However, replicable results have only been reported in two studies in which cocaine effects were found on the habituation cluster and the relevance of this single finding is questionable.

We were also struck by the methodological limitations of the 50 studies that were included. Many important variables were either not controlled or not reported in these articles. In six of the studies (12%), the use of additional drugs other than cocaine was not reported. Of the remaining 44 studies, cocaine use

TABLE 2.1
Summary of Results

	Number of Studies	
Behavior	Significant	Not Significant
Neonatal Behavioral Assessment Scale	7	1
Neonatal Abstinence Score	3	1
Stress/abstinence/withdrawal	1	3
Neurobehavioral status and state organization	1	0
Sucking	1	0
Neonatal Perception Inventory	0	1
Nursing Child Assessment of Feeding	1	1
Cry	2	0
Glabella reflex	2	0
Movement Assessment of Infants	1	0
Bayley Scales	0	1
Fagan Test of Infant Intelligence	1	0
Developmental quotient	1	0
Attachment	1	0
Play	1	0
Behavior/development problems	1	0

was isolated from other drugs in only 2 studies (5%). Typically cocaine was used with tobacco (56%), marijuana (46%), and alcohol (47%). Information on the amount or frequency of drug use was reported in four studies (8%), and the trimester of use was reported in eight studies (16%). The most frequent method for identification of cocaine use was urine toxicology analysis (23, or 46%). Self-report was used in two studies (4%), and urine and/or self-report in 11 studies (22%). Only five studies (10%) reported on the route of administration of cocaine. Primarily, our goal is to relate the pharmacology of cocaine to neurobehavioral effects. To do this, we must account for the presence of other drugs, the frequency and timing, and route of administration. Our current set of studies do not make these distinctions, nor can they conveniently separate users from nonusers (one problem not faced by animal researchers).

Controls for confounding variables were underreported for both demographic and medical factors. Demographic variables such as socioeconomic status (SES) were only reported in 10 studies (20%), maternal age in 22 studies (44%), maternal education in 14 studies (28%), and prenatal care in 32 studies (64%). No attempt was made to control for SES in 33 studies (66%). In 24 studies (48%), no mention was made of whether or not the neurodevelopmental testing was conducted by personnel who were aware of the exposure status of the child. It is also interesting that only 14 studies (28%) mentioned whether or not the mothers or children were part of any intervention program. Medical factors including prenatal care were not controlled in 36 studies (72%), prematurity, birth weight, or gestational age in 34 (68%), 40 (80%), and 30 studies (60%), respectively.

In short, despite the considerable effort that has gone into studying the effects of in utero cocaine exposure on child outcome, surprisingly little is known. What has been reported are largely scattered findings that have not been replicated, as well as studies with serious methodological problems. In addition, most studies have been descriptive and not driven by theoretical models.

RESTATEMENT OF THE PROBLEM

Arguably, the most important contribution to come from the early work in this area is a better understanding of the problem itself (see Fig. 2.3; Lester & Tronick, 1994). We have learned that the problem is far more complicated than had been originally described for two reasons. First, the drug issue is one of polydrug use, not of cocaine alone. Most women who use cocaine also use other drugs, most commonly alcohol, marijuana, and tobacco, but other drugs such as heroin may also be used. There may be women who only use cocaine, but they seem to be more the exception than the rule. Thus, in Fig. 2.3, we assume from the outset that we are dealing with polydrug use.

The second complicating factor is what has been termed *environment* or *lifestyle issues*. Here the term *environment* is used to describe a complex set of interrelated factors including psychological and social factors that lead a mother to use drugs and the neighborhood and general conditions in which drug-exposed children are often raised. These conditions may involve inadequate and even abusive forms of parenting, poverty, high stress, exposure to violence, and a chaotic, disorganized lifestyle. Independent of prenatal drug exposure these factors predict poor developmental outcome. Therefore, drug effects, by which we mean pharmacological effects, are confounded with environmental effects. Thus, we have learned that cocaine seems to be a marker variable for polydrug use and a lifestyle associated with poverty that may jeopardize normal developmental

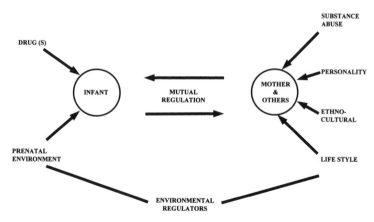

FIG. 2.3. Systems approach to study of cocaine.

outcome. Figure 2.3 shows a systems approach to the problem as we currently understand it. It is reasonable to expect that the combination of prenatal drug exposure and other prenatal factors such as poor prenatal care, poor nutrition, and a poor reproductive history combine to produce, in some cases, an acute neurobehavioral vulnerability or fragility. In the vast majority these infants are probably not permanently damaged. In fact, many appear quite normal. However, there are a significant proportion of these infants who appear stressed and show disorders of behavioral regulation. In a reasonably sound environment, these infants may have every chance for a normal developmental outcome. However, environmental factors can be regulators or disregulators, stabilizers or destabilizers of child development. These factors can exaggerate the child's neurobehavioral vulnerability or help to buffer and regulate child behavior. Unfortunately, all too often these infants do not grow up in environments that facilitate normal development. An infant who is already stressed has that much more to overcome and may recover poorly in a nonsupportive caregiving environment.

As shown in Fig. 2.3, the immediate caretaking of the infant may be compromised by a mother who has a drug problem, by personality disorders possibly related to her use of drugs, and historically based psychopathology. These factors will impinge on the mutual regulatory process of the mother–infant interaction that could disrupt infant regulatory processes. To these proximal factors, add more distal factors including lack of social support and the larger environmental stressors associated with a poverty lifestyle.

In this model, drugs have a direct acute effect and an indirect long-term effect. Drugs have the potential to predispose the infant to a short-term neurobehavioral vulnerability as a direct pharmacological effect on the four A's of infancy. The interaction between the neurodevelopmental vulnerability and the response of the caregiving environment will determine the long-term developmental outcome of the child. The longer term drug effect is indirect, mediated by environmental factors.

We see this model as a reasonable statement of the problem as we now understand it. It enables us to study the effects of cocaine in the context of multiple risk factors that may affect the regulatory capacities of the child and the dyad.

LESSONS FROM THE PAST

There is a certain déjà vu associated with the study of prenatal cocaine exposure (Lester & Tronick, 1994). The study of prenatal influences and insults on child development is a much studied area and it might be useful to consider cocaine exposure as a special case of this larger problem, and in so doing to understand what we can learn from the past as well as what is unique about this particular problem. Arguably, the study of preterm infants provides a good model.

Starting in the 1950s with the National Perinatal Collaborative Study of some 20,000 pregnancy and delivery outcomes, substantial effort was devoted to the effects of prematurity (Niswander & Gordon, 1972). The prevailing *zeitgeist* at that time was that being born prematurely was a form of biological insult likely to effect CNS development and the long-term outcome of the child. Supporting evidence showed that premature infants were overrepresented in many populations of abnormal outcomes, including cerebral palsy and mental retardation (Lilienfeld & Parkhurst, 1951; Pasamanick & Knobloch, 1966). A related movement called for the development of early stimulation programs to help these infants make up for their biological deficits and perhaps prevent poor developmental outcome.

The second generation of studies of the effects of preterm birth told a different story. We were reminded that the evidence (even if it was true) that preterm infants were overrepresented among the handicapped population was based largely on retrospective data. Prospective longitudinal studies began to show that when preterm infants were followed from birth, the majority developed normally. Studies such as the Kauai study (Werner, Bierman, & French, 1971) showed that in fact it was the environments of these children that was predictive of their developmental outcome rather than their medical status at birth. The seminal paper by Sameroff and Chandler (1975) brought these issues to the fore in the form of the transactional model in which the dynamic response of the caretaking environment to the characteristics of the child is seen as the primary determinant of child outcome. Parallel work in the biological domain showed substantial plasticity and mechanisms for recovery of function from insult and injury to the developing nervous system. Doom was replaced by optimism for the developing preterm infant (Waddington, 1966).

We also learned that preterm infants were not a homogeneous group. As babies began to survive at lower and lower birth weights, the medical community distinguished between low birth weight (1,500–2,500 g) and very low birth weight (< 1,500 g). Today we make reference to the "micropreemie" under 900 g. Smaller babies are more at risk not only because they are smaller but also because they are more prone to insult, injury, and illness. Brain injury such as intraventricular hemorrhage and respiratory illness such as bronchopulmonary dysplasia occur mostly in these smaller babies and they often occur together.

Preterm infants also are not homogeneous with respect to their behavior and development. Preterm infants show a wide range of behavioral and developmental trajectories that are multidetermined. The dynamic response of the caregiving environment to the changing behavioral organization of the infant is our best window into the long-term developmental outcome of the preterm infant.

APPLICATION TO DRUG-EXPOSED INFANTS

Like prematurity, drug exposure can be viewed as another *potential* insult or injury to the developing fetus. We do not know if and how drugs affect the fetus, we do not know the effects of polydrug use, and we do not know the effects of timing, dosage, and frequency of use. In some infants there may be true injury, in others there may be any degree of insult, and many infants may escape unscathed. It is also possible that there are effects that we simply do not know how to measure or effects that are not manifest until the child is older. Also, drug effects will interact with other prenatal factors, such as poor nutrition or illness, that may also potentially compromise the infant.

There is a relation between drug exposure and early delivery probably because of the effects of cocaine on labor, although it may also be related to lack of prenatal care. Thus, drug-exposed infants constitute an increasingly large percentage of the infants in the special care nursery. We do not know, however, if the drug-exposed preterm infant is any different from the unexposed preterm infant with a comparable medical history. That is, does drug exposure have an additional, or synergistic effect, when factors such as birth weight, other sicknesses, and insults are taken into account?

One of the major differences between drug exposure and prematurity is that the vast majority of drug-exposed infants are *not* born prematurely. Many are born at term and are otherwise normal and healthy, whereas others are born at term but are growth retarded (IUGR or SGA[1]). As with the preterm, we can say that drug-exposed infants are not a homogeneous group. They are not homogeneous with respect to how they present medically, or with respect to how they present behaviorally. We have just begun to describe some of the different behavioral patterns that drug-exposed infants manifest and it is likely that these different beginnings may result in different developmental trajectories as the exigencies of the caregiving environment come into play.

We also learned from the study of preterm and other high-risk infants that many of our standard developmental tools were not sensitive to the behavioral variations of these infants. Not surprisingly, this is also turning out to be true for the drug-exposed infant. In preterm infants, measures that are more sensitive to behavioral processes such as the Four A's of Infancy are better able to describe the behavioral organization of these infants than tests of gross developmental outcome or milestones.

There has also been a long-standing bias in the research community, influenced in part by funding and public policy issues, that cognitive and intellectual outcomes are of primary importance. Thus, most studies with preterm infants only examined these outcomes, suggesting to readers that developmental consequences were limited to the intellectual domain. But in more recent work with preterm infants, there has been an appreciation for the importance of noncognitive outcomes, including social-emotional development, parent–child relationships, temperament, and peer interaction. These noncognitive outcomes are important in their own right. We have also learned that it is somewhat simplistic to separate cognitive from noncognitive outcomes in the sense that factors such as social-emotional behavior and temperament will influence intellectual achievement and

---

[1]SGA = Small for gestational age.

school performance. A child with emotional or behavior problems may not do well in school even if he or she is intellectually competent.

Not surprisingly, we are already starting to see similar findings with drug-exposed infants. Although the database is very small, studies have shown differences in symbolic play and attachment relationships in drug-exposed infants who score within normal limits on developmental tests (Beckwith et al., 1994). In Chasnoff's 3-year follow-up (Azuma & Chasnoff, 1993) some subtests such as language show significant differences between cocaine-exposed infants and controls but exposed children fall within the normal IQ range.

From the study of preterm and other at-risk populations we have also developed multiple-risk models that should be useful in the study of drug-exposed infants. Cumulative risk models suggest that it is the number of risk factors rather than the nature of specific risk factors that determine developmental outcome (Sameroff, Seifer, Barocas, Zax, & Greenspan, 1987). Other models study the resilient or invulnerable children (those who do well despite the presence of multiple risk factors; Garmezy, Masten, & Tellegen, 1984; Lester et al., 1994). This has led to the study of protective factors that may serve as regulators or reregulators of development and help buffer the effects of high risk factors. These models have yet to be applied to the study of drug-exposed infants.

The study of drug-exposed infants is probably best viewed as a special case of the infant at risk and this suggests that we bring to bear on the study of drug-exposed infants all that we have learned from the study of high-risk infants. This includes the abandonment of preconceived biases that these infants are damaged and doomed to fail and that they are "all alike." Rather, the long-term developmental outcome of these children is likely to be a function of how the caregiving environment responds to the behavioral constellation of the infant with the understanding that both the behavior of the infant and the caregiving environment are making dynamic adjustments to each other, as well as being influenced by other forces. We also need to approach the study of the exposed infant from a holistic perspective in which the full range of child behavior (i.e., cognitive as well as noncognitive) is examined.

UNIQUE ASPECTS OF DRUG-EXPOSED INFANTS

At the same time, as stated elsewhere (Lester & Tronick, 1994), we need to address issues that may be unique to the study of the drug-exposed child. One issue, of course, is whether or not there are specific pharmacological effects of various drugs, and how these interact with other pre-, peri-, and postnatal biological and environmental factors. A second issue is poverty. Although many high-risk infants grow up in impoverished environments, the drug-exposed infants (at least those that we get to study) are almost exclusively from the poorest segment of society. What it means to grow up in poverty is something that we are just beginning to study, let alone understand. There is basic food, nutrition, and health to consider. There may also be homelessness, violence, and crime.

Poverty is also associated with minority status, race, and ethnicity. We have barely begun to address the complexities of these issues but they affect our ability to communicate and establish rapport, and to understand cultural factors that affect use of drugs as well as childrearing practices. There are psychometric concerns that have to do with the appropriateness of tests for minorities that have been developed and standardized based on middle-class U.S. values. How do we determine what behavioral processes to study and how do we interpret our findings if we do not know the meaning of these processes in the local culture? For example, we have a bias in much of the United States that eye contact between mother and infant is important in the development of the mother–child relationship. Some cultures, however, discourage this practice and the relationship is based on other behaviors. Clearly we would not want to penalize a mother from a different culture if she did not look at her baby the way many U.S. mothers do. This requires that cultural issues become part of instrument development when we study families from different cultures.

There are also other subpopulations that need to be studied separately, such as teenage mothers. There is already a parenting risk associated with teenage mothers. There is the belief that the teenage mother using drugs puts her child in double jeopardy, but this is probably too simplistic. Like their infants, teenage mothers are not a homogeneous group. Depending on their level of emotional development some are better parents than others. We need to understand the effects of drug exposure in the context of the phenomenon of teenage parenting.

In the case of the exposed infant we have the potential involvement of the social service and legal community because drug use is illegal and has implications for child abuse and neglect. We have the issue of multiple caretakers and multiple placements. When we want to study the attachment relationship it is not always obvious who is the primary caretaker. What is the role of the biological mother in these cases? We also have the unique problem of maternal drug use and possible addiction. As mentioned earlier, the drug problem of the mother is something that needs to be treated somewhat independently of the child. On the other hand, maternal preoccupation with drugs, associated personality disturbances, perhaps psychopathology, and a chaotic lifestyle will clearly impact on the mother–child mutual regulatory system and on the ability of the child to thrive in this environment.

It is critical that we remain open minded about this problem and that we avoid hitching ourselves to the swinging pendulum, swinging from an emphasis on the harmful effect of the drug to the harmful effect of the environment. We learned from the first generation of research in this area that drug effects were exaggerated and that this led to a misperception by the scientific community as well as the public at large in which a generation of children were seen as doomed. It would be just as dangerous at this point to assume that the maternal lifestyle or larger environment is to blame, making the same mistake in the other direction. At this point in time we know very little about the range of developmental outcomes to expect in drug-exposed children or about the etiology of such outcomes. It is probably fair to say that these children are at increased biological and social risk; that their outcome is undetermined; that the full range of intellectual and social-emotional outcomes are possible; and that neither biological nor environmental factors can be ruled in or out as determinants of the developmental outcome in these infants.

It seems likely that we can expect a wide range of individual differences in patterns of development in these children. These patterns of individual differences will be lawfully but differentially related to the interplay between biological (including drug exposure) and social forces. Biological vulnerability makes a child more sensitive to the effects of a poor caretaking environment. By understanding these patterns of individual differences and their biosocial etiologies, we will be able to understand the developmental outcome of drug-exposed children. This understanding will enable us to develop effective preventive and ongoing treatment programs to facilitate the development of the child.

APPENDIX A: PROPOSED "DRUG" SCORING SYSTEM FOR THE BRAZELTON NEONATAL BEHAVIORAL ASSESSMENT SCALE

Recent research has used the Neonatal Behavioral Assessment Scale to study the effects of prenatal substance abuse, primarily cocaine, on newborn behavior. The effects of cocaine are sometimes difficult to detect due, in part, to methodological problems including determining patterns of cocaine use and confounding with other drug and nondrug effects, but also because some of the effects of cocaine may be relatively subtle.

The traditional seven-cluster scoring system for the Brazelton scale may not be adequate to capture effects due to prenatal cocaine exposure. Specifically, reading of the cocaine literature suggests that at least two patterns of neurobehavioral syndromes can be described in these infants, an excitable pattern and a depressed pattern. The seven-cluster scoring system does not readily lend itself to describing these patterns of behavior. Therefore, the data reduction system described here was developed.

To use this system, the infant is assigned 1 point for each item that he or she meets the criteria for Excitable or Depressed behavior. There are 13 items on both the Excitable and Depressed scales. Therefore, each infant may have a range of 0–13 for the Excitable and Depressed scores. Please note that each infant will have the two scores. If missing data is a problem (some infants do not have all scores) it might be useful to compute the mean (i.e., divide the total Excitable or Depressed score by the number of Excitable or Depressed items that are available for the infant).

Excitable	*Depressed*
Tone > 6	Ball < 4
Motor Maturity < 4	Rattle < 4
Cuddliness < 3	Face < 4
Consolability < 4	Voice < 4
Peak Excitement > 7	Face & Voice < 4
Rapidity Buildup > 6	Alertness < 4
Irritability > 5	Tone < 4
Activity > 6	Pull to Sit < 4
Tremulousness > 5	Defensive < 4
Startles > 4	Peak Excitement < 4
Lability Skin > 7	Rapidity Buildup < 4
Lability State > 3	Irritability < 3
Self Quieting < 3	Activity < 4

REFERENCES

Azuma, S. D., & Chasnoff, I. J. (1993). Outcome of children prenatally exposed to cocaine and other drugs: A path analysis of three-year data. *Pediatrics, 92*(3), 396–402.

Beckwith, L., Rodning, C., Norris, D., Phillipsen, L., Khandabi, P., & Howard, J. (1994). Spontaneous play in two-year-olds born to substance-abusing mothers. In B. M. Lester & E. Z. Tronick (Eds.), *Infant Mental Health Journal* [Special Issue on Prenatal Drug Exposure and Child Outcome], *15*(2), 189–201.

Bingol, N., Fuchs, M., Diaz, V., Stone, R. K., & Gromisch, D. S. (1987). Teratogenicity of cocaine in humans. *Journal of Pediatrics, 110*, 93–96.

Chasnoff, I. J., Griffith, D. R., Freier, C., & Murray, J. (1992). Cocaine/polydrug use in pregnancy: Two year follow-up. *Pediatrics, 89*(2), 284–289.

Cregler, L. L., & Mark, H. (1986). Special report: Medical complications of cocaine abuse. *New England Journal of Medicine, 315*(23), 1495–1500.

Doberczak, T. M., Shanzer, S., Senie, R. T., & Kandall, S. (1988). Neonatal neurologic and electroencephalographic effects of intrauterine cocaine exposure. *Journal of Pediatrics, 113*, 354–358.

Fulroth, R., Phillips, B., & Durand, D. J. (1989). Perinatal outcome of infants exposed to cocaine and/or heroin in utero. *American Journal of Diseases of Childhood, 143*, 905–910.

Garmezy, N., Masten, A., & Tellegen, A. (1984). The study of stress and competence in children: A building block for developmental psychopathology. *Child Development, 55*, 97–111.

Gawin, F. H., & Kleber, H. D. (1988). Evolving conceptualizations of cocaine dependence. *Yale Journal of Biology and Medicine, 61*, 123–136.

Hadeed, A. J., & Siegel, S. R. (1989). Maternal cocaine use during pregnancy: Effect on the newborn infant. *Pediatrics, 84*, 205–210.

Inglass, T. H., Curley, F. J., & Prindle, R. A. (1952). Experimental production of congenital anomalies. *New England Journal of Medicine, 247*, 758–768.

Jacobs, B. L. (1985). Overview of the activity of the brain monoaminergic neurons across the sleep-wake cycle. In A. Wauquier, J. M. Monti, J. M. Gaillard, & M. Radilovacki (Eds.), *Sleep-neurotransmitters and neuromodulators* (pp. 1–14). New York: Raven.

Jones, C. L., & Lopez, R. (1988). *Direct and indirect effects on infants of maternal drug abuse.* Washington, DC: Department of Health and Human Services/National Institute of Health.

Kuhn, T. S. (1962). *The structure of scientific revolutions.* Chicago: University of Chicago Press.

Lauder, J. M. (1988). Neurotransmitters as morphogens. *Progress in Brain Research, 73,* 365–387.

Lester, B. M., & Boukydis, C. F. Z. (1991). No language but a cry. In H. Papousek (Ed.), *Origin and development of nonverbal and vocal communication.* Cambridge: Cambridge University Press.

Lester, B. M., Corwin, M. J., Sepkoski, C., Seifer, R., Peucker, M., McLaughlin, S., & Golub, H. L. (1991). Neurobehavioral syndromes in cocaine exposed newborn infants. *Child Development, 62,* 694–705.

Lester, B. M., Garcia-Coll, C. T., Valcarcel, M., Hoffman, J., & Brazelton, T. B. (1986). Effects of atypical patterns of fetal growth on newborn (NBAS) behavior. *Child Development, 57,* 11–19.

Lester, B. M., McGrath, M. M., Garcia-Coll, C. T., Brem, F. S., Sullivan, M. C., & Mattis, S. B. (1994). Relationship between risk and protective factors, developmental outcome and the home environment at 4-years-of-age in term and preterm infants. In H. Fitzgerald, B. M. Lester, & B. Zuckerman (Eds.), *Children in poverty: Research, health care, and policy issues* (pp. 197–227). New York: Garland.

Lester, B. M., & Tronick, E. Z. (1994). The effects of prenatal cocaine exposure and child outcome: Lessons from the past. [Special issue on prenatal drug exposure and child outcome]. *Infant Mental Health Journal, 15*(2), 107–120.

Lester, B. M., & Zeskind, P. S. (1978). Brazelton scale and physical size correlates of neonatal cry features. *Infant Behavior and Development, 49,* 589–599.

Lilienfeld, A. M., & Parkhurst, E. (1951). A study of the association of factors of pregnancy and parturition with the development of cerebral palsy: A preliminary report. *American Journal of Hygiene, 53,* 262–282.

Lutiger, B., Graham, K., Einarson, T. R., & Koren, G. (1991). Relationship between gestational cocaine use and pregnancy outcome: A meta-analysis. *Teratology, 44,* 405–414.

Mahalik, M. P., Gautieri, R. F., & Mann, D. E. (1984). Mechanisms of cocaine induced teratogenesis. *Research Communications in Substances of Abuse, 5*(4), 279–303.

Mayes, L. C. (1994). Neurobiology of prenatal cocaine exposure, effects on developing monoamine systems. In B. M. Lester & E. Z. Tronick (Eds.), *Infant Mental Health Journal* [Special Issue on Prenatal Drug Exposure and Child Outcome], *15*(2).

Mayes, L. C., Granger, R. H., Bornstein, M. H., & Zuckerman, B. (1992). The problem of prenatal cocaine exposure: A rush to judgment. *Journal of the American Medical Association, 267,* 406–408.

Mirochnick, M., Meyer, J., Cole, J., Herren, T., & Zuckerman, B. (1991). Circulating catecholamine concentrations in cocaine-exposed neonates: A pilot study. *Pediatrics, 88*(3), 481–485.

Moore, T. R., Sorg, J., Miller, L., Key, T., & Clark, K. E. (1986). Hemodynamic effects of intravenous cocaine on the pregnant ewe and fetus. *American Journal of Obstetrics and Gynecology, 155,* 883–888.

Mullen, M. K., Garcia-Coll, C. T., Vohr, B. R., & Oh, W. (1988). Mother–infant feeding interaction in full-term small for gestational age infants. *Journal of Pediatrics, 112,* 143–148.

Niswander, K. R., & Gordon, M. (1972). The collaborative perinatal study of the National Institute of Neurological Diseases and Stroke. In K. R. Niswander & M. Gordon (Eds.), *The women and their pregnancies* (pp. 127–140). Philadelphia: W. B. Saunders.

Pasamanick, B., & Knobloch, H. (1966). Retrospective studies on the epidemiology of reproductive causality: Old and new. *Merrill-Palmer Quarterly, 12,* 7–26.

Richie, J. M., & Greene, N. M. (1985). Local anesthetics. In A. G. Gilman, L. S. Goodman, T. N. Rall, & F. Murad (Eds.), *The pharmacologic basis of therapeutics* (7th ed., pp. 309–310). New York: Macmillan.

Salamy, A., Eldredge, L., Anderson, J., & Bull, D. (1990). Brain-stem transmission time in infants exposed to cocaine in utero. *Journal of Pediatrics, 117*(4), 627–629.

Sameroff, A. J., & Chandler, M. J. (1975). Reproductive risk and the continuum of caretaking casualty. In F. D. Horowitz, M. Hetherington, S. Scarr-Salapatek, & C. Sigel (Eds.), *Review of child development* (Vol. 4, pp. 187–244). Chicago: University of Chicago Press.

Sameroff, A. J., Seifer, R., Barocas, R., Zax, M., & Greenspan, S. (1987). Intelligence quotient scores of 4-year-old children: Social environmental risk factors. *Pediatrics, 79,* 343–350.

Shaul, P. W., Cha, C. M., & Oh, W. (1989). Neonatal sympathoadrenal response to acute hypoxia: Impairment after experimental intrauterine growth retardation. *Pediatric Research, 25,* 472–477.

Spitz, H. L., & Rosecan, J. S. (1987). *Cocaine abuse: New directions in treatment and research.* New York: Brunner/Mazel.

Tarr, J. E., & Macklin, M. (1987). Cocaine. *Pediatric Clinics of North America, 34,* 319–331.

Tronick, E. Z. (1989). Emotions and emotional communication. *American Psychologist, 44,* 112–119.

Tronick, E. Z., Frank, D. A., Cabral, H., & Zuckerman, B. S. (1994). A dose-response effect of in utero cocaine exposure on infant neurobehavioral functioning. *Pediatric Research, 35*(#4), Pt. 2, Abs. #152, p. 28A.

Volpe, J. J. (1992). Effect of cocaine use on the fetus. *Mechanisms of Disease, 327*(6), 399–407.

Waddington, C. H. (1966). *Principles of development and differentiation.* New York: Macmillan.

Werner, E. E., Bierman, J. M., & French, F. E. (1971). *The children of Kauai.* Honolulu: University of Hawaii Press.

Wise, R. (1984). Neural mechanisms of the reinforcing action of cocaine. *National Institute of Drug Abuse Monograph Series* (Vol. 50, pp. 15–53). Washington, DC: U.S. Government Printing Office.

Yoon, J. J., Kim, T., Mac Hee, K., Checola, R. T., & Noble, L. M. (1989). Maternal cocaine abuse and microcephaly. *Pediatric Research, 25,* 79A.

3
▼▼▼▼▼▼▼

Incipient Hazards of Cocaine: Lessons from Environmental Toxicology?

Bernard Weiss
University of Rochester School of Medicine and Dentistry

Imagine that cocaine had been classified and viewed as an environmental pollutant. Suppose it had grasped our attention as an industrial chemical found to contaminate waste dumps, or a toxicant in drinking water supplies, or a new pesticide prompting us to set exposure standards for both workers and consumers. Would its health risks be viewed from a different angle than the one now governing our concerns? The answer to that question would be framed within the process of risk assessment.

Risk assessment might sound like a dilettante's refrain to those of you troubled by the devastation that cocaine abuse has wreaked on this society. You might find it even more troubling, though, to view cocaine through the lens with which the risk assessment process perceives environmental chemicals. We are already aware that some offspring of drug-abusing mothers may be seriously impaired. We see a population of children now surging through the school system who may be burdened by multiple handicaps, only one of which is developmental exposure to cocaine. How serious is such a burden? What should be the scope of the community's concerns? Perhaps only a small proportion of children born to abusing mothers suffer extreme adverse consequences. Perhaps proper therapy and supportive environments can overcome these handicaps. Perhaps some of these handicaps are transitory. But our experience with environmental chemicals argues that a low incidence of visible deficits, even if their bearers are subjected to apparently effective interventions, may seriously underestimate the full cost of this epidemic to society and to its individual casualties. A question posed some years ago in a meeting by David Rall, former director of the National

Institute of Environmental Health Sciences, is a compelling framework for the kinds of risk we confront. He asked: Suppose that thalidomide, instead of causing the birth of children with missing limbs, had instead reduced their intellectual potential by 10%. Would we be aware, even today, of its toxic potency?

The path to an answer for his question courses through the process of risk assessment. The conventional risk assessment process for environmental chemicals (National Research Council, 1983) is defined by four stages: hazard identification, dose–response assessment, exposure assessment, and risk characterization. Hazard identification is the stage at which evidence of adverse health effects is weighed. It is a qualitative exercise based on clinical observations, epidemiologic data, and experiments in animals. The relevance of the latter may be judged by dose–response data, replicability, and metabolic correspondence with humans. Cocaine needs no further documentation to fix it as a developmental neurotoxicant. The succeeding steps in the risk assessment process have yet to elicit much interest from cocaine researchers.

Dose–response and exposure assessment stages provide the information by which the quantitative risks to public health, expressed as risk characterization, are then estimated. Not only are such data mostly lacking for cocaine, but those now available are narrow in scope. The shape of the dose–response function is vague; data available from animal experiments derive from a pharmacological orientation that mainly seeks to produce effects, rather than a toxicological one in which dose extrapolation is a key consideration. We especially lack information about latencies that may stretch over a lifetime and about the total impact of exposure at low levels. Childhood is not the final stage of toxic damage inflicted before birth, nor are overtly identifiable outcomes appropriate measures of risk. Exposure estimates derive largely from interviews whose reliability is suspect. The information on which risk characterization depends, dose–response and exposure assessment, is meager.

LONG-LATENCY DISEASES

Cancer is the prototypical disease upon which health risk assessment was founded. With all its etiological complexities, it is still a far simpler endpoint than any of the multiple dimensions generated by neurotoxicant actions. But risk modeling for cancer provides useful features that neurotoxicology might emulate. Cancer is a disease that typically lurks undiscovered for years, usually decades. Mesotheliomas induced by asbestos, for example, often appear after a latency of as long as 40 years. Neurodegenerative diseases are also marked by long latencies. Most authorities believe that events or processes triggered long before clinical eruption are ultimately responsible. Calne, Eisen, McGeer, and Spencer (1986) proposed that Parkinson's disease, Alzheimer's disease, and motor neuron disease all have roots in early events. Only when the aging nervous system loses its capacity to compensate for this earlier damage does the clinical entity emerge. The following are the parallels between neurodegenerative diseases and cancer (Weiss, 1991):

1. Age-specific incidence rises sharply with age.
2. Clinical signs emerge late in the course of the disease.
3. Marked geographic variations are observed.
4. Events early in life may underlie the progression.

Parkinson's disease (PD) may best exemplify such a view because histology provides quantitative support for it. Also, because its cardinal lesion is deficient dopamine function, it could be more closely linked to cocaine exposure than might other neurodegenerative diseases. Its pathological hallmark is a marked loss of pigmented cells in the pars compacta of the substantia nigra (SN), whose axons convey dopamine to terminals in the caudate and putamen. Cell counts by anatomists (e.g., McGeer, Hagaki, Akiyama, & McGeer, 1988) indicate a gradual loss of this cell population throughout life. Once it declines, say, to 10% or 20% of its original size, some clinical indices of PD may become detectable (Langston, 1989; Marsden, 1990). With such a scenario, early losses in SN would predispose the individual to earlier reduction of cell number to the critical size and earlier onset of clinical deficits. Figure 3.1 depicts three different processes: normal aging, accelerated aging, and aging preceded during postnatal development by a

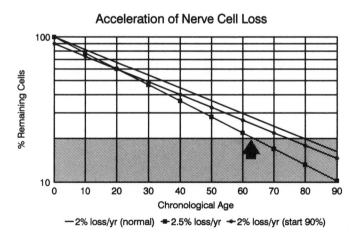

FIG. 3.1. Plot showing decline in neuronal cell density with age in a structure such as the substantia nigra. The hypothetical normal rate is 2% per year. An accelerated rate equal to 2.5% brings cell density into the range of clinical disease (marked by the shaded area) several years earlier, as designated by the arrow. Beginning life with a 10% deficiency in neurons also leads to earlier clinical signs even with a normal rate of decline.

10% erosion of cell number. Assuming that an arbitrary average loss of 2% of remaining cells annually is accelerated by an additional 0.5%, Fig. 3.1 shows that the critical loss level is reached significantly earlier. It also shows that beginning life with a 10% deficit evokes a corresponding shortening of the latency if the rate of progression remains the same.

It also is possible that the original loss provokes more than a simple, parallel decline. The following are the stages of a hypothetical multistage cascade in the etiology of PD.

1. Erosion of cell numbers.
2. Increased transmitter production per cell.
3. Accumulation of toxic products of synthesis.
4. Functional exhaustion.
5. Death.

Zigmond, Abercrombie, Berger, Grace, and Stricker (1990) noted that experimental lesions in animals foment an active compensatory process in which remaining cells, controlled by neurochemical feedback processes, enhance their rate of dopamine synthesis. At the same time, their metabolic products also are created at a higher rate. Figure 3.2 plots the additional output per cell, as the total cell population declines, if production of dopamine is to be held constant. High compensatory rates have been observed experimentally (Zigmond et al., 1990), and the compensatory process seems clinically valid as well (Bernheimer,

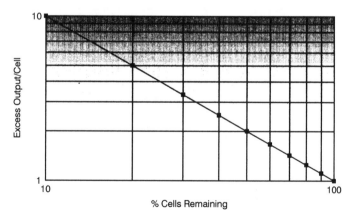

FIG. 3.2. Relationship between cell loss and enhanced requirements imposed on remaining cells. For example, a 50% cell loss means that the surviving cells must produce twice as much neurotransmitter. Such a process actually occurs (Zigmond et al., 1990).

Birkmayer, Hornykiewicz, Jellinger, & Steitelberger, 1973; Jenner, 1989). Even so, striatal dopamine levels fall by about 5% to 8% per decade (Carlsson & Winblad, 1976), indicating limits to compensatory elevations by the remaining SN cells. Schallert's (1988) findings in rats offer additional data about the limits to compensation. Young rats that had received unilateral lesions to areas carrying dopaminergic neurons or pathways apparently recovered after 1 to 3 months. Beginning at about 18 months of age, contralateral sensory deficits reemerged. It is difficult to conceive of any explanation for these findings other than the loss of compensatory capacity with age.

Compensation in this form is not without cost. Increased neurotransmitter production also leads to increased production of free radicals, which current thinking holds to be responsible for some neurodegenerative processes and for many of the adverse consequences of aging. Other toxic products of metabolism, such as quinones, also accumulate. These detrimental corollaries of elevated dopamine production may underlie some of the active neuropathological events detected in PD brains at autopsy (McGeer et al., 1988). Perhaps, then, beginning life with a diminished quota of dopamine synthetic capacity or sensitivity helps accelerate the baseline rate of loss because of the cost of compensation. Individual cells may then reach a stage of functional exhaustion in which they become disabled by the unceasing demands on their synthetic capacity.

Amyotrophic lateral sclerosis (ALS) is another neurodegenerative disease whose origins are speculated to rest in the distant past. Martyn, Barker, and Osmond (1988) correlated the incidence of polio, also a motor neuron disease, with the incidence of ALS several decades later, by examining county-by-county incidence in England and Wales. They noted a significant relationship between rates of polio in the 1930s and rates of ALS in the 1960s. One inference they drew from these data is that subclinical polio infections in childhood, which might have reduced the population of motor neurons without developing into overt disease, left their victims vulnerable to the effects of central nervous system aging and its concomitant depopulation of functional neurons. Such an inference is given force by the postpolio syndrome. Young victims of polio, who apparently recovered, begin to experience a renewal of polio symptoms when they reach middle age or later. Again, most authorities do not ascribe this phenomenon to a latent active process, but to the natural loss of cell numbers that accompanies aging.

One of the more bizarre neurodegenerative diseases is the syndrome known as amyotrophic lateral sclerosis–Parkinsonism dementia (ALS–PD). The native Chamorros of Guam are its most notorious victims. The affliction is thought to arise from the consumption of seeds from the plant *Cycas circinalis* (Spencer, 1990), although some observers contend that dietary mineral imbalances are responsible (Garruto & Yase, 1986). The seeds are ground into a paste and baked into a form resembling a tortilla. Before World War II, processing the seeds through soaking and draining to remove the active but then unidentified toxicant was the usual practice. Under the Japanese occupation, and severe food shortages, the hungry inhabitants shortened the preparation process. After the war, the incidence of ALS–PD began to soar. The U.S. Public Health Service established a station on Guam to study the disease, but could not identify the agent responsible. Spencer (1987), following earlier leads, offered cogent evidence implicating the cycad plant. The gradual conversion of the Chamorro residents of Guam to a conventional U.S. diet parallels a decline in the incidence of the disease.

ALS–PD displays characteristics of three diseases: ALS, Parkinsonism, and dementia of the Alzheimer type. The latter is particularly intriguing. Neuropathological assays reveal the same markers, especially neurofibrillary tangles, seen in the brains of persons diagnosed with Alzheimer's disease. From some viewpoints, the most intriguing aspect of ALS–PD is its sometimes remarkable latency. In one reported case (Zhang, Anderson, Lavine, & Mantel, 1990), the victim had migrated from Guam 45 years earlier and had consumed no cycad products during the intervening years. How can we account for such an extended latency? Is it the culmination of a process set in motion during the subject's early years in Guam? Or, is it a product of a silent lesion, inflicted long before, that flared into clinical disease only with the decline of the brain's reserve capacity?

A NEUROTOXIC PERSPECTIVE

Although neurodegenerative diseases such as PD, ALS, Alzheimer's disease, and Huntington's disease have all been speculated to arise, at least in part, from either exogenous or endogenous neurotoxicants, or both, perhaps the best clues about how to gauge the full developmental impact of cocaine is to review those environmental chemicals that provide the fullest documentation. Lead is an appealing example.

As one of what Hunter (1975) called the ancient metals, lead's poisonous qualities were recognized in antiquity. Lead has been responsible for numerous outbreaks of mass poisoning. It also was recognized as an abortifacient, and, in fact, used surreptitiously for that purpose. Given such a long history, it remains puzzling that its potency as a neurodevelopmental toxicant remained shrouded until rather recently. The beginnings of recognition are often ascribed to a paper published over 50 years ago (Byers & Lord, 1943). It reported that children who had experienced an episode of lead poisoning, contrary to the common belief that recovery is generally complete, subsequently displayed conduct disorders and academic deficiencies.

Not until 1979, however, was compelling evidence presented that, even in the absence of overt lead poisoning, exposed children suffered adverse consequences. Needleman et al. (1979) reported that first- and second-grade children showed differences in IQ and in classroom behaviors as a function of lead concentration in deciduous teeth. Because teeth, like bone, accumulate lead, the shed tooth provides an index of cumulative lead exposure. Blood lead values provide an index only of current exposure. Needleman et al. impelled the regulatory framework to a set of new tenets: Rely, for assessing threats to public health, on psychological test scores and behavior, not on cases of overt poisoning. Newer data from this cohort (Needleman, Schell, Bellinger, Leviton, & Allred, 1990) bolster these tenets. Even in high school, its members displayed evidence of adverse effects attributable to earlier lead exposure. Higher tooth lead values at the beginning of elementary school meant elevated risks of reading difficulties and of failure to graduate from high school.

The 1979 paper also illuminated the defects in cross-sectional studies. Even tooth lead is a rather gross recapitulation of exposure history. It omits the peaks and troughs and other aspects of that history. Neither does it contribute any understanding of fluctuations in behavioral history. Because cross-sectional data posed so many ambiguities, investigators turned to prospective studies. Publications by Bellinger, Leviton, Waternaux, Needleman, and Rabinowitz (1987), Dietrich et al. (1987), and others pointed to early brain development as a major target of lead toxicity. These data demonstrated that prenatal lead levels correlated with standardized indices such as the Bayley Scales of Infant Development administered at age 2. Higher levels in cord blood (Bellinger et al.) or maternal blood (Dietrich et al.) predicted lower scores on these tests. More recent data reveal even more complicated relationships. In further assays of their original sample, Bellinger and Stiles (1993) noted that blood lead levels at age 2 predicted intelligence test scores at age 10. Despite the low lead levels (a mean of about 7 μg/dl), enough variation persisted to provide significant correlations. These data further support the need to pursue latency as a critical variable.

How does the lead story impinge on the risk evaluation of cocaine? Perhaps it can best be illustrated by examining how some critics view the lead findings. What kind of meaning, they ask, can you attach to a 5% IQ difference between higher and lower lead exposure indices when such differences are smaller than the divergence between successive administrations of the same IQ test? Isn't the difference trivial? Aren't there more important hazards confronting children born to mothers who use cocaine? Yes, but risks of different kinds may cumulate.

Risk assessment is merely a precursor to risk management, which is an initiative undertaken on behalf of society and conducted on the basis of many other considerations. Even if we take no action, we should do so only after fully weighing the consequences. In risk assessments for cancer, regulatory agencies such as the EPA calculate exposure levels that presumably would increment the risk by factors of 10^{-5} or 10^{-6}. No one expects that these estimates, based on conservative premises, could be validated in a population in which cancer is a leading cause of death. They drive policy actions nevertheless. Policy actions drawn from the public health impact of cocaine abuse should also be undertaken with full awareness of all the consequences. Lead is a cogent prototype.

Figure 3.3 (Weiss, 1988) is the answer to why a small IQ difference is not trivial. The upper curve depicts the distribution of scores on an intelligence test such as the Stanford–Binet or the Wechsler Intelligence Scale for Children. The mean IQ is 100, with a standard deviation of 15. In a population of 100 million, about 2.3 million will score above 130. If the mean is shifted by 5%, giving a mean IQ of 95, only 990,000 individuals will score above 130 and many more will score below 70, the value that many school systems stipulate as requiring expensive special classrooms and remedial activities. Calculations such as these provided the rationale for the Centers for Disease Control to reduce acceptable blood lead values in children from 25 μg/dl to 10 μg/dl. Even so, the latter value is not a threshold. Statistical modeling has failed to document a convincing threshold.

Lead is a prototype of one sort. Another metal, mercury, expands the latency issue. Methylmercury is an organic form of the element recognized as a potent neurotoxicant. Recognition of that property came during the last century, but its current importance stems from its ecological repercussions. Methylmercury con-

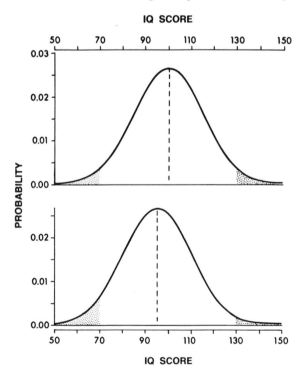

FIG. 3.3.   Consequences of a shift in the IQ distribution. Mean IQ is assumed to be 100, with a standard deviation of 15. In a population of 100 million, 2.3 million individuals will score above 130 (top). A shift of 5%, which produces a mean of 95, means that only 990,000 individuals will score above 130 (from Weiss, 1988).

centrates in the flesh of many fish species, particularly predators at the apex of the food chain, and it can injure the developing brain. Because of its potency, 26 states have issued fish advisories based on elevated mercury levels in fish caught within their borders. Marine species such as shark and swordfish also carry high levels.

The developmental neurotoxicity of methylmercury yielded its first intimations in Japan. In the 1950s, fishermen and their families in the small fishing village of Minamata began to suffer a disabling neurological disease that eventually was confirmed as methylmercury poisoning (Tsubaki & Irukayama, 1977). A higher than usual incidence of cerebral palsy during those years, accompanied by neuropathological findings, seemed to indict methylmercury as a threat to brain development. Prenatal exposure seemed to inflict far greater damage than exposure during adulthood. Without markers of exposure, however, these findings remained ambiguous. The ambiguity was purged in a mass chemical disaster in Iraq.

The arid summer of 1971 seared the Iraqi countryside and ravaged the wheat crop. To restock depleted inventories, the Iraqi government ordered about 80,000 tons of seed grain, mostly wheat of the Mexipak variety, and specified that it be treated with a methylmercury fungicide. Although distributed with warnings that the seeds had been treated with a poison and were suitable only for planting, hungry farm families baked some of the wheat into bread. The result was an epidemic of methylmercury poisoning that exacted about 5,000 deaths in the winter of 1971–1972 (Bakir et al., 1973).

Plunged into crisis, the Iraqi government called on Thomas Clarkson and a team from the University of Rochester, long a center of mercury research, for assistance. Clarkson and his colleagues established a laboratory in Baghdad and embarked on a survey of the Iraqi countryside. By March 1973 the immediate crisis had abated, but its enduring legacy gradually began to surface. Children born to women who had consumed the treated grain during pregnancy exhibited signs of nervous system damage, such as cerebral palsy, much more severe than those of their mothers. Subsequent observations by pediatric neurologists unearthed more subtle defects as the children grew older. Delays in speech and walking were more frequent among the exposed offspring, for example (Marsh et al., 1987).

What made this episode, which exceeded in extent any previous mass chemical disaster, so distinctive was the discovery that the hair follicle takes up methylmercury from blood. The ratio of hair to blood is about 250:1. If you slice scalp hair into segments, you can trace the history of exposure because scalp hair grows at a fairly uniform rate of 1 cm/month. A 12 cm hair shaft yields an exposure history of 1 year. Armed with this technique, it has been possible to provide the most complete dose-response information ever assembled about such an epidemic. Cox, Clarkson, Marsh, and Amin-Zaki (1989) plotted the outcome "delayed walking" (after 18 months of age) against maternal hair levels. These data suggest that even 6 ppm, a level free of any clinical signs, and which could be achieved by the consumption of one swordfish meal per week, may signify the beginnings of a significant increment of risk.

The Iran–Iraq war severed the continuity of the project, but animal experiments probed further into the latent or silent damage possibly provoked by methylmercury. One notable experiment by Cranmer (Spyker, 1975) proved especially cogent. After treating pregnant mice with methylmercury, she maintained the offspring for a lifetime. Her findings are depicted in Fig. 3.4. Many apparently normal mice, once they began to reach middle or advanced age, began to manifest neurobehavioral disturbances of the type pictured in the figure. Others exhibited

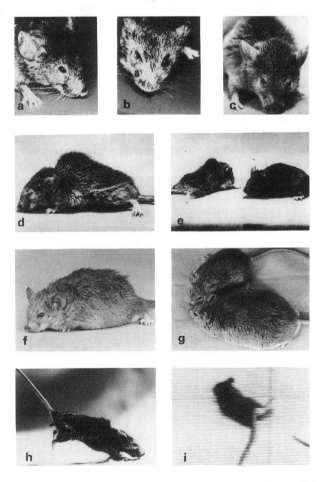

FIG. 3.4. Abnormalities detected in adult mice exposed prenatally to methylmercury. As the mice aged, they began to show purulent exudates from the eyes (a, b, c), kyphosis and hind leg muscular atrophy (d, e), obesity (f, g), debilitation (h), and, when younger, abnormal swimming postures (from Spyker, 1975).

diminished performance on simple behavioral tests. It was almost as if the exposed mice had aged more rapidly than normal mice, except that their disabilities were more flagrant. In monkeys treated earlier in life that had reached their teens, Rice (1989) noted loss of sensation in the hands and impaired coordination. Burbacher, Rodier, and Weiss (1990) observed that monkeys exposed prenatally displayed reduced rates of growth in adolescence.

Lead and methylmercury provide two examples of how the public health implications of cocaine abuse during pregnancy might be pursued. Cocaine presents a more difficult task for several reasons. One is the difficulty in procuring exposure data, most of which come from queries of mothers who are informants of uncertain reliability. Another is the lack of resources that would be necessary to secure such data and to design interventions. Finally, there is a tendency to believe (or hope) that affected children will grow out of their disabilities, or will overcome them with the help of youthful resilience. Isaacson (1975) called this the myth of recovery from early brain damage and marshaled compelling arguments against it. He based his arguments on lesion data, but, as I tried to indicate earlier, they could just as easily have been derived from neurotoxicology.

What appears to be plasticity may simply reflect how difficult it is to ascertain recovery. One of the pioneers in this area, Kennard (1940), lesioned the motor cortex of infant monkeys. Despite apparent compensation soon after surgery, an increasing degree of motor dysfunction began to appear as the monkeys grew older. Goldman (1971) observed analogous phenomena in infant monkeys. With lesions in some cortical locations, deficits seen earlier seemed to fade when the animals were tested at 24 months of age. After lesions in other cortical sites, apparently successful compensation measured at 12 to 18 months of age was succeeded by clear deficits in performance by 24 months of age. Goldman (1974) suggested that these findings might be explained if the lesioned area becomes necessary for function only at a later stage of the maturation process. The process has been described as growing into the lesion.

THE RISK CONNECTION

Because no one doubts that cocaine is a developmental neurotoxicant, the conventional stage of hazard identification in the risk assessment process might now seem superfluous. It would be if we relied on only a single endpoint, as in cancer, and we would then be prepared to undertake the stage of quantitative evaluation labeled as dose–response assessment. For cancer, it describes an attempt to predict incidence at low exposure levels on the basis of data, typically from animal bioassays, obtained at high levels. These predictions take the form of statistical models. A direct passage from hazard identification to dose–response assessment is not feasible in neurotoxicology. Instead of a single endpoint, we have to take into account a plethora of endpoints, mostly based on functional assays rather than pathology. Moreover, we have to consider the role of reversibility, which is not rare for neurotoxicants. The following list describes the elements of what I have called the stage of risk confirmation (Weiss, 1990).

1. Pattern of toxicity.
   a. acute, immediate
   b. chronic, cumulative
   c. delayed
2. Reversibility.
3. Significant endpoints.
   a. behavioral
   b. morphological
   c. neurochemical

Information about several of these components remains at a rather elemental plane in the cocaine literature although the gaps are steadily being filled. They are not being filled thoroughly enough to allow dose–response assessment at a level with which most epidemiologists and statisticians can be comfortable in their extrapolations. It could be argued that our overwhelming concern should be exposures common in abusing mothers and that worries about intermittent use at low doses are an irrelevant luxury. If we viewed cocaine as an environmental toxicant, however, we would insist on risk estimates at low doses no matter how insecure their basis. Recall the question often posed to obstetricians: How much alcohol is it safe to drink during pregnancy? Data gathered by Streissguth and her collaborators (e.g., Streissguth et al., 1986) from their landmark study of fetal alcohol syndrome offer little confidence in the location of a virtual threshold. The equivalent question has been posed for lead, but Wyzga (1990) could not calculate a credible threshold on the basis of data from the study of Bellinger et al. (1987). Thresholds, however, are statistical definitions. A valid risk assessment exercise requires an expanded account of risk versus dose. Even if the current evidence from cocaine research provides little support for significant consequences at low doses, it cannot be dismissed without considerably more data. This is the lesson from ethanol and lead and, perhaps, methylmercury.

The other lesson to be drawn from environmental neurotoxicology is the multiplicity of outcomes we need to consider. These include:

1. Elevated incidence, prevalence.
2. Shift in population distribution.
3. Impaired development.
4. Accelerated aging.

5. Reduced compensatory capacity.
   a. silent toxicity
6. Rate of recovery from reversible effect.

Note their heterogeneity. Is it possible to ignore any of these possibilities when we survey the entire range of possible outcomes? Do we have a reasonable basis for excluding any of them in calculating the ultimate cost of cocaine to the community? Can we even gauge the ultimate cost of blatant abuse? Consequences that may not immediately be apparent to us may assume clandestine disguises until, as Goldman said of surgical lesions, the organism grows into them. How is what Waddington (1993) said about schizophrenia so different from what we face in neurobehavioral teratology? "The neurodevelopmental hypothesis [of schizophrenia] . . . takes as the primary event changes in utero that disrupt the development of fundamental aspects of brain structure and function and that might produce the typical symptoms some two decades later, perhaps only after functional maturation or completion of other, associated, systems or processes—for example, myelination or synaptic pruning" (p. 531).

ACKNOWLEDGMENTS

Preparation of this chapter was supported in part by NIDA Grant DA-07737 and NIEHS Grant ES-01247.

REFERENCES

Bakir, F., Damlugi, S. F., Amin-Zaki, L., Murtadha, M., Khalidi, A., Al-Rawi, N. J., Tikriti, S., Dhahir, H. I., Clarkson, T. W., Smith, J., & Doherty, R. A. (1973). Methylmercury poisoning in Iraq. *Science, 181,* 230–241.

Bellinger, D., Leviton, A., Waternaux, C., Needleman, H., & Rabinowitz, M. (1987). Longitudinal analyses of prenatal and postnatal lead exposure and early cognitive development. *New England Journal of Medicine, 316,* 1037–1043.

Bellinger, D., & Stiles, K. M. (1993). Epidemiologic approaches to assessing the developmental toxicity of lead. *Neurotoxicology, 14,* 151–160.

Bernheimer, H., Birkmayer, W., Hornykiewicz, O., Jellinger, K., & Steitelberger, F. (1973). Brain dopamine and the syndromes of Parkinson and Huntington: Clinical and morphological correlations. *Journal of Neurological Sciences, 20,* 415–455.

Burbacher, T. M., Rodier, P. M., & Weiss, B. (1990). Methylmercury developmental toxicology: A comparison of effects in humans and animals. *Neurotoxicology and Teratology, 12,* 191–202.

Byers, R. K., & Lord, E. E. (1943). Late effects of lead poisoning on mental development. *American Journal of Diseases of Children, 66,* 471–494.

Calne, D. B., Eisen, A., McGeer, E., & Spencer, P. (1986, November 8). Alzheimer's Disease, Parkinson's Disease, and motoneurone disease: Abiotrophic interaction between ageing and environment? *Lancet, 2*(8515), 1067–1070.

Carlsson, A., & Winblad, B. (1976). Influences of age and time interval between death and autopsy on dopamine and 3-methoxytyramine levels in human basal ganglia. *Journal of Neural Transmission, 38,* 271–276.

Cox, C., Clarkson, T. W., Marsh, D. O., & Amin-Zaki, L. (1989). Dose–response analysis of infants prenatally exposed to methylmercury: An application of a single compartment model to single-strand hair analysis. *Environmental Research, 49,* 318–332.

Dietrich, K. N., Kraft, K. M., Bornschein, R. L., Hammond, P. B., Berger, O., Succop, P. A., & Bier, M. (1987). Low-level fetal lead exposure effect on neurobehavioral development in early infancy. *Pediatrics, 80,* 721–730.

Garruto, R. M., & Yase, Y. (1986). Neurodegenerative disorders of the Western Pacific: The search for mechanisms of pathogenesis. *Trends in Neuroscience, 9,* 368–374.

Goldman, P. S. (1971). Functional development of the prefrontal cortex in early life and the problem of neuronal plasticity. *Experimental Neurology, 32,* 366–387.

Goldman, P. S. (1974). An alternative to developmental plasticity: Heterology of CNS structures in infants and adults. In D. G. Stein, J. J. Rosen, & N. Butters (Eds.), *Plasticity and recovery of function in the central nervous system* (pp. 149–174). New York: Academic Press.

Hunter, D. (1975). *The diseases of occupations* (5th ed.). Boston: Little, Brown.

Isaacson, R. L. (1975). The myth of recovery from early brain damage. In N. R. Ellis (Ed.), *Aberrant development in infancy: Human and animal studies* (pp. 1–25). Hillsdale, NJ: Lawrence Erlbaum Associates.

Jenner, P. (1989). Clues to the mechanism underlying dopamine cell death in Parkinson's disease. *Journal of Neurology Neurosurgery and Psychiatry* [Special Supplement], 22–28.

Kennard, M. A. (1940). Relation of age to motor impairment in man and in subhuman primates. *Archives of Neurology and Psychiatry, 44,* 377–397.

Langston, J. W. (1989). Current theories on the cause of Parkinson's disease. *Journal of Neurology Neurosurgery and Psychiatry* [Special Supplement], 13–17.

Marsden, C. D. (1990). Parkinson's disease. *Lancet, 335,* 948–952.

Marsh, D. O., Clarkson, T. W., Cox, C., Myers, G. J., Amin-Zaki, L., & Al-Tikriti, S. (1987). Relationship between concentration in single strands of maternal hair and child effects. *Archives of Neurology, 44,* 1017–1022.

Martyn, C. N., Barker, D. J. P., & Osmond, C. (1988, June 11). Motoneuron disease and past poliomyelitis in England and Wales. *Lancet, 1*(8598), 1319–1322.

McGeer, P. L., Itagaki, S., Akiyama, H., & McGeer, E. G. (1988). Rate of cell death in Parkinsonism indicates active neuropathological process. *Annals of Neurology, 24,* 574–576.

National Research Council. (1983). *Risk assessment in the federal government: Managing the process.* Washington, DC: National Academy Press.

Needleman, H. L., Gunnoe, C., Leviton, A., Reed, M., Peresie, H., Maher, C., & Barrett, P. (1979). Deficits in psychological and classroom performance of children with elevated dentine lead levels. *New England Journal of Medicine, 300,* 689–695.

Needleman, H. L., Schell, A., Bellinger, D., Leviton, A., & Allred, E. N. (1990). The long-term effects of exposure to low doses of lead in childhood. An 11-year follow-up report. *New England Journal of Medicine, 322,* 83–88.

Rice, D. C. (1989). Delayed neurotoxicity in monkeys exposed developmentally to methylmercury. *Neurotoxicology, 10,* 645–650.

Schallert, T. (1988). Aging-dependent emergence of sensorimotor dysfunction in rats recovered from dopamine depletion sustained early in life. *Annals of the New York Academy of Sciences, 515,* 108–120.

Spencer, P. S. (1987). Guam ALS/Parkinsonism-Dementia: A long-latency disorder caused by "slow toxin(s)" in food? *Canadian Journal of Neurological Sciences, 14,* 347–357.

Spencer, P. S. (1990). Chemical time bombs: Environmental causes of neurodegenerative diseases. In R. W. Russell, P. E. Ebert, & A. M. Pope (Eds.), *Behavioral measures of neurotoxicity* (pp. 268–284). Washington, DC: National Academy Press.

Spyker, J. M. (1975). Behavioral teratology and toxicology. In B. Weiss & V. G. Laties (Eds.), *Behavioral toxicology* (pp. 311–344). New York: Plenum.

Streissguth, A. P., Barr, H. M., Sampson, P. D., Parrish-Johnson, J. C., Kirchner, G. L., & Martin, D. C. (1986). Attention, distraction, and reaction time at age 7 years and prenatal alcohol exposure. *Neurobehavioral Toxicology and Teratology, 8,* 721–725.

Tsubaki, F., & Irukayama, K. (Eds.). (1977). *Minamata disease.* New York: Elsevier.

Waddington, J. L. (1993). Schizophrenia: Developmental neuroscience and pathobiology. *Lancet, 341,* 531–537.

Weiss, B. (1988). Neurobehavioral toxicity as a basis for risk assessment. *Trends in Pharmacological Sciences, 9,* 59–62.

Weiss, B. (1990). Risk assessment: The insidious nature of neurotoxicity and the aging brain. *Neurotoxicology, 11,* 305–314.

Weiss, B. (1991). Cancer and the dynamics of neurodegenerative processes. *Neurotoxicology, 12,* 379–386.

Wyzga, R. E. (1990). Towards quantitative risk assessment for neurotoxicity. *Neurotoxicology, 11,* 199–207.

Zhang, Z., Anderson, D. W., Lavine, L., & Mantel, N. (1990). Patterns of acquiring Parkinsonism-Dementia on Guam 1944 through 1985. *Archives of Neurology, 47,* 1019–1024.

Zigmond, M. J., Abercrombie, E. D., Berger, T. W., Grace, A. A., & Stricker, E. M. (1990). Compensations after lesions of central dopaminergic neurons: Some clinical and basic implications. *Trends in Neurological Sciences, 13,* 290–296.

4

▼▼▼▼▼▼▼

Methadone During Pregnancy: A Brief Review of Clinical Outcome and a New Animal Model

Donald E. Hutchings
Ann C. Zmitrovich
New York State Psychiatric Institute

The term *opioids* refers to a family of analgesic compounds, both natural and synthetic, that have morphinelike activity. The natural opioids are obtained from the milky juice contained in the unripe poppy plant *Papaver somniferum*. The juice is dried to a gummy mass, and made into a powder containing a number of alkaloids, chiefly morphine and codeine. There are references to the use of poppy juice in 3rd-century B.C. writings, and by the 16th century the medicinal use of opium to treat pain and diarrhea was well known in Europe.

Heroin or diacetylmorphine, first introduced in 1898, is derived from morphine and produces virtually identical effects. Because of its greater solubility and possibly because it enters the central nervous system (CNS) more rapidly than morphine, it is the major drug of choice among opiate addicts. Although it is still used in Great Britain for the treatment of chronic pain, particularly in cancer patients, it has no general use in medical practice in the United States. Methadone, introduced in 1945, is a completely synthetic opiate. Chemically it is quite different from morphine but it produces nearly identical effects. Although it is being used more frequently in the United States to treat cancer pain, since the late 1960s its major use has been for the treatment of heroin addiction. It is the only drug abuse pharmacotherapy currently approved for the treatment of the pregnant drug abuser.

The following discussion highlights several methodological and interpretive issues that studies of methadone initially brought to light during the formative years of behavioral teratology that have just begun to achieve resolution. Let it be said at the outset that methadone was discovered to be devoid of any teratologic properties; it is neither a structural teratogen nor does it appear to produce brain injury, although there is a suggestion in some studies of effects on motor coordination in children but not in animals. The results of five epidemiological studies have been critically reviewed by Kaltenbach and Finnegan (1984). Overall, despite a host of differences between the studies, there is remarkable agreement on outcome, summarized briefly as follows: First, although there tend to be differences between methadone-exposed and control infants on the Bayley Scales of Infant Development, scores for the methadone-exposed infants are well within the normal range of development. Second, for those children who were tested at 4 years of age, no consistent differences were found on several standard measures of cognitive performance.

Hans (1989) reported that methadone showed no evidence of producing direct effects on cognitive development. Rather, her findings point to a significant interaction of prenatal methadone with socioeconomic class. When drug-exposed children are reared in extremely poor environmental circumstances, they are at greater risk for showing impaired mental development compared with matched controls. She suggested that methadone creates a vulnerability in the exposed children that, in turn, makes them more susceptible to an impoverished environment. This view is consistent with Wilson (1989), who similarly noted that children are equally at risk for a high incidence of behavioral and school-related problems whether they were exposed to heroin prenatally or merely raised in a drug-abuse environment. What, then, are the hazards of prenatal exposure to methadone, and are they best conceptualized using the teratology paradigm?

OPIOID ABSTINENCE IN THE ADULT

The repeated administration of opioids and several other sedative-hypnotic drugs (e.g., alcohol, barbiturates) to adults induces an adaptive physiological state, physical dependence, whereby if drug administration is discontinued, a stereotyped syndrome occurs that is referred to as *withdrawal* or *abstinence*. These symptoms are characterized by rebound effects in those same physiological systems that were initially modified by the drug. For example, the general depressant drugs elevate the threshold for seizures, whereas spontaneous seizures are seen during withdrawal (Jaffe, 1990). Heroin addicts must self-inject at regular intervals—usually 4 to 6 hrs—not only to achieve a state of euphoria but also to avoid abstinence symptoms. Conceptualized in general neuropharmacological terms, this phenomenon can be summarized as follows (World Health Organization, 1981):

1. Exposure to opioids and sedative-hypnotic drugs results in a homeostatic process of neuroadaptation.
2. This neurophysiological process represents a compensatory adaptation induced by a perturbation of the CNS by the presence of the compound in the CNS.

3. Once neuroadaptation has been induced and the compound is no longer present at receptor sites, a neurophysiological state of withdrawal or dysregulation ensues.

The rationale for methadone maintenance is that compared with heroin, methadone is effective when taken orally and has a half-life of approximately 24 hrs, requiring administration only once per day. Maintenance clients administered optimum doses of methadone do not experience euphoria or abstinence and when treated in an effective program of social rehabilitation, are able to resume a relatively normal, and often productive life.

Both heroin and methadone cross the placenta and induce physical dependence in the fetus. At birth, the fetus' supply of maternal opioids is interrupted and the neonate, like the adult, undergoes opioid abstinence. Symptoms may occur at birth or soon after, are characterized by CNS irritability and poor autonomic control, and can include tremors, sleeplessness, seizures, hyperphagia, vomiting, and diarrhea. If severe and untreated (paregoric or diazepam are current drugs of choice), the symptoms can be life threatening. These early symptoms represent acute withdrawal and, depending on time of onset, peak at about 3 to 6 weeks and then slowly subside. Not all infants show all the symptoms and several patterns have been described that differ in time of onset and temporal course depending on the compound and other complex factors (Desmond & Wilson, 1975). Many infants go on to show less severe symptoms of subacute or prolonged withdrawal characterized by restlessness, agitation, fine tremors, and sleep disturbance that resolve around 4 to 6 months of age. Adults too experience a prolonged abstinence characterized by hypersomnia, lowered heart rate, and lowered body temperature, symptoms that are generally mild but nevertheless persist for 6 months or longer (Martin et al., 1973).

PREGNANCY, METHADONE DOSE, AND RISK OF HIV INFECTION

It is well established that daily methadone maintenance doses in the range of 60 to 100 mg are significantly more successful and of optimal rehabilitative benefit for the prevention of relapse to illicit drug use than daily doses of 30 to 50 mg or less (see major review by Hargreaves, 1983). With low-dose regimens, clients begin to complain of withdrawal and are at risk of relapse to excessive alcohol and illicit drug use. A major problem that has evolved in methadone clinics since the late 1970s has been the shift to low maintenance doses in the range of 20 to 40 mg per day (Schuster, 1989). Adding to the problem, if clients become pregnant, it had been strongly recommended that clinics reduce the maintenance dose even further (e.g., 5 to 20 mg/day) in order to minimize symptoms of neonatal abstinence (e.g., Ostrea, Chavez, & Strauss, 1976).

Currently, pregnant clients are routinely maintained at 20 to 30 mg/day or even less. A serious health crisis created by these low maintenance doses is that pregnant clients, particularly during the increased weight gain in the third trimester, begin to experience withdrawal as their low dose results in progressively lower plasma levels. These individuals are thus at high risk for abusing other illicit substances, including intravenous (IV) heroin, alcohol, and cocaine. One result is that with the spread of the human immunodeficiency virus (HIV) since the 1980s, there has been a substantial increase in HIV infection among clients in methadone maintenance programs (Selwyn, Hartel, Wasserman, & Drucker, 1989). Moreover, this problem is growing by alarming proportions and could, in part, be remedied by a higher dosing regimen (Ball, Lange, Meyers, & Friedman, 1988). The sad paradox of the low-dose treatment policy is that pregnant clients are administered suboptimal doses of methadone in order to avoid a manageable risk, that is, the neonatal abstinence syndrome. In this context, *manageable* implies a risk that is readily treated with appropriate pharmacotherapy. The tragedy is that by virtue of the likelihood that these mothers will resort to IV heroin use, they expose themselves as well as their fetuses to the unacceptable risk of HIV infection (Pyun, Ochs, Dufford, & Wedgewood, 1987). Here, *unacceptable* implies a high risk of HIV infection and eventual death for both the mother and child from acquired immunodeficiency syndrome (AIDS). Recent figures from the National Institute on Drug Abuse (NIDA) indicate that 75% of HIV-infected babies are born to IV drug abusers or their sexual partners (*NIDA Notes*, 1990). The pharmacological aspect of treatment is only one of many components of a comprehensive drug treatment program but it does play a major role in the retention of clients in these programs (Ball et al., 1988) so that they remain available for the psychosocial intervention that is so vital for successful rehabilitation.

Despite this serious health menace, methadone clinics are generally reluctant to treat any female client that becomes pregnant, and those that are, are typically placed on a low-dose regimen because of the ill-advised notion that higher doses are harmful to the fetus and newborn. Even in the current climate of fear about HIV infection, there is little interest in reexamining dose–response effects in a treatment population. And although animal studies could provide preclinical risk assessment studies, animal models have been controversial with respect to their adequacy in providing clinically relevant data.

ANIMAL STUDIES OF METHADONE: PHARMACOLOGICAL ISSUES

One of the more interesting developments that occurred as methadone researchers attempted to develop animal models beginning in the 1970s was the eruption of a debate over their pharmacological relevance. Sparber (1983) raised a key issue that focused on differences between humans and rats with respect to the half-life and duration of action of methadone. In the human, as mentioned earlier, the plasma half-life of methadone is about 24 hrs. When administered once daily in humans, physical dependence is maintained over the 24 hrs before the next daily dose and the patient does not experience opioid withdrawal. But in the rat, the half-life is only about 90 min in nongravid animals and 3 to 5 hrs in gravid animals. Sparber (1983) contended that the dams and fetuses undergo daily withdrawal after each dose so that those experimental paradigms that used administration once daily, rather than producing chronic dependence produced daily withdrawal, and it was this feature of the treatment that produced the adverse effects that some workers were reporting. Because these animal paradigms did not adequately model the human methadone regimens, he considered the data to be irrelevant and the conclusions misleading.

In the early 1980s when this debate occurred, others expressed various points of disagreement with Sparber but they were merely offering alternate guesses in the absence of definitive data and the issue could only be resolved with new research. By this time, however, methadone was generally accepted as a safe and effective treatment, including its use during pregnancy, and there was little incentive to carry out the needed research. Two major events changed the existing priorities: A sudden increase in the use of cocaine began sweeping the country in the mid-1980s and the drug abuse research and treatment community became preoccupied with trying to assess the public health hazard and formulate remedies. Any residual concern about heroin abuse and methadone programs was entirely eclipsed by the "crack" cocaine epidemic. And in the midst of this, public health authorities, as well as public reaction, was being overtaken by the growing AIDS epidemic, and survey data revealed that a disproportionately large number of HIV-positive individuals were IV drug users who shared dirty needles to inject cocaine and heroin. Along with other preventative measures, a renewed emphasis on the importance of methadone maintenance programs was launched by NIDA in the hope of providing a treatment intervention to stop the rapid spread of AIDS. These events also provided a new rationale and impetus to develop animal models that would study dose–response effects of methadone, particularly if there was any special hazard produced at high doses. Such studies would first require, however, the development of an animal model that was clinically relevant.

New Animal Studies

Beginning in 1986, animal studies began to appear that effectively solved the pharmacological problems that plagued the earlier research. These studies used the newly developed osmotic minipump to administer methadone (e.g., Darmani, Saady, Scholl, & Martin, 1991; Enters, Guo, Pandey, Ko, & Robinson, 1991; Wang, Pasulka, Perry, Pizzi, & Schnoll, 1986), a technique that has the important advantage of delivering a fixed flow rate of methadone so that physical dependence is produced in the dam, but with a minimum of maternal and fetal toxicity. Our laboratory carried out a study to compare the effects of methadone administered by the osmotic minipump (Hutchings et al., 1992) with previous findings from our laboratory that used once daily dosing (Hutchings, Feraru, Gorinson, & Golden, 1979; Hutchings, Hunt, Towey, Rosen, & Gorinson, 1976).

Two doses of methadone were administered by osmotic minipump from Day 8 of gestation through parturition. Nontreated (NT) and pair-fed (PF) dams served as controls and all litters were fostered at birth to untreated dams. Naloxone, an opiate antagonist, was administered to the dams immediately after parturition and by virtue of the abstinence symptoms observed (e.g., weight loss, teeth chattering, diarrhea), physical dependence was clearly demonstrated. As to effects on the offspring, compared to once daily dosing, we observed the following: First, fewer resorptions were produced at comparable dose levels, suggesting that the daily high peak concentrations associated with once daily dosing were embryotoxic. Second, the high dose produced a transitory delay in postnatal weight gain, an effect we had not previously observed with once daily dosing. Finally, the behavioral effects—a critical aspect of the study that we describe directly— were virtually identical to those previously reported for once daily dosing.

The behavioral endpoint used in this study is one that we had developed in our laboratory for the purpose of assessing prenatal methadone effects (Hutchings et al., 1979). Testing is carried out at 22 days of age by placing groups of three littermates from each of the treated and control groups in cages and measuring their activity on electronic activity monitors during an 8-hr observation period. No behavioral effects were observed for either the control group or the low-dose methadone group. The high-dose methadone offspring, however, spent less time resting, showed disrupted rhythmicity, and showed poor state regulation. They were also more active and significantly more state-labile; that is, they showed more frequent shifts from low to high activity.

The activity data for two groups of 22-day-old pair-fed/vehicle controls and high-dose animals are shown in Fig. 4.1. From direct behavioral observations, it was determined that counts of 0 represent periods during which the test group was huddled and sleeping; these 0 counts are referred to as *sleep-rest periods.* The brief spikes that range from 0 to 50 were typically produced by periods of waking of one or more of the three test animals and repositioning within the group. Active exploration by the entire group of three produced counts of approximately 50 and higher. As shown in the top panel of Fig. 4.1, at the outset of the observation period, the control groups showed active exploration for about 30 min, followed by a sleep-rest period. Following this, they tended to show a distinct rhythmicity in their rest–activity cycle. By comparison, the 15 mg/kg groups shown in the lower panel revealed striking differences; they remained active throughout virtually the entire 8-hr observation period and their activity patterns were marked by relatively rapid oscillations from low to high levels, with a complete absence of any prolonged sleep-rest periods.

The rest–activity cycles measured at postnatal Day (PND) 22 for the NT and PF control offspring are identical to control data previously published from our

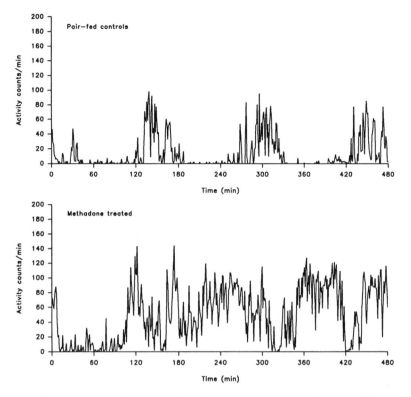

FIG. 4.1. Activity for offspring of methadone-treated (lower panel) and pair-fed control rats (upper panel) at 22 days of age.

laboratory (Hutchings et al., 1979; Hutchings, Miller, Gamagaris, & Fico, 1989). The findings of the irregular rest–activity cycle, increased changes in activity level and less time spent in rest periods that we report here among the 15 mg/kg exposed offspring are also the same as the behavioral effects we previously described (Hutchings et al., 1979). Moreover, they bear a striking resemblance to similar persistent effects observed among opiate-exposed human infants and may provide an animal model of prolonged abstinence. Again, the earlier research used a once daily dosing schedule, yet the behavioral effects seen in the offspring were virtually the same as those found here. We have no explanation for the similarity of effects using such different dosing techniques and can only conclude that the pharmacological mechanism in both the dams and offspring remains poorly understood. Clearly, however, the results are not simply related to the maternal toxicity associated with once daily dosing or the dependence produced by continuous methadone infusion.

Related to the controversy over an adequate animal model, these results provide some resolution to the assertion of Sparber (1983) that the daily withdrawal associated with once daily administration was the likely cause of adverse effects in the offspring. Comparing the earlier work that used once daily dosing with the findings using the minipump, it is clear that methadone, whether administered once daily or under conditions that produced steady state blood levels in the dams, produces disrupted rest–activity scores in 22-day-old offspring.

Further studies from our laboratory using the minipump model have provided important additional information regarding the relevance of this model to the clinical description of opiate abstinence. Using the same treatment and control procedures described earlier, acoustic startle amplitude, used as a measure of CNS hyperexcitability, was measured for each treated and control animal at PND 22. Because prenatal methadone exposure resulted in reduced body weight at the time of testing, it was necessary to analyze startle amplitude using weight as a covariate. This analysis showed that the methadone-treated offspring had a significantly enhanced mean startle amplitude compared with the controls, suggesting that prenatal exposure to methadone produces a prolonged state of CNS hyperexcitability similar to clinical descriptions of human infants undergoing opiate abstinence.

To determine if the rest–activity and startle effects seen at PND 22 diminish over time as they do in opiate-exposed human infants, treated and control animals were tested either for changes in acoustic startle amplitude or the rest–activity cycle at PND 30. Methadone-treated offspring were no different from the controls on either measure, suggesting that prenatal exposure to methadone produces a prolonged but transitory opioid abstinence. Therefore, startle amplitude and a disturbed rest–activity cycle peak at approximately 3 weeks of age, and are no longer evident at 4 weeks of age. Together, these findings define a state of hyperexcitability in the young rat that resolves by 1 month of age. This transitory state parallels clinical descriptions of human infants undergoing opiate abstinence.

METHADONE SUMMARY

It now seems clear that acute withdrawal is directly related to the rate at which the drug is cleared from plasma—the more rapid the clearance, the more severe the symptoms (Rosen & Pippenger, 1976). The mechanism underlying prolonged withdrawal is unknown; it occurs, however, after pharmacologically active concentrations of the compound have cleared from the CNS. Adults also experience a prolonged abstinence characterized by hypersomnia, lowered heart rate, and lowered body temperature, symptoms that are generally mild but nevertheless persist for 6 months or longer (Martin et al., 1973).

We reported that rat offspring prenatally exposed to methadone during the last 2 weeks of gestation show a disrupted rest–activity cycle and an enhanced acoustic startle response at PND 22, findings we interpret as representing prolonged abstinence. However, offspring prenatally exposed to methadone and tested at PND 30 were no different from controls on these same outcome variables.

These findings support the interpretation that the behavioral disturbances observed at PND 22 are transitory and represent a state of prolonged opiate abstinence. Moreover, these effects parallel similar observations for human neonates prenatally exposed to opioids.

Finally, we reported that neither prenatally administered cocaine (Zmitrovich, Hutchings, Dow-Edwards, Malowany, & Church, 1992) nor delta-9-tetrahydrocannabinol (Hutchings et al., 1989) disrupt the rest–activity cycle of the 3-week-old rat, findings consistent with the clinical view that these compounds do not appear to produce neonatal abstinence. Perhaps the disruption of the rest–activity cycle that we have found for methadone is specific to opioids and/or other sedative-hypnotic compounds. Thus, testing for changes in the rest–activity cycle as well as acoustic startle in 3- to 4-week-old rats may be useful screening techniques to detect compounds that have the potential to produce neonatal abstinence. Both the acoustic startle and rest–activity measure are readily automated and yield straightforward results that are relatively easy to analyze and interpret.

ACKNOWLEDGMENTS

Research for this chapter was supported by grant DA07822 from the National Institute on Drug Abuse. Portions of this chapter were adapted from Hutchings, D. E. (1993). A contemporary overview of behavioral teratology: A perspective from the field of substance abuse. In H. Kalter (Ed.), *Issues and reviews in teratology* (pp. 125–167). New York: Plenum.

REFERENCES

Ball, G. C., Lange, W. R. R., Meyers, C. P., & Friedman, S. R. (1988). Reducing the risk of AIDS through methadone maintenance treatment. *Journal of Health and Social Behavior, 29,* 214–226.

Darmani, N. A., Saady, J. J., Schnoll, S. H., & Martin, B. R. (1991). Demonstration of physical dependence following chronic continuous methadone delivery via osmotic minipumps in pregnant rats. *Neurotoxicology and Teratology, 13,* 627–630.

Desmond, M. M., & Wilson, G. S. (1975). Neonatal abstinence syndrome: Recognition and diagnosis. In R. D. Harbison (Ed.), *Perinatal addiction* (pp. 113–121). New York: Spectrum.

Enters, E. K., Guo, H., Pandey, U., Ko, D., & Robinson, S. E. (1991). The effects of prenatal methadone exposure on development and nociception during the early postnatal period of the rat. *Neurotoxicology and Teratology, 13,* 161–166.

Hans, S. L. (1989). Developmental consequences of prenatal exposure to methadone. *Annals of the New York Academy of Sciences, 562,* 195–207.

Hargreaves, W. A. (1983). Methadone dose and duration of treatment. In J. R. Cooper, F. Altman, B. S. Brown, & D. Czechowicz (Eds.), *Research on the treatment of narcotic addiction: State of the art* (DHHS Pub. No. ADM 83-1281, pp. 19–79). Rockville, MD: National Institute on Drug Abuse.

Hutchings, D. E., Feraru, E., Gorinson, H. S., & Golden, R. (1979). The effects of prenatal exposure to methadone on the rest-activity cycle of the preweanling rat. *Neurobehavioral Toxicology and Teratology, 1*, 33–40.

Hutchings, D. E., Hunt, H. F., Towey, J. P. Rosen, T. S. & Gorinson, H. S. (1976). Methadone during pregnancy in the rat: Dose level effects on maternal and perinatal mortality and growth in the offspring. *Journal of Pharmacology and Experimental Therapeutics, 197*, 171–179.

Hutchings, D. E., Miller, N., Gamagaris, Z., & Fico, T. A. (1989). The effects of prenatal exposure to delta-9-tetrahydrocannabinol on the rest-activity cycle of the preweanling rat. *Neurotoxicology and Teratology, 11*, 353–356.

Hutchings, D. E., Zmitrovich, A., Brake, S. C., Malowany, D., Church, S., & Nero, T. J. (1992). Prenatal administration of methadone using the osmotic minipump: Effects on maternal and offspring toxicity, growth, and behavior in the offspring. *Neurotoxicology and Teratology, 14*, 65–71.

Jaffe, J. H. (1990). Drug addiction and drug abuse. In A. G. Gilman, T. W. Rall, A. S. Nies, & P. Taylor (Eds.), *The pharmacological basis of therapeutics* (8th ed., pp. 522–573). New York: Pergamon.

Kaltenbach, K., & Finnegan, L. P. (1984). Developmental outcome of children born to methadone maintained women: A review of longitudinal studies. *Neurobehavioral Toxicology and Teratology, 6*, 271–275.

Martin, W. R., Jasinski, D. R., Haertzen, C. A., Kay, D. C., Jones, B. E., Mansky, P. A., & Carpenter, R. W. (1973). Methadone: A reevaluation. *Archives of General Psychiatry, 28*, 286–295.

NIDA notes. (1990, Summer). Rockville, MD: National Institute on Drug Abuse.

Ostrea, E. M., Chavez, C. J., & Strauss, M. E. (1976). A study of factors that influence the severity of neonatal narcotic withdrawal. *Journal of Pediatrics, 88*, 642–645.

Pyun, K. H., Ochs, H. D., Dufford, M. T. W., & Wedgewood, R. J. (1987). Perinatal infection with human immunodeficiency virus. *New England Journal of Medicine, 317*, 611–614.

Rosen, T. S., & Pippenger, C. E. (1976). Pharmacological observations on the neonatal withdrawal syndrome. *Journal of Pediatrics, 88*, 104.

Selwyn, P. A., Hartel, D., Wasserman, W., & Drucker, E. (1989). Impact of the AIDS epidemic on morbidity and mortality among intravenous drug users in a New York City methadone maintenance program. *American Journal of Public Health, 79*, 1358–1362.

Schuster, C. R. (1989, Spring/Summer). Methadone maintenance: An adequate dose is vital in checking the spread of AIDS. In *NIDA Notes*. Rockville, MD: National Institute on Drug Abuse.

Sparber, S. B. (1983). Preclinical perinatal and developmental effects of methadone: Behavioral and biochemical aspects. In J. R. Cooper, F. Altman, S. Brown, & D. Czechowicz (Eds.), *Research on the treatment of narcotic addiction: State of the art* (DHHS Pub. No. ADM 83-1281, pp. 318–346). Rockville MD: National Institute on Drug Abuse.

Wang, C., Pasulka, P., Perry, B., Pizzi, W. J., & Schnoll, S. H. (1986). Effects of perinatal exposure to methadone on brain opioid and a2-adrenergic receptors. *Neurobehavioral Toxicology and Teratology, 8*, 399–402.

Wilson, G. S. (1989). Clinical studies of infants and children exposed prenatally to heroin. *Annals of the New York Academy of Sciences, 562*, 183–194.

World Health Organization Expert Committee on Addiction-Producing Drugs. (1981). *Bulletin of the World Health Organization, 39*, 225.

Zmitrovich, A. C., Hutchings, D. E., Dow-Edwards, D. L., Malowany, D., & Church, S. (1992). The effects of prenatal exposure to cocaine on the rest-activity cycle of the preweanling rat. *Pharmacology, Biochemistry, and Behavior, 43*, 1059–1064.

METHODS

The authors in this section agree that the study of prenatal cocaine exposure presents a number of difficult methodological challenges. Methodologically sound studies are critical. Claims about the consequences of exposure to cocaine during gestation, or lack thereof, have extended beyond the scientific literature. The popular media have declared exposure to cocaine during gestation to be a present-day scourge with long-term, devastating consequences to the children, as well as societal resources. Angry scientists have responded to these claims by emphasizing the lack of well-conducted, longitudinal research, and the sparse support at this time for such declarations. This is an issue fraught with consequences for individuals as well as social policy. Erroneous negative findings can be as dangerous as invalid positive ones. The failure to detect an effect might be interpreted to mean that cocaine exposure is safe. This could lead to a lax public health policy that would result in the failure to try to prevent what might be avoidable prenatal damage. Reporting deficits resulting from cocaine exposure that turn out to be mistaken can lead to stigmatization and inappropriate direction of intervention resources. By enumerating the difficulties of this research endeavor, the chapters in this section point the way to the most methodologically valid study designs that can best inform the scientific community, public policymakers, and the public about the effects of this societal problem.

Vorhees reviews the animal research of the last decade on effects of cocaine exposure. He focuses his inquiry on how well these studies have established that cocaine is, in fact, a hazard, as all other questions follow from this. Vorhees points out the many limitations of the efforts he has reviewed. These include the small number of species studied, the paucity of research in rats that is comparable to third-trimester exposure in humans, concerns about the comparability to human exposure of route of administration and pharmacokinetics, and issues of the appropriateness of control groups. The author expresses his uncertainty as to whether the large number of negative reports is due to the relative safety of cocaine exposure or to the possibility that cocaine has very specific effects. The widely cast nets of the early studies have turned up relatively few hits compared to misses. Several other critical research issues are raised in this chapter, including the need to control for maternal carryover effects, whether peak exposure or total exposure has greater consequences, and whether there are critical periods of exposure. These are questions most easily addressed by animal studies.

Neuspiel describes the problems of identifying and controlling the effects of confounding variables. It is clear that cocaine use is not an isolated event. Neuspiel enumerates several ways in which cocaine users differ from nonusers. In particular, use is associated with many other toxic exposures, such as alcohol and nicotine; the social environment probably differs in significant ways; and both the physical and mental health of users is likely to be worse. The concern is that findings attributed to cocaine exposure may actually be the result of differences between the groups on some other, confounding variable. Therefore, it is crucial to take this issue into account when designing studies.

J. Jacobson and S. Jacobson identify several additional methodological difficulties they have gleaned from their experience studying prenatal alcohol exposure. Issues of the validity of the procedures used to assess exposure levels, and the sensitivity of the developmental outcome measures are discussed, as well as the appropriate handling of confounding and mediating variables. This chapter raises the very difficult question of how to determine accurately the amount and timing of prenatal exposure to cocaine. The issue is critical, because a teratogen may be tolerated at low levels but be problematic once a threshold is exceeded. The authors suggest that studies must recognize the threshold problem, which necessitates obtaining some measure of extent of exposure. Unstable and inconsistent findings thus far may be the result of "positive" samples being heterogeneous for exposure level.

Olson and colleagues call our attention to still other difficulties of studying this problem. Using the Seattle Cocaine and Pregnancy Study as a model, they point out the necessity of recruiting an appropriate sample, with an unbiased comparison group, that has sufficient power to answer the questions of interest. They bring up the difficulty of maintaining a sample of drug-using women for longitudinal study of their children, and the importance of adopting a developmental perspective of the potential toxicity of cocaine exposure. The authors discuss the need to assess specific functions thought to be sensitive to prenatal cocaine exposure, with age-appropriate measures at the proper ages. The questions of confounding variables, and the complexities of measuring the timing and extent of exposure are discussed as well.

The final chapters in this section address two of the specific concerns discussed by the previous authors. Bendersky and colleagues discuss the need for multiple, sensitive, and predictive outcomes in assessing the impact of prenatal exposure. A study of developmental effects of intraventricular hemorrhage in children born prematurely is presented as a model for examining the impact of an early biological perturbation. The authors suggest that the measurement of other early medical complications associated with the biological insult, as well as multiple environmental risks, is crucial. Analysis that evaluates the interactions among the biological and environmental risks over time is applicable to the cocaine-exposed child. Criteria for choosing appropriate functional outcomes are suggested, and one such measure, contingency learning and its emotional concomitants, is discussed in detail. Findings to date indicate that prenatal cocaine exposure may specifically influence arousal, engagement in a learning task, and emotional responsivity in the first year of life.

Finally, Ostrea presents the case for one answer to the problem of identifying drug exposure. The author presents a compendium of studies that ascertain the usefulness of meconium drug screening. He reviews the studies that established the relation between dosage and timing of drug administration and the concentration of metabolites in the meconium, the precision of radioimmunoassay techniques, the best method for collecting and storing meconium, and confirmation of the utility of the technique in clinical studies. Ostrea concludes by reporting exciting recent developments, including using meconium assays to establish the amount and timing of drug use, the detection of meconium as early as the 16th week of gestation, and the ability to assay nicotine metabolites in this matrix.

The chapters of this section powerfully convey the difficulties of conducting research in this area. Problems include multiple pre- and postnatal confounding variables; a lack of reliable methods for determining the extent and timing of prenatal exposure; a need for sensitive, specific, and developmentally appropriate outcome measures; and the difficulty of recruiting and maintaining a sample of children of chemically dependent women. The authors draw on their enormous combined experience to illuminate a path toward achieving a true understanding of the effects of prenatal cocaine exposure.

5

▼▼▼▼▼▼▼

A Review of Developmental Exposure Models for CNS Stimulants: Cocaine

Charles V. Vorhees
University of Cincinnati

In the 1980s the illicit use of cocaine in North America became a recognized health issue and shortly thereafter newborns appeared in hospitals with apparent cocaine-related symptoms born to women using cocaine during pregnancy. Initial clinical studies suggested several adverse effects in such neonates, including possible cerebral hemorrhages (Dixon & Bejar, 1989), increase in SIDS frequency (Chasnoff, Hunt, Kletter, & Kaplan, 1989), increased congenital malformation rates (Bingol, Fuchs, Diaz, Stone, & Gromisch, 1987), lowered birth weight and head circumference (Chasnoff, Griffith, MacGregor, Dirkes, & Burns, 1989; MacGregor et al., 1987; Zuckerman et al., 1989; and see Neuspiel & Hamel, 1991), and neurobehavioral symptoms (Anday, Cohen, Kelley, & Leitner, 1989; Chasnoff, Burns, & Burns, 1987; Chasnoff, Burns, Schnoll, & Burns, 1985; Chasnoff, Griffith, Freier, & Murray, 1992; Chasnoff, Hunt, et al., 1989; Lester et al., 1991). Subsequent to these reports, several studies were published suggesting fewer or no effects (Coles, Platzman, Smith, James, & Falek, 1992; Neuspiel, Hamel, Hochberg, Greene, & Campbell, 1991; Richardson & Day, 1991). Lutiger, Graham, Einarson, and Koren (1991) published a meta-analysis of previous clinical studies. In this analysis, intrauterine death and increased genitourinary defects were the only effects that emerged with consistency and even these effects were only weakly associated with cocaine exposure. Subsequent studies continued to report reductions in birth weight, but other changes have been difficult to link to cocaine exposure. Furthermore, the presence of multiple confounding variables in the populations under investigation led some investigators to suggest that the deleterious developmental effects of cocaine had been overstated and that the effects observed were as strongly associated with a cluster of other risk factors as they were with cocaine (Mayes, Granger, Bornstein, & Zuckerman, 1992; Zuckerman & Frank, 1992). More recently, the association between intrauterine cocaine exposure and genitourinary tract abnormalities has been questioned (Koren, 1993).

However, the recent rising tide of skepticism by some investigators (Koren, Glasdonte, Robeson, & Robieux, 1992) has also been mingled with several new reports of cocaine-associated effects. One has shown residual head circumference deficits at 2 years of age (Chasnoff et al., 1992) and another has shown neurobehavioral effects in neonates exposed prenatally to cocaine, finding deficits in the habituation cluster on the Brazelton Neonatal Behavioral Assessment Scales (Mayes, Granger, Frank, Schottenfield, & Bornstein, 1993).

In the midst of this, other investigators have attempted to develop animal models of developmental cocaine exposure in order to determine if cocaine is hazardous (i.e., to establish causality), to establish exposure parameters (route and pattern of exposure), to characterize dose–response patterns, to investigate pathophysiology, and to determine mechanism of action. All of the steps in this process depend on the first, and the question addressed by this chapter is the extent to which causality has been established for cocaine as a developmental neurotoxin and the types of models used thus far to explore this possibility.

TYPES OF RESEARCH ON PRENATAL COCAINE

This review was restricted to prenatal and/or neonatal cocaine exposure studies in animals published between 1982 and early 1993. No nonhuman primate studies were identified. The search identified 51 published articles. In an effort to categorize these, they were sorted into six major types; the number of each type is shown in Table 5.1. It is evident that there is a heterogeneous distribution of

TABLE 5.1
Summary of Experiments on Developmental Exposure to Cocaine
1982–1993

Area	No. of Articles[a]	Percentage
Behavioral teratologic	22.5	45
Teratologic	3	6
Pharmacokinetic	5.5	11
Developmental toxicity	6	12
Neurochemical	11	22
Neurophysiologic	2	4
Total	50	100

[a]Some experiments were difficult to classify and were therefore divided and half placed in two separate categories. Table 5.6 contains 51 citations because the results of one experiment were reported in two separate papers.

TABLE 5.2
Summary of Experiments on Developmental Exposure to Cocaine
1982–1993

		No.[a]	Percentage
Species	Rat	49	90.7
	Mouse	5	9.2
Strain (rat)	SD	28	57.1
	LE	16	32.6
	W	5	10.2

[a]Total sums to more than 50 because some articles reported results from multiple experiments and one experiment reported in two separate articles.
SD = Sprague-Dawley, LE = Long-Evans, W = Wistar.

focus areas. The largest has been on cocaine's potential effects on neurobehavioral outcomes, followed by neurochemical, developmental toxicity/teratogenicity, pharmacokinetic, and neurophysiologic studies. Because the pharmacokinetic experiments are aimed at determining exposure conditions, rather than assessing offspring outcome, these experiments were excluded from some of the comparisons discussed here.

SPECIES USED IN ANIMAL MODELS

Table 5.2 shows the species, and for the predominantly investigated species, the strains that have been used. Experiments in rats predominate, and the two strains of rats used most, the Sprague–Dawley (SD) and Long–Evans (LE) together represent nearly 90% of the published rat experiments. One may wonder whether this represents an adequate range of potentially useful cocaine models and it is probably worthwhile for investigators to widen the spectrum of species considered in future research.

EXPOSURE PERIODS USED

Table 5.3 summarizes the experiments with outcome measures in terms of exposure period. The preponderance of prenatal-only experiments is striking. Only about 7% of articles have focused on early postnatal exposure periods, despite the fact that in rodents early postnatal development corresponds to human second- and third-trimester development. To give but one example, the brain growth spurt occurs during the third trimester in humans and during the first 10 days of postnatal life in the rat (Dobbing, 1968; Dobbing & Sands, 1979). This may be important because a review of the early postnatal exposure studies shows that all of them have reported significant drug-related effects. These studies have focused on changes in brain glucose metabolism and behavior (Dow-Edwards,

TABLE 5.3
Summary of Experiments on Developmental Exposure to Cocaine
1982–1993

Exposure Period	No.[a]	Percentages
Prenatal	38	84.4
Pre- & Postnatal	4	8.9
Postnatal	3	6.7
Total	45	

[a]Total number excludes five articles that were pharmacokinetic experiments.

1989; Dow-Edwards, Freed, & Milhorat, 1988; Dow-Edwards, Freed-Malen, & Hughes, 1993; Hughes, Pringle, Scribani, & Dow-Edwards, 1991) and support the concept that late gestational exposure to cocaine is associated with long-term functional changes.

EXPOSURE ROUTES

As in any modeling of risk, exposure parameters, and therefore route of exposure, is an important consideration. Humans primarily ingest cocaine intranasally or by inhalation of the pyrolized product. It is not essential that animal models mimic exactly the details of human routes, but it is important that the models reflect the internal dose and dose pattern observed in humans. Table 5.4 shows the exposure routes that have been used in the subset of articles classified as behavioral teratologic experiments. The first thing worth noting is that 19 of the 23 experiments in this category (83%) have administered the drug subcutaneously and the remainder have administered the drug by oral gavage (per oral or p.o. in the table). Several pharmacokinetic experiments have reported on the maternal and fetal plasma and brain concentrations of cocaine and its principal metabolite obtained by these two routes of exposure (Dow-Edwards, 1990; Dow-Edwards, Fico, Osman, Gamagaris, & Hutchings, 1989; Spear, Frambes, & Kirstein, 1989; Wiggins, Rolsten, Ruiz, & Davis, 1989). What has emerged is that gavage produces a higher peak and more rapid elimination phase of drug exposure than does subcutaneous administration. However, because of species differences in predominant metabolic pathways and rate of metabolism, comparing routes of administration is best made by examining the time to peak, peak (C_{max}), and elimination curves of the drug in maternal and fetal plasma. On a theoretical basis, intravenous or intraperitoneal routes would appear more similar to human exposure patterns because they are known from many experiments on other drugs to produce rapid drug absorption, distribution, and elimination rates. Of these two, intravenous would be the most rapid and intraperitoneal the second most rapid. Intraperitoneal experiments with prenatal cocaine have been reported, and all are teratologic, pharmacokinetic, or biochemical experiments (DeVane, Simp-

TABLE 5.4
Summary of Positive and Negative Behavioral Teratologic Experiments
on the Effects of Prenatal Cocaine in Relation to Route of Exposure
1982–1993

Route	Findings	No.	Percentage
P.O.[a]	+	1	25.0
	–	3	75.0
S.C.[b]	+	15	78.9
	–	4	21.1
Total		23	

[a]All p.o. experiments involved prenatal exposure. [b]Of the positive s.c. experiments, 14 were prenatal and 1 was postnatal.

kins, Miller, & Braun, 1989; El-Bizri, Guest, & Varma, 1991; Fantel & MacPhail, 1982; Finnell, Toloyan, VanWaes, & Kaliva, 1990; Tyrala, Mathews, & Rao, 1992; Weaver, Rivkees, & Reppert, 1992; Webster, Brown-Woodman, Lipson, & Ritchie, 1991), and none are behavioral teratologic. To the extent that one would predict central nervous system (CNS) effects from cocaine exposure, this anomaly in the published literature stands out. Although the teratologic experiments have generally found only low frequencies of malformations associated with high-dose cocaine exposure, these experiments have reported little on the pharmacokinetics of the intraperitoneal route of exposure. Given the importance of this and the likelihood that intraperitoneal administration should produce sharper and higher peak maternal cocaine concentrations in plasma than from subcutaneous administration, further investigation of the intraperitoneal route appears warranted.

In all of the prenatal outcome experiments reviewed, a majority have reported two observations: Prenatal cocaine exposure reduces maternal weight gain during gestation and decreases offspring birth weight. Because cocaine has well-established anorectic effects, these findings are not surprising. They suggest, however, that having experimental controls for reduced food intake and body weight gain are important. A few investigators have reported that the doses and dose regimens they have used do not induce significant maternal weight gain reductions. In these instances, controls have been feed ad libitum. Obviously, when no deviation in maternal weight gain occurs, the need for a nutritionally matched (pair-fed) control group is obviated. Thus, the need for pair-fed controls depends on the model being investigated. Under no circumstances, however, would an uninjected or ungavaged control group be sufficient, regardless of feeding conditions. This becomes important because a number of published articles have appeared in which both pair-fed-injected and untreated controls have been included. If all comparisons are based on the pair-fed-injected controls, then no misinterpretations are likely, but when an untreated group is included in the experiments, comparisons to this group are often performed. Such comparisons can be misleading and are not justified as indicating cocaine-related effects.

Another point illustrated in Table 5.4 is the number of behavioral teratologic experiments in which a cocaine-related effect was described (indicated as positive experiments) compared to those in which no cocaine effects were found (negative experiments). Although there are more positive than negative studies, one must be concerned that reporting biases may contribute to this imbalance. Despite this probable bias, what is surprising is that seven negative studies have been published. This is high for a suspected behavioral teratogen, leading one to wonder whether the field will become less biased in reporting negative studies. It is too early to know the answer, but the existence of so many negative studies raises some questions about the apparent potency of cocaine as a developmental neurotoxin. Are all these negative reports erroneous or is cocaine not neurotoxic? Alternatively, is cocaine a potent behavioral teratogen, but does it produce a narrow spectrum of effects causing many investigations into its effects to have missed its effects? I suggest as a working hypothesis that the latter is the case, not only because some more recent data have begun to turn up reliable effects, but also on theoretical grounds, that until more diverse, thorough models are developed and tested, it is premature to assume otherwise.

So why have so many negative reports been published on cocaine compared to other suspected teratogens? One possibility is that there is a reverse bias at work here, stemming from the fact that cocaine has received so much attention that any paper on cocaine, positive or negative, is more likely to be accepted by journals than are reports on less attention-getting compounds. Although it is difficult to know, this certainly appears to be the case.

BEHAVIORAL TERATOLOGIC EXPERIMENTS
REPORTING COCAINE-ASSOCIATED EFFECTS

Table 5.5 presents a summary of the 14 positive subcutaneous and 1 positive gavage behavioral teratologic experiments. The experiments are listed chronologically. Several experiments were published as a numbered series. In the case of Church and Overbeck (1990a) only Study II was behavioral and therefore only this one was included in this table. Also, the experiment that appears as Goodwin et al. (1992) was the second of two papers based on a single experiment. The first one reported on effects in the dams (Heyser, Molina, & Spear, 1992), and therefore was not included in Table 5.5. Two articles appear by Johns, Means, Anderson, Means, and McMillen (1992) and Johns, Means, Means, and McMillen (1992), but both papers report on the results of a single experiment.

Only those effects reported to be statistically significant between cocaine-treated and pair-fed controls (where such controls were included) are shown in Table 5.5 and all articles included in this review are listed in Table 5.6. Perhaps the three most noteworthy characteristics of the information in Table 5.5 are:

TABLE 5.5
Summary of Positive Behavioral Teratologic Experiments on Prenatal Cocaine
1982–1993

Article	Route	Dose	Exposure	Effect
Hutchings, Fico, & Dow-Edwards (1989)	po	30,60	7–21[a]	↑Locomotor activity at P20 & 23 only in the 60 mg/kg prenatal cocaine group only
Smith, Mattran, Kurkjian, & Kurtz (1989)	sc	10	3–17[a]	↓Spontaneous alternation frequency (males only)
				↓Open-field activity (males only)
				↑DRL-20 response rate
				↓Tail-flick latency
				↑T-water maze latency (early trials males only)
				↓Shock sensitivity
Spear, Kirstein, Bell et al. (1989)	sc	40	7–19[a]	↓Odor conditioning
				↓Shock-induced wall climbing
				↑Activity during shock-induced wall climbing
Church & Overbeck (1990b)	sc	20,30,40,50	7–20	↓Left bias in spontaneous alternation
				↓Passive avoidance retention at 50 mg/kg dose
Henderson & McMillen (1990)	sc	15	1–birth	↓Surface righting development
				↑Locomotor activity at P30; no effect at P60
Heyser, Chen, Miller, Spear, & Spear (1990)	sc	40	7–19[a]	↓Sensory preconditioning at P8 & P12; no effect at P21
				↓1st order conditioning at P8; no effect at P12 or P21
Raum, McGivern, Peterson, Sryne, & Gorski (1990)	sc	10,30	15–20	↓Scent marking in males
				↓Latency to intromission
Sobrian et al. (1990)	sc	20	14–20[a]	↑Surface righting & cliff avoidance development
				↑Startle development
				↓Response on locomotor activity to d-amphetamine & cocaine challenges

(Continued)

TABLE 5.5
(Continued)

Article	Route	Dose	Exposure	Effect
Church, Holmes, Overbeck, Tilak, & Zajac (1991)	sc	30	7–20	↓Locomotor activity
Heyser, Miller, Spear, & Spear (1992)	sc	40	7–19[a]	↓Conditioned place preference ↑Number of chamber entries
Johns, Means, Means et al. (1992)	sc	15	1–20 (Coc-D) or 2–3,8–9, 14–15, 19–20 (Coc-I)	↑Locomotor activity at P30 during 1st 15 min. in Coc-D group ↓Locomotor activity at P30 during dark cycle in Coc-I group
Johns, Means, Anderson et al. (1992)	sc	15	Ibid	↑Open-field non-entries in Coc-D group ↑Open-field activity in Coc-I group
Bilitzke & Church (1992)	sc	40	7–20	↓Immobility time on Porsolt forced-swim test
Goodwin et al. (1992)	sc	40	7–19[a]	↓Odor conditioning at P7 in coc-coc group on the 2–4 training trial conditions & in the fos-coc group on the 2 & 3 training trial condition No effect on auditory conditioning at P17; no effect on odor conditioning on P17 ↓Latency to 1st attack on shock-induced aggression in coc-coc & fos-coc groups
Meyer, Sherlock, & MacDonald (1992)	sc	20	10–19[a]	Effects tested using cocaine challenge: ↑wall climbing at all challenge doses in controls, but ↑ wall climbing at high challenge dose only in prenatal cocaine group

[a]Adjusted for evidence of conception as embryonic (E) day 0.

TABLE 5.6
Summary of 51 Articles Representing 50 Experiments on Developmental Exposure to Cocaine Presented in Chronological Order

Authors	Dose	Species	Rate	Exposure	Route	Conc.	Controls
Fantel & MacPhail (1982)	50,60,75	Rat:SD	1/d	E8–12	i.p.	n.g.	AL
	60	M:SW	1/d	E7–16	i.p.	n.g.	PF
Church, Dincheff, & Gessner (1988a)	20,25,30 35,40,45	Rat:LE	2/d	E7–19	s.c.	20	AL
Church, Dincheff, & Gessner (1988b)	20,25,30 35,40,45	Rat:LE	2/d	E7–19	s.c.	20	AL
Dow-Edwards et al. (1988)	25	Rat:SD	2/d	P1–2	s.c.	n.g.	AL
	50		1/d	P3–10			
DeVane et al. (1989)	30 (base)	Rat:SD	1/d	E18 or 19	i.p.	30	None
Dow-Edwards et al. (1989)	40,80	Rat:SD	1/d	E0–16	p.o.	26–32	AL
	20,40				s.c.	20,40	AL
Fung, Reed, & Lau (1989)	30 (base)	Rat:SD	Contuous	E2–birth	mini-pump	n.a.	S-Fost.
Hutchings, Fico, & Dow-Edwards (1989)†	30,60	Rat:W	1/d	E7–21[a]	p.o.	6,12	AL PF S-Fost.
Smith et al. (1989)	10	Rat:LE	1/d	E3–17[a]	s.c.	10	AL
Spear, Kirstein, et al. (1989)	40	Rat:SD	1/d	E7–19[a]	s.c.	13.3	AL PF
Spear, Frambes, & Kirstein (1989)	10,20,40	Rat:SD	1/d	E7–19[a]	s.c.	13.3	AL
Wiggins et al. (1989)	10,60	Rat:LE	1/d	E19 or 20	p.o.	n.g.	None
Church, Overbeck, & Andrzejczak (1990)	20,30, 40,50	Rat:LE	2/d	E7–20	s.c.	20	AL PF
Church & Overbeck (1990a)	20,30, 40,50	Rat:LE	2/d	E7–20	s.c.	20	AL PF
Church & Overbeck (1990b)	20,30, 40,50	Rat:LE	2/d	E7–20	s.c.	20	AL PF

(Continued)

TABLE 5.6
(Continued)

Authors	Dose	Species	Rate	Exposure	Route	Conc.	Controls
Dow-Edwards (1990)	30,60	Rat:W	1/d	E7-21[a]	p.o.	n.g.	—
Dow-Edwards, Freed, & Fico (1990)	60	Rat:W	1/d	E7-20[a]	p.o.	12	PF
							S-Fost.
Finnell et al. (1990)	20,40,60	DBA/2J SWV	1/d	E6-8 E8-10	i.p.	n.g.	AL
Giordano et al. (1990)	30	Rat:SD	1/d	E12-21	s.c.	30	AL
Henderson & McMillen (1990)	15 (base)	Rat:SD	2/d	E1-birth	s.c.	n.g.	AL S-Fost.
Heyser et al. (1990)	40	Rat:SD	1/d	E7-19[a]	s.c.	13.3	AL
Raum et al. (1990)	10	Rat:SD	single	P0	s.c.	n.g.	AL
	10,30		2/d	E15-20			AL &
	3		2/d	E15-20 & P1-5			S-Fost.
Scalzo, Ali, Frambes, & Spear (1990)	40	Rat:SD	1/d	E7-19[a]	s.c.	13.3	AL
Sobrien et al. (1990)	40	Rat:SD	1/d	E14-20[a]	s.c.	n.g.	AL
Barron, Foss, & Riley (1991)	60	Rat:LE	1/d	E13-20[a]	p.o.	13.3	AL
Church et al. (1991)	30	Rat:LE	2/d	E7-20	s.c.	20	AL PF S-Fost.
Church & Overbeck (1991)	30,40	Rat:LE	2/d	E7-20	s.c.	20	AL PF S-Fost.
Clow, Hammer, Kirstein, & Spear (1991)	10,20,40	Rat:SD	1/d	E7-19[a]	s.c.	3.33 6.66 13.3	AL PF S-Fost.
El-Bizri et al. (1991)	2.1,4.2, 8.5,17, 34	Rat:SD	1/d	E0-19	i.p. s.c.	n.g.	AL

Reference							
Hughes et al. (1991)	50	Rat:SD	1/d	P1–10 P11–20	s.c.	n.g.	AL
Rodriguez-Sanchez, Alvaro, & Arilla (1991)	40	Rat:W	1/d	E7–19 E7–19,PO–15 PO–15	s.c.	n.g.	AL
Seifert & Church (1991)	40,50	Rat:LE	2/d	E7–20	s.c.	n.g.	AL PF S-Fost.
Webster et al. (1991; based on Webster & Brown-Woodman, 1990)	70 (1) 60 (1) 50 (2)	Rat:SD	1/d	E16	i.p.	n.g.	AL
Foss & Riley (1991a)	60 40	Rat:LE	1/d	E13–20[a] E7–20[a]	p.o. s.c.	13.3 13.3	AL PF
Foss & Riley (1991b)	40	Rat:LE	1/d	E13–20[a]	s.c.	13.3	AL PF
Riley & Foss (1991a)	60 40	Rat:LE	1/d	E13–20[a] E7–20[a]	p.o. s.c.	13.3 13.3	AL PF
Riley & Foss (1991b)	60	Rat:LE	1/d	E13–20[a]	p.o.	13.3	AL PF
Akbari, Kramer, Whitaker-Azmitia, Spear, & Azmitia (1992)	40 40,10	Rat:SD	1/d	E13–22 E13–22 & P1–5	s.c.	13.3	AL
Akbari & Azmitia (1992)	40	Rat:SD	1/d	E13–22	s.c.	13.3	AL S-Fost.
Bilitzke & Church (1992)	40	Rat:LE	2/d	E7–20	s.c.	20	AL PF S-Fost.
Church & Rauch (1992)	50	Mouse: BALB/c xSJL	1/d	E7–18	s.c.	20	AL PF
Goodwin et al. (1992)	40	Rat:SD	1/d	E7–19[a]	s.c.	13.3	AL S-Fost.

(Continued)

81

TABLE 5.6
(Continued)

Authors	Dose	Species	Rate	Exposure	Route	Conc.	Controls
Heyser, Molina et al. (1992)	40	Rat:SD	1/d	E7–19[a]	s.c.	13.3	AL S-Fost.
Heyser, Miller et al. (1992)	40	Rat:SD	1/d	E7–19[a]	s.c.	13.3	AL PF S-Fost.
Johns, Means, Means et al. (1992)	15	Rat:SD	2/d	E1–20 E2–3,8–9, 14–15,19–20	s.c.	n.g.	PF S-Fost.
Johns, Means, Anderson et al. (1992)	15	Rat:SD	2/d	E1–20 E2–3,8–9, 14–15,19–20	s.c.	n.g.	PF S-Fost.
Meyer et al. (1992)	20	Rat:SD	2/d	E10–19[a]	s.c.	6.6	AL PF S-Fost.
Minabe, Ashby, Heyser, Spear, & Wang (1992)**	40	Rat:SD	1/d	E7–19[a]	s.c.	13.3	AL PF S-Fost.
Tyrala et al. (1992)	10	Mouse: ICR	1/d	E6–14	i.p.	n.g.	AL
Weaver et al. (1992)	10,20	Rat:SD	1/d	E20	i.p.	n.g.	AL
Dow-Edwards et al. (1993)	50	Rat:SD	1/d	P11–20	s.c.	10	AL
Factor, Hart, & Jonakait (1993)**	10,40	Rat:SD	Continuous	E7–21	minipump	n.a.	AL Some S-Fost.
Seidler & Slotkin (1993)**	10,33.3	Rat:SD	3/d	E8–20,18–20	s.c.	3.3	AL

[a]Adjusted for evidence of conception as embryonic day E0.
**Articles obtained too late to be included in Tables 5.1–5.4 or 5.7–5.11 but are similar in design.
  n.a. = not applicable.
  n.g. = not given by authors.
  See Table 5.2 for explanation of rat strains.

82

1. Few of the experiments include any attempt to construct dose–effect profiles of the effects of prenatal cocaine, even though this is fundamental to characterizing a drug's effects (only 3 of the 14 articles reported using more than a single dose of cocaine).

2. There has been little variation in the prenatal exposure periods used; fully 12 of the 14 studies used exposure periods spanning the last two thirds of gestation. No attempt to investigate stage-specific effects has occurred, a curious result in a field in which vulnerability is defined in ontogenetic terms. Two experiments used more focused exposures, examining late gestational administration, but because only one stage was examined no stage-specific comparisons were possible. The only article reporting any exposure pattern effects of any kind was the pair of papers by Johns, Means, Anderson, et al. (1992) and Johns, Means, Means, et al. (1992), in which an intermittent cocaine exposure pattern (Coc-I) was compared to a daily cocaine administration pattern (Coc-D). However, this design is conceptually distinct from a stage-specific approach and had an entirely different conceptual orientation. Given that all known teratogens demonstrate stage-specific effects this point warrants further attention.

3. Finally, an examination of Table 5.5 in the *Effect* column reveals that the effects observed differ widely from experiment to experiment. They differ not only in their findings, but also in their test methods. Consequently, no common thread runs through them. It is apparent that these early experiments fall within a screening domain, with investigators casting a wide and rather nonspecific net in the hope of discovering whether cocaine produces any form of neurobehavioral teratogenicity.

What is not illustrated in Table 5.5, but is every bit as important, is the substantial number of tests (not counting entire experiments) in which no effects of cocaine were found. In fact, across all the behavioral teratologic studies published thus far, there are a larger number of no-effect findings when examined on a test-by-test basis compared to positive findings. One interpretation of this is that cocaine has very specific effects, hence widely cast nets tend to turn up relatively few hits compared to misses. An alternative explanation is that cocaine has no long-term effects, therefore the few positive findings reported represent Type I errors. The literature is insufficiently developed at this time to determine which of these alternatives is correct.

CONTROLS FOR NUTRITIONAL AND MATERNAL FACTORS

Returning to the issue of appropriate controls for investigations of prenatal cocaine, a summary of the two major types of controls for each reviewed article is presented in Table 5.7. Of all 51 articles, approximately 40% included pair-fed controls. As

TABLE 5.7
Summary of Experiments on Developmental Exposure to Cocaine
1982–1993

Type of Experimental Controls	No.	Percentage
Pair-fed controls		
W/	21	42.0
W/O	29	55.0
Total	50	
Surrogate fostered controls		
W/	16	47.1
W/O	18	52.9
Total	34[a]	

[a]Includes only those experiments with prenatal exposure and postnatal outcomes.

discussed earlier, to the extent that control for undernutrition is one of the most salient confounders in animal experiments using cocaine, this suggests that much of the early published work in this field has not included the most important type of control group.

A related issue has to do with possible carryover effects of the drug on postnatal maternal rearing behavior or maternal drug or metabolite residues that might continue to be passed to the progeny during lactation. The principal control used for this confounder is fostering, in which the progeny exposed to the drug prenatally are transferred to untreated, recently parturient foster dams shortly after birth. In order to balance for the effect of fostering per se, control litters are usually also fostered. This leads to the fostering–crossfostering design (Vorhees, 1986). In its simplest form the design consists of experimental dams (E) and progeny (e) and control dams (C) and progeny (c). The two maternal treatment groups produce four rearing–offspring combinations: Ee, Ec, Ce, Cc. Exchanging litters within a treatment condition is termed *fostering*, whereas exchanging litters across treatment conditions is termed *crossfostering*. An even more complete design includes experimental dams and progeny that are left undisturbed and control dams and progeny that are left undisturbed. In this way one can theoretically sort the influence of intrauterine drug exposure from maternal drug exposure effects, which in turn can be sorted from the direct effects of fostering. However, the logic behind this approach is linear and it assumes that by subtracting the influence of each of the identified contributions, these factors can be separated in stepwise fashion from one another.

There is little doubt that the fostering–crossfostering design has its place in helping to resolve some interpretational problems that arise in prenatal drug investigations, but it is not a complete solution. One problem is that interactions may not be linear; therefore, the isolation of factors may not be absolute. Another problem is that fostering usually occurs over a window of 24 to 48 hrs postdelivery.

This is a significant interval for maternal–infant interaction and may be long enough to alter the course of development, regardless of subsequent conditions.

As noted in Table 5.7, less than half of the developmental cocaine studies have included any control for maternal carryover effects. Of those that have included some control, only one has attempted to sort the factors systematically. All the others were what is termed *surrogate fostering* designs (Vorhees, 1986), in which experimental and control progeny were all fostered to a third set of untreated, recently parturient dams. This design attempts to eliminate maternal carryover effects without trying to measure them. The design succeeds in requiring fewer groups and being less complex than the fostering–crossfostering design, but the gain is short term because this design never resolves the crucial question: Is there any carryover effect and if so what is it? If another study is performed, then the issue of fostering again arises, and because no estimate of its effects was obtained in the first experiment, the tendency is to include surrogate fostering again in order to ensure comparability. Henceforth, all experiments with positive effects from a lab that starts with surrogate fostering must continue to include it or run the risk of not repeating the original effect.

Accordingly, I argued (Vorhees, 1986) that it may be preferable to conduct initial experiments without fostering in order to: (a) determine if a hazard exists, (b) map the range of possible effects, and (c) characterize dose–effect relationships. The latter study cannot possibly be conducted as a fostering–crossfostering study in any case, because the size of the experiment would be prohibitive. If a drug is found to produce effects, and they are replicable and dose dependent, then a single-dose fostering–crossfostering experiment is in order (usually at the dose found to be most efficacious of those tested in the dose–response experiment). If substantial maternal carryover effects are uncovered, then these must be considered in all future designs on that drug. If on the other hand, only minor or no maternal carryover effects are obtained, then this control procedure may be omitted from future investigations. The cocaine field has not yet resolved this point, but it is getting closer.

One experiment has been published in an attempt to deal with maternal carryover effects. This experiment was not designed quite like the model case described earlier. Heyser, Molina, and Spear (1992) treated rats prenatally with either 40 mg/kg of cocaine (C40) or saline (LC). At birth, some dams raised their own litters producing the groups LC/LC and C40/C40. Others were fostered (FOS) to untreated surrogate dams producing four additional combinations: two groups raised by foster dams (FOS/LC and FOS/C40) and two groups of offspring from the foster dams that were raised by cocaine- or saline-treated dams (LC/FOS and C40/FOS). The logic was similar to that of the full fostering–crossfostering design, inasmuch as each nominal factor (maternal carryover, fostering, and drug treatment) was represented in the design. The authors of this investigation reported the effects of the various conditions on maternal behavior in one paper and the effects on offspring behavior in another. They examined the dams on measures of home cage behavior, pup retrieval, and intruder aggression. They found a difference in aggression between LC/LC and C40/C40 dams, in which cocaine dams appeared more aggressive. The implications of such a difference are unclear and no effects were found on other behaviors such as on offspring retrieval and home cage maternal–infant interactions. In the second article, the authors (Goodwin et al., 1992) reported on the effects on the offspring. They examined the progeny on tests of odor aversion conditioning (Day 7), odor or auditory aversion conditioning (Day 17), and shock-induced and intruder aggression (Day 60). They found no differences in aversive odor or auditory conditioning at Day 17. At Day 7, both the C40/C40 and FOS/C40 groups performed poorly on aversive odor conditioning compared to controls, but the C40/C40 group was worse than the FOS/C40 group, suggesting that some portion of the cocaine effect might be accentuated by maternal carryover effects. Shock-induced aggression in the progeny at Day 60 showed that the C40/FOS and C40/C40 groups had slightly shorter latencies to attack than controls or the FOS/C40 group. This curious pattern implicates maternal carryover effects as the primary determinant of altered aggression in the adult progeny, and as such, raises the issue of whether effects attributed to intrauterine cocaine might be indirect or nonspecific. However, these data must be interpreted with caution because they are the only ones found thus far of this kind and it is unknown how changes in shock-induced aggression fit into the overall pattern of cocaine-associated developmental effects. Moreover, the magnitude of the effect was small and significant only by planned comparison statistical methods. The data provide a hint of the potential for misattribution of cocaine-induced neurotoxicity and suggest that this issue may deserve further attention.

Table 5.8 shows a summary of all the positive cocaine behavioral teratogenic studies covered in this review with respect to the two principal controls of pair-feeding and fostering. As can be seen, every combination has been reported, making this set of experiments difficult to sort out. Of the 15 articles listed in Table 5.8, 9 included pair-fed controls, and 11 included fostering controls. The convergence of both of these two types of controls occurred in seven articles, representing six experiments. These are shown in Table 5.9. It can be seen that no clear pattern of neurobehavioral effects is evident, but in fairness it must be emphasized that doses, test apparatus, test procedures, exposure periods, and ages of assessment in these experiments were all quite different. Nevertheless, there may be some beginnings of consistency emerging. Table 5.10 lists those articles that report intralaboratory replication of findings. As can be seen, Spear's laboratory published three experiments in which early postnatal deficits in aversive odor conditioning were found after prenatal exposure to cocaine at 40 mg/kg given subcutaneously once per day on Days 7 through 19 of gestation. That represents the good news. The bad news is that no instances of interlaboratory replication of neurobehavioral findings could be found in the published literature thus far.

TABLE 5.8
Summary of Behavioral Teratologic Experiments on Prenatal Cocaine
1982–1993

Article	Route	Dose	Exposure Period	Pair-Fed Controls	Surrogate Fostering
Smith et al. (1989)	sc	10	3–17[a]	No	No
Spear, Kirstein, et al. (1989)	sc	40	7–19[a]	Yes	No
Church & Overbeck (1990a)	sc	20,30,40,50	7–20	Yes	No
Henderson & McMillen (1990)	sc	15	1–birth	No	Yes
Heyser et al. (1990)	sc	40	7–19[a]	No	Yes
Raum et al. (1990)	sc	10,30	15–20	No	Yes
Sobrian et al. (1990)	sc	20	14–20[a]	No	No
Church et al. (1991)	sc	30	7–20	Yes	Yes
Heyser et al. (1992)	sc	40	7–19[a]	Yes	Yes
Johns, Means, Means, et al. (1992)	sc	15	1–20 2–3,8–9, 14–15,19–20	Yes	Yes
Johns, Means, Anderson, et al. (1992)	sc	15	Ibid.	Yes	Yes
Bilitzke & Church (1992)	sc	40	7–20	Yes	Yes
Goodwin et al. (1992)	sc	40	7–19[a]	No	Yes
Meyer et al. (1992)	sc	20	10–19[a]	Yes	Yes
Hutchings et al. (1989)	po	30,60	7–21[a]	Yes	Yes

[a]Adjusted for evidence of conception as embryonic (E) day 0.

TABLE 5.9
Behavioral Teratologic Experiments Having Both Pair-Fed
and Surrogate Fostered Controls
1982–1993

Article	Route	Dose	Exposure Period	Effect
Hutchings et al. (1989)	po	30,60	7–21[a]	↑ Locomotor activity on P20 & 23 only at 60 mg/kg dose
Church et al. (1991)	sc	30	7–20	↓ Locomotor activity
Heyser et al. (1992)	sc	40	7–19[a]	↓ Conditioned place preference ↑ Number of chamber entries
Johns, Means, Means et al. (1992)	sc	15	1–20 2–3,8–9, 14–15,19–20	↑ Locomotor activity at P30 for 1st 15 min in Coc-D group ↓ Locomotor activity at P30, dark cycle in Coc-I group
Johns, Means, Anderson et al. (1992)	sc	15	Ibid.	↑ Open-field non-entries in Coc-D group ↑ Open-field activity in Coc-I group
Bilitzke & Church (1992)	sc	40	7–20	↓ Immobility time on Porsolt forced-swim test
Meyer et al. (1992)	sc	20	10–19[a]	Effects tested using cocaine challenge: ↑ wall climbing at all challenge doses in AL & PF groups ↑ wall climbing at high challenge dose only in prenatal cocaine group

[a]Adjusted for evidence of conception as embryonic (E) day 0.

TABLE 5.10
Replication of Effects from Positive Behavioral
Teratologic Experiments on Prenatal Cocaine
1982–1993

Article	Route	Dose	Exposure	Effect
Intralaboratory Replication				
Spear, Kirstein, et al. (1989)	sc	40	7–19[a]	↓ Odor conditioning
Heyser et al. (1990)	sc	40	7–19[a]	↓ Sensory preconditioning at P8 & P12; no effect at P21 ↓ 1st order conditioning at P8; no effect at P12 or P21
Goodwin et al. (1992)	sc	40	7–19[a]	↓ Odor conditioning at P7 in coc-coc group on the 2–4 training trial condition & in the fos-coc group on the 2 & 3 training trial condition
Interlaboratory Replication				
None				

[a]Adjusted for evidence of conception as embryonic (E) day 0.

DOSE RATE AND ROUTE OF EXPOSURE

Important factors in addition to drug dose are dose rate and (as mentioned previously) route of exposure. Table 5.11 summarizes these points. For dose rate, almost 70% of the published studies used once per day administration. This is curious given that: (a) some people are reported to use the drug multiple times per day, and (b) cocaine has a short elimination half-life. Short-lived drugs in humans

TABLE 5.11
Summary of Experiments on Developmental Exposure to Cocaine
1982–1993

Dose Rate/Route	No.	Percentage
Dose Rate		
1/d	34	68.0
2/d	15	30.0
>2/d	0	0
Continuous	1	2.0
Total	50	
Route of Administration		
S.C.	38	69.1
I.P.	7	12.7
P.O.	9	16.4
I.V.	0	0
Infusion	1	1.8
Total	55[a]	

[a]Total exceeds 50 because several articles report experiments using more than one route of administration and one experiment was reported in two separate papers.

are often even shorter lived in rodents. Thus, duration of drug exposure emerges as a point needing further scrutiny. For example, Dow-Edwards et al. (1989) showed that oral cocaine produced peak maternal plasma concentrations of cocaine approximately 15 min after drug administration. She further showed that such exposure produced a maternal elimination half-life of 23 min (Dow-Edwards, 1990). Hence, the drug is better than 87% cleared from maternal plasma in about 1 hr. Thus, for the remaining 23 hrs of development on that day (which in the rodent is extensive) there is no exposure. If cocaine is selective in the developmental processes it affects, once-daily exposure regimens will miss many embryological events. Even if once-daily dosing did hit a critical event in one litter it could miss it in the next, producing large variability in the outcomes seen. The situation is similar for subcutaneous administration. Dow-Edwards et al. (1989) showed that with this route, lower cocaine plasma peak concentrations were produced than by oral administration, suggesting slower absorption, distribution, and elimination. However, these investigators only sampled up to 45 min postinjection. Nevertheless, they found little decline in maternal plasma concentrations after a dose of 40 mg/kg. Spear, Frambes, and Kirstein (1989) also reported rising maternal plasma cocaine after subcutaneous cocaine administration, and noted that the values had not peaked by 2 hrs after doses of 20 and 40 mg/kg, although they had begun to decline by 2 hrs after a dose of 10 mg/kg. In this experiment, the elimination phase was not followed, but even if it lasted several hours, this may produce only a few hours of drug exposure each day. If a day in rodent development represents roughly 1 week in human development, missing a large fraction of a day in rats represents a significant portion of embryogenesis. Indeed more of development is unexposed than is exposed. This would be acceptable if we knew the most susceptible developmental events for cocaine, but we do not; therefore, the most critical events could be being consistently missed. Obviously, more pharmacokinetic data on rats after different routes of exposure is needed to clarify the exposure pattern. As for other routes, only a few intraperitoneal studies have been done, none are neurobehavioral, and no intravenous or inhalation developmental experiments could be found for cocaine. Overall, the literature appears overly weighted to the subcutaneous route of administration.

Closely related to duration of exposure per dose is the number of doses administered. As can be seen in Table 5.11, single-dose models predominate in the literature with twice per day making up the remainder, save one article that reported using miniosmotic pump infusion administration. No experiments could be found using more than 2 daily treatments despite the theoretical relevance of such a regimen to some human use patterns and to the pharmacokinetics of the drug. This represents a gap in the models of cocaine explored thus far.

The work of Nau, Sierer, Spielmann, Neubert, and Gansau (1981) on valproic acid reminds us that duration of drug exposure may not be the only critical factor in determining developmental toxicity. Peak drug concentration is also a crucial factor for some drugs. Nau et al. (1981) showed that large doses of valproic acid were teratogenic in mice, whereas steady infusion of an equivalent total dose of the drug daily was not. Thus, some drugs have been suggested to be toxic based on total exposure (an area under the exposure-time curve type of effect), whereas others appear to depend on peak concentration (Nau, 1988). If cocaine is a significant developmental toxin, it will need to be determined whether it is a peak effect or total exposure effect type of agent. None of the published experiments appear to be trying to determine which of these key factors applies to cocaine.

Finally, the existing literature has done little searching for possible critical periods of exposure. Because this is one of the cornerstones of developmental toxicology, it is apparent that this represents a major gap in our existing knowledge. In this regard, the work of Dow-Edwards, who has reported on two postnatal cocaine exposure periods, represents perhaps the most forward-looking set of experiments (Dow-Edwards et al., 1988; Dow-Edwards et al., 1993; Hughes et al., 1991). These investigations are shedding light on the possible effects of second- and third-trimesterlike exposures, which may be especially susceptible times in development for the action of a dopamine agonist such as cocaine.

IMPLICATIONS FOR FUTURE RESEARCH

In conclusion, the early cocaine animal literature has developed a distinct but somewhat restricted set of experimental approaches to modeling human cocaine exposure during pregnancy. These have been dominated by high, single-daily-dose approaches administered by the subcutaneous route and given throughout most of gestation to Sprague–Dawley rats. Given that little consensus exists concerning cocaine's developmental toxicity from these models, there is ample reason to believe that a wider range of models might prove revealing. At this juncture, the jury is out on whether cocaine is a significant developmental neurotoxin, but a few promising neurobehavioral and neurochemical studies have appeared that tentatively suggest that there may be cocaine-specific effects on the developing mammalian brain. Replication across laboratories along with investigations of mechanisms of drug action will be crucial steps in determining the significance of the more promising recent findings (Table 5.5).

ACKNOWLEDGMENTS

The author wishes to thank Lisa Ehrman, Alissa Hock, and Chad Messer for assistance in compiling the literature for this review. Supported in part by Public Health Service grant DA06733 from NIH.

REFERENCES

Akbari, H. M., & Azmitia, E. C. (1992). Increased tyrosine hydroxylase immunoreactivity in the rat cortex following prenatal cocaine exposure. *Developmental Brain Research, 66,* 277–281.

Akbari, H. M., Kramer, H. K., Whitaker-Azmitia, P. M., Spear, L. P., & Azmitia, E. C. (1992). Prenatal cocaine exposure disrupts the development of the serotonergic system. *Brain Research, 572*, 57–63.

Anday, E. K., Cohen, M. E., Kelley, N. E., & Leitner, D. S. (1989). Effect of in utero cocaine exposure on startle and its modification. *Developmental Pharmacology and Therapeutics, 12*, 137–145.

Barron, S., Foss, J. A., & Riley, E. P. (1991). The effect of prenatal cocaine exposure on umbilical cord length in fetal rats. *Neurotoxicology and Teratology, 13*, 503–506.

Bilitzke, P. J., & Church, M. W. (1992). Prenatal cocaine and alcohol exposures affect rat behavior in a stress test (the Porsolt swim test). *Neurotoxicology and Teratology, 14*, 359–364.

Bingol, N., Fuchs, M., Diaz, V., Stone, R. K., & Gromisch, D. S. (1987). Teratogenicity of cocaine in humans. *Journal of Pediatrics, 110*, 93–96.

Chasnoff, I. J., Burns, K. A., & Burns, W. J. (1987). Cocaine use in pregnancy: Perinatal morbidity and mortality. *Neurotoxicology and Teratology, 9*, 291–293.

Chasnoff, I. J., Burns, W. J., Schnoll, S. H., & Burns, K. A. (1985). Cocaine use in pregnancy. *New England Journal of Medicine, 313*, 666–669.

Chasnoff, I. J., Griffith, D. R., Freier, C., & Murray, J. (1992). Cocaine/polydrug use in pregnancy: Two-year follow-up. *Pediatrics, 89*, 284–289.

Chasnoff, I. J., Griffith, D. R., MacGregor, S., Dirkes, D., & Burns, K. A. (1989). Temporal patterns of cocaine use in prenany: Perinatal outcome. *Journal of the American Medical Association, 261*, 1741–1744.

Chasnoff, I. J., Hunt, C. E., Kletter, R., & Kaplan, D. (1989). Prenatal cocaine exposure is associated with respiratory pattern abnormalities. *American Journal of Diseases of Children, 143*, 583–587.

Church, M. W., Dincheff, B. A., & Gessner, P. K. (1988a). Dose-dependent consequences of cocaine on pregnancy outcome in the Long–Evans rats. *Neurotoxicology and Teratology, 10*, 51–58.

Church, M. W., Dincheff, B. A., & Gessner, P. K. (1988b). The interactive effects of alcohol and cocaine on maternal and fetal toxicity in the Long–Evans rat. *Neurotoxicology and Teratology, 10*, 355–361.

Church, M. W., Holmes, P. A., Overbeck, G. W., Tilak, J. P., & Zajac, C. S. (1991). Interactive effects of prenatal alcohol and cocaine exposures on postnatal mortality, development and behavior in the Long–Evans rats. *Neurotoxicology and Teratology, 13*, 377–386.

Church, M. W., & Overbeck, G. W. (1990a). Prenatal cocaine exposure in the Long–Evans rat: II. Dose-dependent effects on offspring behavior. *Neurotoxicology and Teratology, 12*, 335–343.

Church, M. W., & Overbeck, G. W. (1990b). Prenatal cocaine exposure in the Long–Evans rat: III. Developmental effects on the brainstem auditory-evoked potential. *Neurotoxicology and Teratology, 12*, 345–351.

Church, M. W., & Overbeck, G. W. (1991). Sensorineural hearing loss as evidenced by the auditory brainstem response following prenatal cocaine exposure in the Long–Evans rat. *Teratology, 43*, 561–570.

Church, M. W., Overbeck, G. W., & Andrzejczak, A. L. (1990). Prenatal cocaine exposure in the Long–Evans rat: I. Dose-dependent effects on gestation, mortality, and postnatal maturation. *Neurotoxicology and Teratology, 12*, 327–334.

Church, M. W., & Rauch, H. C. (1992). Prenatal cocaine exposure in the laboratory mouse: Effects on maternal water consumption and offspring outcome. *Neurotoxicology and Teratology, 14*, 313–319.

Clow, D. W., Hammer, R. P., Kirstein, C. L., & Spear, L. P. (1991). Gestational cocaine exposure increases opiate receptor binding in weanling offspring. *Developmental Brain Research, 59*, 179–185.

Coles, C. D., Platzman, K. A., Smith, I., James, M. E., & Falek, A. (1992). Effects of cocaine and alcohol use in pregnancy on neonatal growth and neurobehavioral status. *Neurotoxicology and Teratology, 14*, 23–33.

DeVane, C. L., Simpkins, J. W., Miller, R. L., & Braun, S. B. (1989). Tissue distribution of cocaine in the pregnant rat. *Life Sciences, 45*, 1271–1276.

Dixon, S. D., & Bejar, R. (1989). Echoencephalographic findings in neonates associated with maternal cocaine and methamphetamine use: Incidence and clinical correlates. *Journal of Pediatrics, 115*, 770–778.

Dobbing, J. (1968). Vulnerable periods in developing brain. In A. N. Davison & J. Dobbing (Eds.), *Applied neurochemistry* (pp. 287–316). Philadelphia: F. A. Davis.

Dobbing, J., & Sands, J. (1979). Comparative aspects of the brain growth spurt. *Early Human Development, 3*, 79–83.

Dow-Edwards, D. L. (1989). Long-term neurochemical and neurobehavioral consequences of cocaine use during pregnancy. *Annals of the New York Academy of Sciences, 562*, 280–289.

Dow-Edwards, D. L. (1990). Fetal and maternal cocaine levels peak rapidly following intragastric administration in the rat. *Journal of Substance Abuse, 2*, 427–437.

Dow-Edwards, D. L., Fico, T. A., Osman, M., Gamagaris, Z., & Hutchings, D. E. (1989). Comparison of oral and subcutaneous routes of cocaine administration of behavior, plasma drug concentration and toxicity in female rats. *Pharmacology, Biochememistry and Behavior, 33*, 167–173.

Dow-Edwards, D. L., Freed, L. A., & Fico, T. A. (1990). Structural and functional effects of prenatal cocaine exposure in adult rat brain. *Developmental Brain Research, 57*, 263–268.

Dow-Edwards, D. L., Freed, L. A., & Milhorat, T. H. (1988). Stimulation of brain metabolism by perinatal cocaine exposure. *Developmental Brain Research, 42*, 137–141.

Dow-Edwards, D. L., Freed-Malen, L. A., & Hughes, H. E. (1993). Long-term alterations in brain function following cocaine administration during the preweaning period. *Developmental Brain Research, 72*, 309–313.

El-Bizri, H., Guest, I., & Varma, D. R. (1991). Effects of cocaine on rat embryo development *in vivo* and in cultures. *Pediatric Research, 29*, 187–190.

Factor, E. M., Hart, R. P., & Jonakait, G. M. (1993). Neurochemical development of the raphe after continuous prenatal cocaine exposure. *Brain Research Bulletin, 31*, 49–56.

Fantel, A. G., & MacPhail, B. J. (1982). The teratogenicity of cocaine. *Teratology, 26*, 17–19.

Finnell, R. H., Toloyan, S., VanWaes, M., & Kalivas, P. W. (1990). Preliminary evidence for a cocaine-induced embryopathy in mice. *Toxicology and Applied Pharmacology, 103*, 228–237.

Foss, J. A., & Riley, E. P. (1991a). Elicitation and modification of the acoustic startle reflex in animals prenatally exposed to cocaine. *Neurotoxicology and Teratology, 13*, 541–546.

Foss, J. A., & Riley, E. P. (1991b). Failure of acute cocaine administration to differentially affect acoustic startle and activity in rats prenatally exposed to cocaine. *Neurotoxicology and Teratology, 13*, 547–551.

Fung, Y. K., Reed, J. A., & Lau, Y.-S. (1989). Prenatal cocaine exposure fails to modify neurobehavioral responses in the striatal dopaminergic system in newborn rats. *General Pharmacology, 20*, 689–293.

Giordano, M., Moody, C. A., Zubrycki, E. M., Dreshfield, L., Norman, A. B., & Sanberg, P. R. (1990). Prenatal exposure to cocaine in rats: Lack of long-term effects on locomotion and stereotypy. *Bulletin of the Psychonomic Society, 28*, 51–54.

Goodwin, G. A., Heyser, C. J., Moody, C. A., Rajachandran, L., Molina, V. A., Arnold, H. M., McKinzie, D. L., Spear, N. E., & Spear, L. P. (1992). A fostering study of the effects of prenatal cocaine exposure: II. Offspring behavioral measures. *Neurotoxicology and Teratology, 14*, 423–432.

Henderson, M. G., & McMillen, B. A. (1990). Effects of prenatal exposure to cocaine or related drugs on rat developmental and neurological indices. *Brain Research Bulletin, 24*, 207–212.

Heyser, C. J., Chen, W.-J., Miller, J., Spear, N. E., & Spear, L. P. (1990). Prenatal cocaine exposure induces deficits in Pavlovian conditioning and sensory preconditioning among infant rat pups. *Behavioral Neuroscience, 104*, 955–963.

Heyser, C. J., Miller, J. S., Spear, N. E., & Spear, L. P. (1992). Prenatal exposure to cocaine disrupts cocaine-induced conditioned place preference in rats. *Neurotoxicology and Teratology, 14*, 57–64.

Heyser, C. J., Molina, V. A., & Spear, L. P. (1992). A fostering study of the effects of prenatal cocaine exposure: I. Maternal behaviors. *Neurotoxicology and Teratology, 14*, 415–421.

Hughes, H. E., Pringle, G. F., Scribani, L. A., & Dow-Edwards, D. L. (1991). Cocaine treatment in neonatal rats affects the adult behavioral response to amphetamine. *Neurotoxicology and Teratology, 13*, 335–339.

Hutchings, D. E., Fico, T. A., & Dow-Edwards, D. L. (1989). Prenatal cocaine: Maternal toxicity, fetal effects and locomotor activity in rat offspring. *Neurotoxicology and Teratology, 11*, 65–69.

Johns, J. M., Means, L. W., Means, M. J., & McMillen, B. A. (1992). Prenatal exposure to cocaine I: Effects on gestation, development, and activity in Sprague–Dawley rats. *Neurotoxicology and Teratology, 14*, 337–342.

Johns, J. M., Means, M. J., Anderson, D. R., Means, L. W., & McMillen, B. A. (1992). Prenatal exposure to cocaine II: Effects on open-field activity and cognitive behavior in Sprague–Dawley rats. *Neurotoxicology and Teratology, 14*, 343–349.

Koren, G. (1993). Cocaine and the human fetus: The concept of teratophilia. *Neurotoxicology and Teratology, 15*, 310–304.

Koren, G., Glasdonte, D., Robeson, C., & Robieux, I. (1992). The perception of teratogenic risk of cocaine. *Teratology, 46*, 567–571.

Lester, B. M., Corwin, M. J., Sepkoski, C., Seifer, R., Peucker, M., McLaughlin, S., & Golub, H. L. (1991). Neurobehavioral syndromes in cocaine-exposed newborn infants. *Child Development, 62*, 694–705.

Lutiger, B., Graham, K., Einarson, T. R., & Koren, G. (1991). Relationship between gestational cocaine use and pregnancy outcome: A meta-analysis. *Teratology, 44*, 405–414.

MacGregor, S. N., Keith, L. G., Chasnoff, I. J., Rosner, M. A., Chisum, R. N., Shaw, P., & Minogue, J. (1987). Cocaine use during pregnancy: Adverse perinatal outcome. *American Journal of Obstetrics and Gynecology, 157*, 686–690.

Mayes, L. C., Granger, R. H., Bornstein, M. H., & Zuckerman, B. (1992). The problem of prenatal cocaine exposure: A rush to judgment. *Journal of the American Medical Association, 267*, 406–408.

Mayes, L. C., Granger, R. H., Frank, M. A., Schottenfield, R., & Bornstein, M. H. (1993). Neurobehavioral profiles of neonates exposed to cocaine prenatally. *Pediatrics, 91*, 778–783.

Meyer, J. S., Sherlock, J. D., & MacDonald, N. R. (1992). Effects of prenatal cocaine on behavioral responses to a cocaine challenge on postnatal day 11. *Neurotoxicology and Teratology, 14*, 183–189.

Minabe, Y., Ashby, C. R., Jr., Heyser, C., Spear, L. P., & Wang, R. Y. (1992). The effects of prenatal cocaine exposure on spontaneously active midbrain dopamine neurons in adult male offspring: An electrophysiological study. *Brain Research, 586*, 152–156.

Nau, H. (1988). Species differences in pharmacokinetics, drug metabolism, and teratogenesis. In H. Nau & W. J. Scott (Eds.), *Pharmacokinetics in teratogenesis: Vol. 1, Interspecies comparison and maternal/embryonic-fetal drug transfer* (pp. 81–106). Boca Raton, FL: CRC Press.

Nau, H., Sierer, R., Spielmann, H., Neubert, D., & Gansau, C. (1981). A new model for embryotoxicity testing: Teratogencity and pharmacokinetics of valproic acid following constant-rate administration in the mouse using human therapeutic drug and metabolite concentrations. *Life Sciences, 29*, 2803–2814.

Neuspiel, D. R., & Hamel, S. C. (1991). Cocaine and infant behavior. *Journal of Developmental and Behavioral Pediatrics, 12*, 55–64.

Neuspiel, D. R., Hamel, S. C., Hochberg, E., Greene, J., & Campbell, D. (1991). Maternal cocaine use and infant behavior. *Neurotoxicology and Teratology, 13*, 229–233.

Raum, W. J., McGivern, R. F., Peterson, M. A., Sryne, J. H., & Gorski, R. A. (1990). Prenatal inhibition of hypothalamic sex steroid uptake by cocaine: Effects on neurobehavioral sexual differentiation in male rats. *Developmental Brain Research, 53*, 230–236.

Richardson, G. A., & Day, N. L. (1991). Maternal and neonatal effects of moderate cocaine use during pregnancy. *Neurotoxicology and Teratology, 13*, 455–460.

Riley, E. P., & Foss, J. A. (1991a). The acquisition of passive avoidance, active avoidance, and spatial navigation tasks by animals prenatally exposed to cocaine. *Neurotoxicology and Teratology, 13,* 559–564.

Riley, E. P., & Foss, J. A. (1991b). Exploratory behavior and locomotor activity: A failure to find effects in animals prenatally exposed to cocaine. *Neurotoxicology and Teratology, 13,* 553–558.

Rodriguez-Sanchez, M. N., Alvaro, I., & Arilla, E. (1991). Effect of prenatal and postnatal cocaine exposure on somatostatin content and binding in frontoparietal cortex and hippocampus of developing rat pups. *Peptides, 12,* 951–956.

Scalzo, F. M., Ali, S. F., Frambes, N. A., & Spear, L. P. (1990). Weanling rats exposed prenatally to cocaine exhibit an increase in striatal D2 dopamine binding associated in an increase in ligand affinity. *Pharmacology, Biochemistry and Behavior, 37,* 371–373.

Seidler, F. J., & Slotkin, T. A. (1993). Prenatal cocaine and cell development in rat brain regions: Effects on ornithine decarboxylase and macromolecules. *Brain Research Bulletin, 30,* 91–99.

Seifert, M. F., & Church, M. W. (1991). Long term effects of prenatal cocaine exposure on bone in rats. *Life Sciences, 49,* 569–574.

Smith, R. F., Mattran, K. M., Kurkjian, M. F., & Kurtz, S. L. (1989). Alternations in offspring behavior induced by chronic prenatal cocaine dosing. *Neurotoxicology and Teratology, 11,* 35–38.

Sobrian, S. K., Burton, L. E., Robinson, N. L., Ashe, W. K., James, H., Stokes, D. L., & Turner, L. M. (1990). Neurobehavioral and immunological effects of prenatal cocaine exposure in rat. *Pharmacology, Biochemistry and Behavior, 35,* 617–629.

Spear, L. P., Frambes, N. A., & Kirstein, C. L. (1989). Fetal and maternal brain and plasma levels of cocaine and benzoylecgonine following chronic subcutaneous administration of cocaine during gestation in rats. *Psychopharmacology, 97,* 427–431.

Spear, L. P., Kirstein, C. L., Bell, J., Yoottanasumpun, V., Greenbaum, R., O'Shea, J., Hoffmann, H., & Spear, N. E. (1989). Effects of prenatal cocaine exposure on behavior during the early postnatal period. *Neurotoxicology and Teratology, 11,* 57–63.

Tyrala, E. E., Mathews, S. V., & Rao, G. S. (1992). Effect of intrauterine exposure to cocaine on acetylcholinesterase in primary cultures of fetal mouse brain cells. *Neurotoxicology and Teratology, 14,* 229–233.

Vorhees, C. V. (1986). Principles of behavioral teratology. In E. P. Riley & C. V. Vorhees (Eds.), *Handbook of behavioral teratology* (pp. 23–48). New York: Plenum.

Weaver, D. R., Rivkees, S. A., & Reppert, S. M. (1992). D1-dopamine receptors activate c-*fos* expression in the fetal suprachiasmatic nuclei. *Proceedings of the National Academy of Sciences (USA), 89,* 9201–9204.

Webster, W. L., & Brown-Woodman, P. D. C. (1990). Cocaine as a cause of congenital malformations of facsular origin: Experimental evidence in the rat. *Teratology, 41,* 689–697.

Webster, W. S., Brown-Woodman, P. D. C., Lipson, A. H., & Ritchie, H. E. (1991). Fetal brain damage in the rat following prenatal exposure to cocaine. *Neurotoxicology and Teratology, 13,* 621–626.

Wiggins, R. C., Rolsten, C., Ruiz, B., & Davis, C. M. (1989). Pharmacokinetics of cocaine: Basic studies of route, dosage, pregnancy and lactation. *Neurotoxicology, 10,* 367–382.

Zuckerman, B., & Frank, D. A. (1992). "Crack kids": Not broken. *Pediatrics, 89,* 337–339.

Zuckerman, B., Frank, D. A., Hingson, R., Amaro, H., Levenson, S. M., Kayne, H., Parker, S., Vinci, R., Aboagye, K., Fried, L. E., Cabral, H., Timperi, R., & Bauchner, H. (1989). Effects of maternal marijuana and cocaine use on fetal growth. *New England Journal of Medicine, 320,* 762–768.

6

▼▼▼▼▼▼▼

The Problem of Confounding in Research on Prenatal Cocaine Effects on Behavior and Development

Daniel R. Neuspiel
Albert Einstein College of Medicine

Does prenatal use of cocaine cause behavioral or developmental harm after the birth of an exposed child? Whether such effects occur and, if they do, to what degree they are associated with cocaine use per se is an increasingly controversial question. Some of the earliest published human and animal studies reported damage to cocaine-exposed offspring, and this view of severe effects has received a lot of play among both professionals and the lay public. However, this image of severe or lasting damage from cocaine is inconsistent with the experience of many professionals involved in the clinical care of these infants and children. In addition, recent studies raise numerous questions about the magnitude of risk associated with cocaine. Despite these newer observations, the earlier view is still popular, and may be termed the *mythology of severe risk* (Neuspiel, 1993a). A discussion of the roots and consequences of this mythology concludes this chapter.

The main emphasis of this review is on issues in designing and conducting research studies in this area, especially the problem of confounding, that is, the co-occurrence of other variables with cocaine exposure that may cause effects that are erroneously attributed to cocaine. Other difficulties in study design may also have serious implications; these include how cocaine-exposed groups are sampled, measurement of exposure, cohort retention, and selection of dependent variables (Neuspiel & Hamel, 1991). Further, Koren, Graham, Shear, and Einarson (1989) demonstrated that there is a bias that leads to a greater likelihood of reporting and publishing studies showing adverse effects of cocaine. The same bias results in underreporting or not publishing those studies failing to show such

95

effects. Additionally, it is especially difficult to recruit and retain drug-exposed children and their families for follow-up studies.

The reasons for considering confounding factors in these studies include:

- Cocaine use has been associated with many other toxic exposures (e.g., tobacco, alcohol, other illicit and licit drugs).
- The social environment of cocaine users may differ substantially from that of nonusers (e.g., access to prenatal care, housing).
- The physical and emotional health of cocaine users may differ from that of nonusers (e.g., nutrition, stress, sexually transmitted diseases).

Confounding effects are of extreme importance in any type of research on the causes of health problems, but the effects of concurrent exposures are of particular importance in studies of drug use because of the high frequency of many other potential risk factors among cocaine users—all of which are known to cause harm to the fetus and child. This review begins with a general discussion of this problem, followed by some examples of confounding in cocaine-related infant behavior studies, and the examination of some simulated data that further demonstrate this problem.

WHAT IS CONFOUNDING?

The term *confounding* has its origins in the Latin *confundere*, meaning to pour, mingle, or mix together. In a broad sense, confounding is the mixing of the effect of one exposure under study with the effect of other variables on the disease or outcome, leading to a biased or distorted estimate of the impact of that exposure (Hennekens, Buring, & Mayrent, 1987; Rothman, 1986). A confounder, also known as a confounding variable, must meet three conditions:

1. It must itself be a risk factor for the disease or condition under study, regardless of whether cocaine exposure has occurred.
2. It must co-occur with the exposure under study, disproportionately from its frequency among unexposed subjects.
3. It must not be directly caused by exposure to cocaine; that is, it should not be an intermediate or intervening factor in the causal pathway between cocaine exposure and developmental or behavioral outcome.

At times it is difficult or impossible to determine whether a specific variable is a confounder, an intervening factor, or a chance association with the exposure and outcome. Further understanding requires knowledge about the biological relationship between the study exposure, suspected confounder, and outcome

(Kelsey, Thompson, & Evans, 1986). Behavioral researchers are typically unaware of or uncertain about the exact ways that causes lead to effects. In this situation, available information from prior research and known physiology may help decide whether or not a given factor is a confounder.

A confounder should be identified as such before data collection, not after statistical analysis (Kleinbaum, Kupper, & Morgenstern, 1982; Schlesselman, 1982). Some investigators examine their data for significant group differences in covariates before deciding which to consider as confounders. There are several reasons *not* to screen for confounding by statistical testing:

1. In a cohort study, a statistical association between the exposure and purported confounder does not denote a necessary relationship between the confounder and outcome; thus, confounding may not really exist.
2. In a case-control study, an association between the possible confounder and group status does not mean there is a relationship with exposure.
3. A nonsignificant difference may be due to small sample size, yet may be accompanied by important differences in risk estimates.
4. The significance test only addresses sampling variability, and ignores study bias and errors of interpretation. The real question of interest in an observational study should not be whether an observation is due to chance, but what is the most accurate estimate of the effect of exposure on outcome.

The three conditions characterizing confounding may be further examined to shed more light on this problem:

1. *A confounder must be a risk factor for the outcome condition of interest.* The confounding variable need not cause the condition, but it must at least be a marker or surrogate for the cause (Breslow & Day, 1980). As an example, age and social class or status are frequent confounders, but they rarely are actual direct causes. The key aspect here is that the confounder's association with the outcome must not come only from its association with the exposure, but should be clinically related to the outcome, even among subjects free of the exposure under study.

Can we determine whether a possible confounder is a risk factor for the study outcome by simply examining our study data? Not according to current epidemiologic theory: It is the actual relation between the variable and outcome from prior knowledge, not the observed relationship in the data of our study, that determines whether confounding exists. Observed data relationships may be particularly distorted in studies with few subjects, and such studies may falsely identify a statistically significant risk factor due to Type I error.

2. *A confounder must be associated with the main exposure of interest in the study population.* The association between the confounder and the exposure must

not be solely from the association of the exposure with the outcome. It follows that the confounder must be distributed in unequal proportions between exposure groups. When matching is used as a technique to select a comparison unexposed group based on the same level of a confounder, the distribution of the confounder is artificially equalized between exposure groups, and the association between the confounder and exposure should be removed. Assuming that the matching is done using accurate measurement of the confounder, this particular confounding effect is controlled and no longer exists within the study groups.

3. *A confounder must not be an intervening or intermediate variable in the causal pathway between exposure and outcome.* Prior information and knowledge from previous research separate from the study data are required to determine this criterion. In some cases, it may make sense to treat a variable both as a confounder and intermediate factor in separate analyses (Rothman, 1986). Birth weight and gestational age may be considered both as potential confounders and intervening variables in studies of the behavioral consequences of prenatal cocaine exposure. This occurs because low birth weight and prematurity may be causally linked to cocaine exposure, and these factors in turn may confer higher risk for adverse behavioral or developmental outcome. Cocaine exposure may lead to higher risk for low birth weight and prematurity, which may then lead to increased risk for less optimal development. In this sense, birth weight and gestation are intervening variables, not confounders. Because cocaine may act through other pathways, and because these variables are not necessarily causally linked with cocaine, they could also be confounders.

Misclassification of Confounders: Some Examples in Other Areas of Research

An understanding of causal relationships may be seriously compromised by misclassification of confounding variables (Miettinen, 1985; Rothman, 1986). When a strong confounder coexists with a weak relationship between exposure and outcome, results may deviate substantially from the truth. Rothman illustrated this situation in research on the relationship between coffee drinking and bladder cancer, where smoking is a strong confounder. To control this confounding effect, accurate smoking measurement is needed. Because such measurement is often not fully possible, some residual confounding remains. When dichotomous measures of smoking such as "ever smoked" versus "never smoked" are used, this residual confounding effect is exaggerated, because both dose differences and passive tobacco exposure are ignored. Many readers of such research may believe that confounding is controlled here, despite these limitations.

In another example, Miettinen (1985) described how the risk of laryngeal cancer associated with alcohol consumption persists even after control for smoking. Because the association between alcohol and smoking is strong, and smoking is a strong risk factor for cancer of the larynx, it is possible that the observed association between alcohol and cancer is a biased result, due to the inaccurate measurement of tobacco exposure. Accurate measurement of smoking is also of key importance in studies of cocaine effects, as the following discussion elucidates. Miettinen discussed some occasions when the operational consideration of confounding is so difficult that a satisfactory epidemiological investigation is not possible. At these times, he continued, the optimal study size may be zero.

What Can Be Done About Confounding?

Adjustments can be made for the problem of confounding in the design phase of an investigation, via the selection of comparison subjects matched for the potential confounder. Such matching can be done on a group or, preferably, on an individual basis. Other approaches to consideration of confounding rely on analytical methods, including stratification, analysis of variance, and various multivariable methods. Further discussion of control for confounding may be found in many epidemiological texts (e.g., Breslow & Day, 1980; Hennekens et al., 1987; Kelsey et al., 1986; Rothman, 1986; Schlesselman, 1982).

STUDIES OF COCAINE EFFECTS ON INFANT AND TODDLER BEHAVIOR: THE IMPACT OF CONFOUNDING

Research on the relationship of prenatal cocaine exposure with infant and child behavioral outcomes has been limited in quantity and quality. Cocaine effects on newborns have been examined in eight extant publications using the Brazelton Neonatal Behavioral Assessment Scale (NBAS), and these reported conflicting results. Although this review is limited to issues of confounding, it is fully recognized that many other methodological problems exist in this work, including my own (Hutchings, 1993).

The eight pertinent studies are summarized in Table 6.1 (Chasnoff, Burns, Schnoll, & Burns, 1985; Chasnoff, Griffith, MacGregor, Dirkes, & Burns, 1989; Coles, Platzman, Smith, James, & Falek, 1992; Eisen et al., 1991; Mayes, Granger, Frank, Schottenfeld, & Bornstein, 1993; Neuspiel, Hamel, Hochberg, Greene, & Campbell, 1991; Richardson & Day, 1991; Woods, Eyler, Behnke, & Conlon, 1993). Many potential confounders were considered, using varying units of measurement and methods of control. Often, the units of measurement of these variables were not specified. Methods for control of confounding included group or individual matching for each potential confounder between exposure groups, and analytic methods included multiple linear regression and analysis of covariance (ANCOVA).

The eight studies considered a range of between 3 and 13 possible confounders each, with a median of 5 per study. The results of these studies were evenly split: Four showed cocaine effects on varying aspects of NBAS scores, and four showed

TABLE 6.1

Cocaine Effects on Neonatal Behavioral Assessment Scale

Study	Confounders	Method	NBAS Findings
Chasnoff et al. (1985)	maternal age, gravidity, smoking (yes/no), alcohol (+ or − 2/month)	group matching	cocaine effect
Chasnoff et al. (1989)	maternal age, SES, smoking (cigarettes/day)	group matching	cocaine effect
Neuspiel et al. (1991)	examination (3),* perinatal (6),* exposures (4)*	multiple linear regression	no effect
Coles et al. (1992)	parity, race, examiner, age at exam, first trimester alcohol (3 categories), marijuana (yes/no), tobacco (yes/no), tobacco (pack/day)	group matching (ANCOVA for pack/day tobacco)	no effect
Eisen et al. (1991)	gender, ethnicity, gestational age, birth weight	group matching (other unnamed variables by multiple linear regression)	cocaine effect
Richardson & Day (1991)	alcohol, marijuana, tobacco (all duration and dose, smoking cigarettes/week), obstetric complications, examiner	multiple linear regression (gender, gestational age, maternal age, age at exam "considered" by unstated method)	no effect
Woods et al. (1993)	race, parity, smoking (yes/no), birth weight/gestational age, delivery type	individual matching	no effect
Mayes et al. (1993)	birth weight, gestational age, race, prenatal care, gravidity	matching (birth weight, gestational age, race) Unclear regarding other variables	cocaine effect

*Confounders entered in groups (N of variables).

no effects compared with unexposed infants. NBAS items are commonly clustered into seven distinct aspects of behavior (Lester, 1984). The four studies reporting cocaine effects were inconsistent in the specific cluster of NBAS items affected.

The potential confounders considered in this research are presented in Table 6.2, along with the number of studies including each variable. Twenty different possible confounding variables were considered, although none of the variables were utilized in every study. Tobacco smoke exposure was the most frequently considered confounder, in six of the eight studies. Arguably, several of these might be considered as intervening variables, rather than or in addition to being confounders. These mediating or intervening variables are birth weight, gestational age, obstetric complications, and prenatal care. Each of these factors could be considered part of the causal pathway between cocaine exposure and behavioral or developmental outcome.

Smoking may be a strong predictor of outcome in these studies (Rush, 1992). If tobacco smoke is also related to cocaine exposure, which it usually is, then accurate measure of the former must be used to control for and avoid residual confounding effects. In three of the NBAS studies, the unit of measurement of tobacco exposure was dichotomous: Smoking during pregnancy was simply indicated as present or absent (Chasnoff et al., 1985; Neuspiel et al., 1991; Woods et al., 1993). A fourth study also used dichotomous smoking in matching during initial analysis, but after it was determined that the exposure groups differed in packs per day smoked, this quantitative measure was used in analysis of covariance (Coles et al., 1992). Two studies measured tobacco use by cigarettes per day or per week, respectively.

Interestingly, the two studies that did not even consider smoking as a confounder reported that cocaine was associated with less optimal NBAS scores (Eisen et al., 1991; Mayes et al., 1993). These findings could represent inaccurate results, due to confounding by the uncontrolled effects of smoking, as well as to other confounding effects. The three studies that used dichotomous smoking

TABLE 6.2
Confounders Considered in Cocaine NBAS Studies

# Studies Considering Each Confounder				
6	*4*	*3*	*2*	*1*
Tobacco	Maternal age	Examiner	SES	Time since fed
	Race or ethnicity	Parity	Gravidity	Delivery type
	Alcohol	Infant age		Prenatal care
		Child gender		Type feeding
		Birth weight		Obstetric complications
		Marijuana		Weight/gestation
		Gestational age		Opiates

Note. Total studies = 8.

measures may have incompletely controlled for this confounding effect (Chasnoff et al., 1989; Coles et al., 1992; Richardson & Day, 1991), because cocaine users may smoke more cigarettes than nonusers. Even the three studies using number of cigarettes or packs per day or week may not have accurately considered tobacco smoke exposure, because this measurement does not account for exposure of the mother to others smoking in her environment. Exposure to passive smoke and other environmental toxins may be higher in a drug-using environment (Neuspiel, Markowitz, & Drucker, 1994).

Neonatal measures have not been predictive of later child behavior (McCall, 1979), and cocaine effects may not be evident until a later age. For both of these reasons, long-term studies are needed. However, developmental and behavioral follow-up studies of cocaine-exposed infants beyond the newborn period are extremely limited in number and quality. Published studies are summarized here by child age at latest observation (Table 6.3).

At follow-up of infants studied with the NBAS, we observed these babies and their mothers at 2 to 3 months of age (Neuspiel et al., 1991). There were no differences in mother–infant interaction between cocaine-exposed and unexposed

TABLE 6.3
Follow-Up Studies of Cocaine Effects Beyond the Newborn Period

Study	Age	Measure	Confounders	Findings
Neuspiel et al. (1991)	2–3 months	NCAFS[a]	None	No effect
Schneider & Chasnoff (1992)	4 months	MAI[b]	Race (in analysis)	Cocaine effect
Rodning et al. (1989a, 1989b)	13 months	Gesell (+) BSID[c] (−)	None	Cocaine effect
Graham et al. (1992)	18 months	BSID[c], Vineland	Group matched: marital status tobacco alcohol ethnicity maternal age gravidity parity	No effect
Chasnoff et al. (1992)	24 months	BSID[c]	Group matched: maternal age race SES	No effect > 6 months
Azuma & Chasnoff (1993)	36 months	SB IQ[d]	Group matched: maternal age race SES	No crude effect[e]
Singer et al. (1994)	16–18 months	BSID	Group matched: race SES	Cocaine effect

[a]Nursing Child Assessment of Feeding Scale. [b]Movement Assessment of Infants. [c]Bayley Scales of Infant Development. [d]Stanford–Binet IQ Test. [e]Some drug effect on IQ noted after path analysis.

mother–infant pairs during an observed feeding interaction using the Barnard Nursing Child Assessment of Feeding Scale. No confounders were considered because of the absence of crude effects.

Schneider and Chasnoff (1992) examined 74 cocaine- and polydrug-exposed infants and 50 unexposed infants at 4 months of age with the Movement Assessment of Infants. This instrument evaluates muscle tone, primitive reflexes, automatic reactions, and volitional movement from 4 through 12 months and provides a risk assessment score for motor dysfunction. The mean total risk scores in this study were higher in the cocaine and polydrug group. However, the tests were done by an examiner who may have been biased by being aware of infant group assignment. Furthermore, there was inadequate control for confounding in this study, as the only variable considered was race.

Rodning, Beckwith, and Howard (1989a, 1989b) reported a study of 18 polydrug-exposed infants, 14 of whom were exposed to cocaine, compared with 57 high-risk preterm infants. The groups differed in prenatal care, gestational age, birth weight, and child-care custody. At 13 months of age, the Gesell developmental exam was done in the drug-exposed group, while the Bayley Scales of Infant Development (BSID) was used in the high-risk preterm group. The authors reported significantly lower scores in the drug-exposed group, although both groups performed in the average range. Among several problems with this study were that scores between these two different exams may not be comparable, no consideration of confounding was made, and the examiners were not blind to study group assignment. In this study, a separate observation of free play was done at 18 to 20 months, and the drug-exposed group had fewer representational play events.

In an investigation of the children of 30 social cocaine users, defined as nonaddicted women who stopped use of cocaine after discovery of pregnancy, compared with the offspring of 20 cannabis users and 30 drug-free women, Graham et al. (1992) employed group matching to control for marital status, tobacco, alcohol, ethnicity, maternal age, gravidity, and parity. At 18 months, examiner-blinded evaluations with the BSID and Vineland Adaptive Behavior Scales were performed. No differences between groups in either scale were noted.

Chasnoff, Griffith, Freier, and Murray (1992) administered the BSID at 3, 6, 12, 18, and 24 months of age in cocaine- and polydrug-exposed children compared with unexposed controls. Groups were matched on maternal age, race, and socioeconomic status. Cocaine- and polydrug-exposed infants had lower mental and psychomotor developmental indices at 6 months of age, but not at later exams, and all BSID scores were greater than 100. Drug-exposed children had persistent smaller head circumferences through 2 years of age, but this finding was not accompanied by developmental deficit.

At 3 years of age, this same cohort was reevaluated with the Stanford–Binet Intelligence Scale (Azuma & Chasnoff, 1993). IQ scores for each group were in the normal range and not statistically distinguishable, although the drug-exposed children continued to have smaller mean head circumference. Using path analytic procedures, drug exposure had both direct and indirect effects on cognitive functioning. However, environmental factors contributed similarly to IQ results, and this analysis did not account for several important confounders.

A separate report from the same investigators (Griffith, Azuma, & Chasnoff, 1994), with a smaller follow-up sample, found some group differences in Stanford–Binet scores. However, the selection factors in this smaller sample complicate its interpretation.

Singer et al. (1994) studied 41 cocaine-exposed very low birth weight (VLBW) infants compared with 41 nonexposed VLBW infants. The cocaine-exposed group had lower BSID scores at follow-up ages of 16.6 months (exposed) and 18.5 months (unexposed). These findings are problematic due to lack of control for alcohol, marijuana, tobacco, and foster care, all of which were greater in the cocaine group. Additionally, these investigators used single-tailed statistical testing with questionable justification.

This brief overview of the methodologic problems in this research, focusing on problems of confounding, demonstrates that because of these confounders, little can be currently concluded with much confidence about the impact of prenatal cocaine exposure on the developing human brain. Other methodological problems not considered in this discussion add further uncertainties to research in this area.

EXAMINATION OF CONFOUNDING
IN A SIMULATED DATA SET

This section further illustrates and quantifies the potential effects of confounding in this area of research. A sample of 100 subjects was simulated, 50 exposed to cocaine and 50 unexposed, with the two groups having equal random normally distributed scores on a behavioral measure designed to be similar to an NBAS cluster score. A confounder (substance X), modeled after tobacco exposure, is assumed to be a strong causal predictor of a decrement in this same score, with a population mean of 5.0 in X-exposed and 7.0 in the unexposed groups, both with standard deviations of 1 unit. On the basis of our previous research data on smoking rates in cocaine users and nonusers, 80% of the cocaine group are estimated to be exposed to X and 20% unexposed (Neuspiel et al., 1991). It is assumed that there is no statistical interaction between cocaine and X exposures.

SYSTAT statistical software (SYSTAT, 1992) was used to generate a sample distribution of this behavioral measure, which will be called Z. The sample means are in Table 6.4a and show crude differences between cocaine exposure groups. Two-way analysis of variance (ANOVA) was used to control simultaneously for cocaine and X exposure, with the main effects shown in Table 6.4b. Here, it is demonstrated that X is a confounder for the apparent crude relationship between

TABLE 6.4a
Crude Values of Z by Substance Exposure

Substance	Exposed	Unexposed	P
Cocaine	5.23	6.36	< .0005
X	4.98	6.60	< .0005

TABLE 6.4b
Two-Way ANOVA for Substance Effects on Z

Substance	F	P
Cocaine	1.1	.30
X	38.2	< .0005

TABLE 6.4c
Misclassified X Exposure: Crude Effects on Z

Substance	Exposed	Unexposed	P
Cocaine	5.23	6.36	< .0005
X	5.12	6.08	< .0005

TABLE 6.4d
Misclassified X Exposure: Two-Way ANOVA

Substance	F	P
Cocaine	7.53	.007
X	5.72	.019

cocaine and the Z score. That is, even though we know that there is no effect of cocaine by design here, an apparent cocaine effect is due to the unbalanced distribution of a strong confounder (X) between the groups.

In order to demonstrate the effect of misclassification of the confounding variable, the next analysis starts with the same data set, but 40% of the X-exposed subjects are randomly misclassified as unexposed. The level of 40% is based on our data (Neuspiel et al., 1994), where 39% of smokers were misclassified as nonsmokers by reliance on self-report. The crude relationships are depicted in Table 6.4c. Whereas there are not great differences here from the previous table, the ANOVA is more striking (Table 6.4d). This demonstrates that in the presence of a strong confounder with no main effect of exposure to the primary independent variable, inaccurate or misclassified measurement of the confounder at a plausible level can lead to systematic deviation from the truth.

Conclusions from these simulated data should be made cautiously, however. The magnitude of effect on this artificial Z score may be greater than what truly occurs in relation to either tobacco or cocaine effects on children. The simulated score is assumed to be normally distributed, yet in truth neither NBAS clusters nor most other behavioral scores meet the assumptions of normality. It was also assumed that misclassification of exposure to the confounder was independent of the Z score in each subject, which may not be the case in humans. Despite these reservations, the simulated data demonstrate the importance of the relationships of confounders that bear on work in this area.

WHERE DO WE GO FROM HERE?

Clearly there are adverse effects of the most common correlates of drug use. Many factors besides cocaine in the environments of pregnant women, often continuing through infancy and early childhood, may also impact on development and behavior, and may be differentially distributed between cocaine users and nonusers. These include poor access to health care, parenting difficulty, family violence, incarceration, nutrition, chronic illness, inadequate housing, unemployment, stress, alcohol, and other social and environmental exposures. A one-dimensional emphasis on cocaine use is therefore an unsatisfactory causal explanation because it deconstructs the reality in which the exposure occurs and leads to inappropriate public health responses to these complex problems.

Rush (1992) reviewed the developmental and behavioral effects of smoking in pregnancy, and suggested that the main problem in interpreting observational studies of these effects is the failure to control adequately for social differences between smokers and nonsmokers. He cautioned that full control for such social effects is probably impossible, and that the behavioral and social status differences associated with both smoking and child development have not been well considered in prior research. This interpretation may be generalizable to studies of outcomes related to cocaine and other substance exposures.

Cocaine is not innocuous in its effects, and beyond potential teratogenicity, its intoxicating actions after birth may impair the parent–child relationship. But other behaviors related to drug dependency may also compromise the health of the fetus and child. Studies to date seem to show that only a small proportion of cocaine-exposed pregnancies result in negative outcomes of clinical significance and, when adverse outcomes are observed, other factors besides cocaine exposure are clearly implicated.

Why then is there such a persistent mythology of belief in very severe effects of gestational cocaine exposure? The tenacity of this belief may result from societal attitudes, media practices, and government policy. Blaming the behavior of mothers for adverse gestational outcomes is used to justify more social control over women's actions in pregnancy, and this approach has been gaining in popularity (Pollitt, 1990). Chasnoff, Landress, and Barrett (1990) in a study including all socioeconomic and ethnic groups in Pinellas County, Florida, reported that non-White women are more likely to be identified as drug users, despite toxicological evidence of comparable levels of use in both Whites and non-Whites. African-American women have been particularly victimized by the criminal justice system in drug prosecutions (Roberts, 1991). In recent data from our hospital, African-American women were also at greater risk of losing their cocaine-exposed newborns to foster care (Neuspiel, Zingman, Templeton, DiStabile, & Drucker, 1993).

In these times, it appears to be more politically expedient to attribute childhood problems to the individual behavior of drug-using women than to examine and remediate the social factors that lead to family dysfunction, persistent untreated addiction, and pervasive poverty. The former victim-blaming approach is consonant with a new form of biological determinism that has emerged in recent years, emphasizing allegedly constitutional determinants for violent, criminal, and antisocial behavior. To some who support this line of "violence research," early cocaine exposure has become one of the major purported risk factors for a life of crime. In a society where disproportionately more non-White infants are identified as cocaine exposed, this line of reasoning leads to further racial discrimination and stigmatization directed against both mothers and children. Terms such as *crack babies* and *crack kids* have become virtual racial epithets.

Thus, the consequences of overestimating the risks of intrauterine cocaine exposure go far beyond mere epidemiological theory. Blaming this exposure alone for adverse infant outcomes may have negative consequences for the mother, such as unnecessary termination of pregnancy, as demonstrated recently by Koren, Gladstone, Robeson, and Robieux (1992). Additionally, the labeling of cocaine-exposed children with or without developmental impairments as "crack kids" who are "irreparably damaged" may confer a self-fulfilling prophecy of failure and may lead to inattention to other sources of developmental risk (Mayes, Granger, Bornstein, & Zuckerman, 1992; Neuspiel, 1993b). Cocaine users and their children face many risks, and all of these need more accurate consideration in future research.

ACKNOWLEDGMENTS

This work was presented, in part, at the College on Problems of Drug Dependence in Toronto, Canada on June 13, 1993. It was supported by Grant No. R18-DA06925 from the National Institute on Drug Abuse. Helpful comments on the manuscript were made by Dr. Ernest Drucker.

REFERENCES

Azuma, S. D., & Chasnoff, I. J. (1993). Outcome of children prenatally exposed to cocaine and other drugs: A path analysis of three-year data. *Pediatrics, 92,* 396–402.

Breslow, N. E., & Day, N. E. (1980). *Statistical methods in cancer research, Volume 1: The analysis of case-control studies.* Lyon, France: International Agency for Research on Cancer.

Chasnoff, I. J., Burns, W. J., Schnoll, S. H., & Burns, K. A. (1985). Cocaine use in pregnancy. *New England Journal of Medicine, 313*, 666–669.

Chasnoff, I. J., Griffith, D. R., Freier, C., & Murray, J. (1992). Cocaine/polydrug use in pregnancy: Two-year follow-up. *Pediatrics, 89*, 284–289.

Chasnoff, I. J., Griffith, D. R., MacGregor, S., Dirkes, K., & Burns, K. A. (1989). Temporal patterns of cocaine use in pregnancy: Perinatal outcome. *Journal of the American Medical Association, 261*, 1741–1744.

Chasnoff, I. J., Landress, H. J., & Barrett, M. E. (1990). The prevalence of illicit drug or alcohol use during pregnancy and discrepancies in mandatory reporting in Pinellas County, Florida. *New England Journal of Medicine, 322*, 1202–1206.

Coles, C. D., Platzman, K. A., Smith, I., James, M. E., & Falek, A. (1992). Effects of cocaine and alcohol use in pregnancy on neonatal growth and neurobehavioral status. *Neurotoxicology and Teratology, 14*, 23–33.

Eisen, L. N., Field, T. M., Bandstra, E. S., Roberts, J. P., Morrow, C., Larson, S. K., & Steele, B. M. (1991). Perinatal cocaine effects on neonatal stress behavior and performance on the Brazelton scale. *Pediatrics, 88*, 477–480.

Graham, K., Feigenbaum, A., Pastuszak, A., Nulman, I., Weksberg, R., Einarson, T., Goldberg, S., Ashby, S., & Koren, G. (1992). Pregnancy outcome and infant development following gestational cocaine use by social cocaine users in Toronto, Canada. *Clinical Investigations in Medicine, 15*, 384–394.

Griffith, D. R., Azuma, S. D., & Chasnoff, I. J. (1994). Three-year outcome of children exposed prenatally to drugs. *Journal of the American Academy of Child and Adolescent Psychiatry, 33*, 20–27.

Hennekens, C. H., Buring, J. E., & Mayrent, S. L. (1987). *Epidemiology in medicine.* Boston: Little, Brown.

Hutchings, D. E. (1993). The puzzle of cocaine's effects following maternal use during pregnancy: Are there reconcilable differences? *Neurotoxicology and Teratology, 15*, 281–286.

Kelsey, J. L., Thompson, W. D., & Evans, A. S. (1986). *Methods in observational epidemiology.* New York: Oxford.

Kleinbaum, D. G., Kupper, L. L., & Morgenstern, H. (1982). *Epidemiologic research: Principles and quantitative methods.* Belmont, CA: Lifetime Learning Publications.

Koren, G., Gladstone, D., Robeson, N., & Robieux, I. (1992). The perception of teratogenic risk of cocaine. *Teratology, 46*, 567–571.

Koren, G., Graham, K., Shear, H., & Einarson, T. (1989). Bias against the null hypothesis: The reproductive hazards of cocaine. *Lancet, 2*, 1440–1442.

Lester, B. M. (1984). Data analysis and prediction. In T. B. Brazelton (Ed.), *Neonatal Behavioral Assessment Scale* (2nd ed., pp. 85–96). Philadelphia: J. B. Lippincott.

Mayes, L. C., Granger, R. H., Bornstein, M. H., & Zuckerman, B. (1992). The problem of prenatal cocaine exposure: A rush to judgment. *Journal of the American Medical Association, 267*, 406–408.

Mayes, L. C., Granger, R. H., Frank, M. A., Schottenfeld, R., & Bornstein, M. H. (1993). Neurobehavioral profiles of neonates exposed to cocaine prenatally. *Pediatrics, 91*, 778–783.

McCall, R. B. (1979). The development of intellectual functioning in infancy and the prediction of later IQ. In J. D. Osofsky (Ed.), *Handbook of infant development* (pp. 707–741). New York: Wiley.

Miettinen, O. S. (1985). *Theoretical epidemiology: Principles of occurrence research in medicine.* New York: Wiley.

Neuspiel, D. R. (1993a). Cocaine and the fetus: Mythology of severe risk. *Neurotoxicology and Teratology, 15*, 305–306.

Neuspiel, D. R. (1993b). On pejorative labeling of cocaine exposed children. *Journal of Substance Abuse Treatment, 10*, 407.

Neuspiel, D. R., & Hamel, S. C. (1991). Cocaine and infant behavior. *Journal of Developmental and Behavioral Pediatrics, 12,* 55–64.

Neuspiel, D. R., Hamel, S. C., Hochberg, E., Greene, J., & Campbell, D. (1991). Maternal cocaine use and infant behavior. *Neurotoxicology and Teratology, 13,* 229–233.

Neuspiel, D. R., Markowitz, M., & Drucker, E. (1994). Intrauterine cocaine, lead, and nicotine exposure and fetal growth. *American Journal of Public Health, 84,* 1492–1495.

Neuspiel, D. R., Zingman, T. M., Templeton, V. H., DiStabile, P., & Drucker, E. (1993). Determinants of discharge custody of cocaine-exposed newborns. *American Journal of Public Health, 83,* 1726–1729.

Pollitt, K. (1990). "Fetal rights": A new assault on feminism. *Nation, 250,* 409–418.

Richardson, G. A., & Day, N. L. (1991). Maternal and neonatal effects of moderate cocaine use during pregnancy. *Neurotoxicology and Teratology, 13,* 455–460.

Roberts, D. E. (1991). Punishing drug addicts who have babies: Women of color, equality, and the right of privacy. *Harvard Law Review, 104,* 1419–1482.

Rodning, C., Beckwith, L., & Howard, J. (1989a). Characteristics of attachment and play organization in prenatally drug-exposed toddlers. *Developmental Psychopathology, 11,* 277–289.

Rodning, C., Beckwith, L., & Howard, J. (1989b). Prenatal exposure to drugs: Behavioral distortions reflecting CNS impairment? *Neurotoxicology, 10,* 629–634.

Rothman, K. J. (1986). *Modern epidemiology.* Boston: Little, Brown.

Rush, D. (1992). Exposure to passive cigarette smoking and child development: An updated critical review. In D. Poswillo & E. Alberman (Eds.), *Effects of smoking on the fetus, neonate, and child* (pp. 150–170). New York: Oxford.

Schlesselman, J. J. (1982). *Case-control studies: Design, conduct, analysis.* New York: Oxford.

Schneider, J. W., & Chasnoff, I. J. (1992). Motor assessment of cocaine/polydrug exposed infants at age four months. *Neurotoxicology and Teratology, 14,* 97–101.

Singer, L. T., Yamashita, T. S., Hawkins, S., Cairns, D., Baley, J., & Kliegman, R. (1994). Increased incidence of intraventricular hemorrhage and developmental delay in cocaine-exposed, very low birth weight infants. *Journal of Pediatrics, 124,* 765–771.

SYSTAT. (1992). *SYSTAT for Windows* (Version 5). Evanston, IL: Author.

Woods, N. S., Eyler, F. D., Behnke, M., & Conlon, M. (1993). Cocaine use during pregnancy: Maternal depressive symptoms and infant neurobehavior over the first month. *Infant Behavior and Development, 16,* 83–98.

7

▼▼▼▼▼▼▼

Strategies for Detecting the Effects of Prenatal Drug Exposure: Lessons from Research on Alcohol

Joseph L. Jacobson
Sandra W. Jacobson
Wayne State University

An urban crack cocaine epidemic during the late 1980s coupled with reports of learning disabilities and behavioral disturbances in the offspring of cocaine-using mothers ("crack kids") have led to numerous prospective, longitudinal investigations of the effects of in utero cocaine exposure (e.g., Chasnoff, Griffith, Freier, & Murray, 1992; Coles, Platzman, Smith, James, & Falek, 1992; Hurt, Malmud, Brodsky, & Giannetta, 1992; Mayes, Granger, Frank, Schottenfeld, & Bornstein, 1993; Richardson & Day, 1991; Singer, Arendt, & Yamashita, 1992; Zuckerman et al., 1989). These are complex studies with unique methodological problems, including ascertainment of exposure from multiple biological measures, yet they share many of the research design problems encountered in studies of prenatal exposure to alcohol and other drugs that have been ongoing for almost 20 years (e.g., Coles et al., 1991; Fried & Watkinson, 1988; Hans, Henson, & Jeremy, 1992; Streissguth, Bookstein, Sampson, & Barr, 1989). The alcohol and drug studies, together with others on effects of exposure to environmental contaminants (e.g., J. L. Jacobson, S. W. Jacobson, & Humphrey, 1990; Needleman et al., 1979) have spawned a new subdiscipline known as *human behavioral teratology*, the study of effects of intrauterine toxic exposure on cognitive and behavioral development. This chapter reviews several methodological issues the earlier studies have dealt with that may warrant consideration in contemporary research on cocaine.

The alcohol studies were initiated in response to the discovery of fetal alcohol syndrome (FAS) in the offspring of alcohol-abusing mothers. FAS is characterized by intrauterine growth retardation, central nervous system impairment,

111

and distinctive craniofacial dysmorphology (Jones & Smith, 1973). The distinctive physiognomy and severity of functional impairment made FAS relatively easy to identify, but documenting the developmental effects of lower level intrauterine alcohol exposure has proven considerably more difficult. Because the effects can be relatively subtle, their detection depends to a considerable degree on the validity of the procedures used for assessing exposure, the sensitivity of the developmental outcomes evaluated, and the appropriateness of methodologies for controlling for confounding influences.

The principal methodological challenge in any prospective, longitudinal study is reducing the risk of spurious correlation. Because random assignment is not possible in human studies, it is critically important to assess a broad range of potential confounding influences and to control for them statistically as outlined later. Studies of prenatal exposure differ from many other developmental studies in that, in addition to the risk of spuriously attributing an observed effect to prenatal exposure (Type I error), failure to detect a real effect (Type II error) is also of particular concern. Despite our caveats that no inference should be made from a null finding, the need by policymakers and the general public to evaluate the risks associated with a potentially toxic exposure will inevitably lead negative findings to be interpreted to mean that the exposure is "safe." Thus, a failure to detect real risks associated with an exposure may prevent necessary public health precautions and warnings from being implemented. Type I error is, of course, also of concern in these studies. One risk associated with erroneously inferring a teratogenic effect is that exposed children may be pejoratively labeled and stigmatized by lowered expectations by teachers and parents (Mayes, Granger, Bornstein, & Zuckerman, 1992).

ASSESSMENT OF EXPOSURE
AND SAMPLE SELECTION

In contrast to cocaine, opiates, marijuana, and other illicit drugs, which can be measured in urine, meconium, and hair, alcohol is rapidly metabolized and therefore must be assessed on the basis of maternal report. In the first prospective study of this exposure, Streissguth and associates interviewed each mother once during the fifth month of gestation about her consumption of beer, wine, and liquor both during pregnancy and prior to pregnancy recognition (Streissguth, D. C. Martin, J. C. Martin, & Barr, 1981). In two subsequent studies (Day et al., 1989; Fried & Watkinson, 1988), mothers were interviewed three times— during the fourth and seventh prenatal months and within 24 hrs of delivery—to provide alcohol consumption reports for each trimester. Coles, Smith, Lancaster, and Falek (1987) administered two interviews, one at the onset of prenatal care, the second postpartum. One of the most elaborate interview procedures was developed by Sokol, Martier, and Ernhart (1983) in Cleveland and also used in our recent study of 480 African-American, inner-city Detroit infants (J. L. Jacobson et al., 1993). This procedure involves interviewing the mother at every prenatal clinic visit and asking her to recall each episode of drinking during the previous 2 weeks. An effort is made to aid the mother's recall by encouraging her to remember specifically whom she spent time with and what activities she engaged in during this period.

In most of these studies, exposure has been quantified in terms of average ounces of absolute alcohol per day (AA/day). Absolute alcohol is computed by multiplying the volume of each type of alcoholic beverage consumed (beer, wine, etc.) by its proportionate alcohol content (Bowman, Stein, & Newton, 1975). Although detailed measures of pattern of alcohol consumption, such as "bingeing" (e.g., more than five drinks per occasion) or chronicity (e.g., drinking days per month) are often collected, they are not usually included in published reports,[1] because the summary AA/day measure is usually more reliable and allows for comparison between studies. Many women drink at low levels during gestation, but few developmental effects have been found in relation to pregnancy drinking at levels of less than 0.5 oz AA/day, the equivalent of one drink per day (J. L. Jacobson & S. W. Jacobson, 1994). Given these data, a dichotomous yes/no measure will not adequately assess the risks associated with pregnancy drinking. Because most women who drink consume less than 0.5 oz/day, grouping the large number of light drinkers together with the relatively small number whose drinking would put their infants at serious risk is likely to make it difficult to detect the true effects of the alcohol exposure.

DETECTING TERATOGENIC EFFECTS IN INFANCY

Virtually all prospective studies of the effects of prenatal alcohol exposure have used the Bayley (1969) Scales of Infant Development to assess neurobehavioral development in infancy. The Bayley, which provides both a Mental Development Index (MDI) and a Psychomotor Development Index (PDI), focuses primarily on the rate at which the infant attains age-appropriate developmental skills. The Bayley has proven sensitive to a broad range of prenatal exposures, including alcohol (O'Connor, Brill, & Sigman, 1986; Streissguth, Barr, Martin, & Herman, 1980), lead (Bellinger et al., 1984; Dietrich et al., 1987), methadone (Hans et al., 1992), and polychlorinated biphenyls (PCBs; Gladen et al., 1988; Rogan & Gladen, 1991). Although predictive validity for school-age cognitive function is poor for children

---

[1]The principal exception is Streissguth and associates, who used a partial least squares approach (Sampson, Streissguth, Barr, & Bookstein, 1989) to analyze their data. This approach utilizes multiple correlated pregnancy drinking measures (e.g., number of drinking occasions per month, average number of drinks per drinking occasion, and maximum drinks on any occasion) to compute the weighted sum of exposure measures most strongly related to a weighted sum of outcome measures. In their analyses, binge drinking is frequently found to relate most strongly to outcome.

performing within the normal range (McCall, Hogarty, & Hurlburt, 1972), most neurotoxic exposures detected by the Bayley are also associated with poorer cognitive performance at school age. Thus, the Bayley may be sufficiently sensitive to detect group differences associated with neurotoxic exposure even if it is not sufficiently reliable to predict differences for individual children.

Although measurement of alcohol exposure has varied considerably from study to study, drinking during pregnancy has been linked repeatedly to poorer Bayley Scale performance. In Seattle, Streissguth et al. (1980) found a relationship between maternal drinking prior to pregnancy recognition and 8-month MDI and PDI. Golden, Sokol, Kuhnert, and Bottoms (1982) found poorer MDI and PDI performance in 12 infants identified at risk for fetal alcohol effects based on heavy pregnancy drinking and a neonatal examination for dysmorphic features. Smith, Coles, and Falek (1987) found poorer 12-month MDI performance in the offspring of 28 Atlanta heavy drinkers who continued to drink during pregnancy although not in the offspring of 13 heavy drinkers who abstained during the second and third trimesters. In Detroit, we found an association between moderate-to-heavy drinking during pregnancy and poorer 13-month MDI performance (J. L. Jacobson et al., 1993). By contrast, no effects were seen on the Bayley in Greene et al.'s (1991) Cleveland study or Richardson and Day's (1991) Pittsburgh study.

In the Detroit study, we performed a contingency table analysis in which the bottom 10th percentile of the distribution was used to indicate "poor performance" on the MDI. This analysis showed an increased incidence of poor performance above a threshold of 0.5 oz AA/day during pregnancy (Table 7.1). An examination of the Cleveland data revealed that the sample included only 7 infants whose mothers drank more than that threshold, compared with 45 in Detroit, suggesting that the Cleveland cohort contained too few infants exposed in the range in which the MDI effect is clearly seen. When we randomly deleted all but seven of the infants whose mothers drank more than the 0.5 oz threshold in Detroit, the zero-order correlation of alcohol with the MDI dropped from −.17 to −.05, making it similar to the −.06 correlation reported in Cleveland.

TABLE 7.1
Infants Scoring in the Bottom 10th Percentile on the Bayley MDI
by Pregnancy Drinking Level ($N = 375$)

Descriptor	oz AA/Day	N	(%)
Abstainer	.00	4	(6.7)
Very light	.01–.24	22	(9.4)
Light	.25–.49	2	(5.4)
Moderate	.50–.99	6	(23.1)
Heavy	1.00–1.99	2	(15.4)
Very heavy	2.00+	1	(16.7)
Total sample		37	(9.9)

Note. The bottom 10th percentile used was after adjustment for potential confounders.

These data underscore the importance of overrepresenting more highly exposed individuals in teratological studies to reduce the risk of failing to detect real effects. Although all the major alcohol studies have used oversampling, sample selection in Cleveland was based on the Michigan Alcoholism Screening Test (MAST; Seltzer, 1971), which assesses alcohol-related social problems, rather than on self-report of drinking during the index pregnancy. The Cleveland sample did not adequately overrepresent moderate-to-heavy drinkers because many women with a history of alcohol abuse who score positive on the MAST abstain during pregnancy. In Detroit, for example, 22.9% of the women who scored positive reported very little drinking (< 0.1 oz AA/day) during pregnancy, and only 32.4% of the women who reported drinking heavily (≥ 1.0 oz AA/day) were MAST positive. In the Pittsburgh study, which had pregnancy drinking levels similar to those in Cleveland and also failed to detect effects on the Bayley, moderate-to-heavy drinkers may not have been adequately represented due to the decision to oversample from too broad a range of moderate drinkers (≥ 3 drinks/week, the equivalent of 0.2 oz AA/day).

The Bayley is an apical test; successful performance on a single item usually depends on the integrity of multiple elements of cognitive and fine motor function, as well as attention to the task and motivation to perform. The principal advantage of apical tests is sensitivity. Because the infant's performance on a given item can be affected by deficits in any of several domains, the Bayley is sensitive to a broad range of impairments. The principal weakness of an apical test is lack of specificity; no information is provided about which aspects of cognitive function have been compromised. Given the Bayley's sensitivity, it is probably advisable to include it in any assessment of the effects of a previously unstudied exposure. Selection of additional, more specific tests should be based on what is known or suspected about the nature of the deficits associated with the exposure in question.

The most consistent finding regarding the effects of prenatal alcohol exposure in older children relates to attention. Deficits in sustained attention have been documented in both retrospective (Aronson, Kyllerman, Sabel, Sandin, & Olegard, 1985; Shaywitz, Cohen, & Shaywitz, 1980) and prospective (Brown et al., 1991; Streissguth, Barr et al., 1986; Streissguth, Martin et al., 1984) studies. Streissguth, Barr, and Sampson (1990) also suggested there may be an alcohol-related deficit in speed of information processing. Although no tests of sustained attention have been developed for use during infancy, two measures of processing speed have recently become available for infants—fixation duration (Colombo & Mitchell, 1990) and reaction time (RT; Haith, Hazan, & Goodman, 1988). The use of mean duration of visual fixation to index infant processing speed is supported by evidence that shorter fixations are associated with more rapid encoding of visual information in infancy (Colombo, Mitchell, Coldren, & Freeseman, 1991) and predict higher childhood IQ scores (Sigman, Cohen, Beckwith, Asarnow, & Parmelee, 1991; Sigman, Cohen, Beckwith, & Parmelee, 1985).

Fixation duration and infant RT measures were both used in the Detroit alcohol study, which was the first to document a direct relationship between them, indicating that they reflect a common domain of function (S. W. Jacobson et al., 1992).

Fixation duration data can be obtained on any paired comparison test, such as Fagan and Singer's (1983) Visual Recognition Memory Test or the Cross-modal Transfer Test (Gottfried, Rose, & Bridger, 1977). In addition to scoring preference for the novel stimulus to assess recognition memory or cross-modal transfer of information, mean fixation duration can easily be tabulated by dividing total duration looking time by number of looks. Haith et al. (1988) assessed reaction time in their new paradigm for assessing infant visual expectation in the context of processing dynamic visual information. The infant, seated on the mother's lap, views a videotape of moving geometric designs and schematic faces. After a baseline of randomly placed presentations, 60 stimuli appear in a predictable left–right alternation. The infant's eye movements are recorded on videotape, which is coded to determine speed of response, defined as latency between the onset of the stimulus and the time the infant's eye begins to move toward it.

One of the principal findings from the Detroit alcohol study is that maternal drinking during pregnancy is associated with slower, less efficient cognitive processing in infancy, as indicated by both longer fixation duration (S. W. Jacobson, J. L. Jacobson, Sokol, Martier, & Ager, 1993), and slower RT (S. W. Jacobson, J. L. Jacobson, & Sokol, 1994). By contrast to PCBs and methylmercury, prenatal exposure to which has been linked to lower novelty preference (i.e., poorer recognition memory) on the Fagan test (Gunderson, Grant, Burbacher, Fagan, & Mottet, 1986; S. W. Jacobson, Fein, J. L. Jacobson, Schwartz, & Dowler, 1985), there was no effect of prenatal alcohol on either of the novelty preference measures. The effect of alcohol on processing speed was seen in three separate domains—recognition memory, cross-modal transfer, and visual expectation—and at two different ages—6.5 and 12 months. These data, therefore, suggest a specific effect of in utero alcohol exposure on speed or efficiency of information processing, which is consistent with data on newborns and older children reported by Streissguth et al. (1990). Given that fixation duration appears to be predictive of cognitive function in childhood, this processing speed deficit could play an important role in the learning problems seen in older children exposed prenatally to alcohol (Coles et al., 1991; Shaywitz et al., 1980; Streissguth et al., 1990).

Where the specific effects of a prenatal exposure are not known in advance or deficits are suspected in multiple domains, the investigator may want to assess a large number of developmental outcomes. Given the high cost of recruiting and maintaining a prenatally exposed cohort and of assessing the necessary potential confounders, it makes sense to obtain as comprehensive a picture as possible of the nature of the impairment. However, a comprehensive test battery with a large number of outcome measures raises the concern that, where many outcomes are assessed simultaneously, a certain proportion will be significant by chance. One traditional approach for dealing with multiple comparisons is the Bonferroni correction. Instead of using $p < .05$ as the criterion to reject the null hypothesis, .05 is divided by the number of outcomes assessed, so that if 20 outcomes are tested, a $p < .0025$ criterion would be used, making chance findings much less likely. The principal problem with the Bonferroni correction is an increased risk of Type II error. Reliable effects can easily be missed if all those between $p < .0025$ and .05 are considered nonsignificant. A better solution is to assess a broad range of outcomes in terms of the usual $p < .05$ criterion, recognizing that the use of multiple measures will increase the risk of Type I error in the short run. Any unpredicted finding from a single study can and should be treated as tentative until replicated.

CONTROLLING FOR CONFOUNDING INFLUENCES

One of the most difficult issues in human behavioral toxicology is controlling for confounding influences. Although some investigators assess only a few potential confounders, most try to measure as many factors as possible known or suspected of impacting the outcomes of interest. Table 7.2 lists the principal

TABLE 7.2
Control Variables Tested Routinely in the Detroit Prenatal Alcohol Exposure
and Infant Cognition Study

Demographic background
   Maternal age[a]
   Marital status[a]
   Welfare recipient[a]
   Parity
   Child's sex
Prenatal
   Number of clinic visits
Socioenvironmental
   Maternal education (years)[a]
   Maternal vocabulary[a]−Peabody Picture Vocabulary Test−Revised (Dunn & Dunn, 1981)
   HOME Inventory (Caldwell & Bradley, 1979)
   Maternal depression[a]−Beck Depression Inventory (Beck, Ward, Mendelson, Mock, &
     Erbaugh, 1961)
   Maternal ego development[a] (Loevinger & Wessler, 1970)
Maternal drug use during pregnancy
   Smoking (cigarettes/day)
   Cocaine (days/month)
   Opiates (days/month)
   Marijuana (days/month)
Situational
   Child's age at testing
   Examiner

---

[a]Mother or primary caregiver.

control variables assessed in the Detroit infant alcohol study. The number of prenatal clinic visits was used as an indicator of quality of prenatal care. Maternal vocabulary was assessed on the Peabody Picture Vocabulary Test–Revised (PPVT–R; Dunn & Dunn, 1981) to control for parental intelligence, which influences infant cognitive performance both through genetic endowment and quality of intellectual stimulation. The PPVT–R is strongly correlated with standardized tests of adult IQ and, although minority subjects often score low, the test has been validated for use with lower class African-American mothers in relation to several relevant demographic and personality variables (S. W. Jacobson, J. L. Jacobson, & Frye, 1991).

Quality of parenting was assessed on the HOME Inventory (Caldwell & Bradley, 1979), which combines a semistructured parental interview with informal observation of parent–child interaction to evaluate quality of intellectual stimulation and emotional responsiveness provided by the parent.[2] Although designed to be administered in the home, considerations of personal safety in poor neighborhoods may preclude home visits by project staff members. The validity of administering the HOME in the laboratory has been demonstrated at 24 months by Barnard, Bee, and Hammond (1984) and at 12 months by our finding that the correlations of a laboratory-administered HOME with the 13-month Bayley were midway between those reported by investigators who performed the assessment at home (Barnard et al., 1984; Siegel, 1984).

It is important that control variables be measured as accurately as possible. In a multivariate analysis, unreliable measurement will lead to an underestimate of the effect of the control variable, which may, in turn, artificially inflate the variance attributed to the substance in question. In the Detroit alcohol study, mothers were asked to report illicit drug use at each prenatal clinic visit in terms of the number of days per month they used each of the following: cocaine, opiates (heroin, methadone, or codeine), marijuana, depressants, and other stimulants.[3] Although detailed drug dose information would have been of interest, dosage data were not collected because they were considered unreliable due to the wide variability in the degree of purity of illicit street drugs.

Given the high rate of denial associated with illicit drug use, it is critical to confirm maternal self-report by urine screen, meconium, or hair testing, whenever possible. Zuckerman et al. (1989) found that birth size was not related to prenatal

---

[2]Caldwell and Bradley (1979) recommended that the information required for the HOME Inventory protocol be elicited informally and spontaneously from the mother. S. W. Jacobson (1987) prepared scripts for the infant, preschool, and elementary school versions of the HOME, based on the probes suggested by Caldwell and Bradley, which reorganize and standardize the presentation of the interview material to facilitate this approach.

[3]Because use of depressants and other stimulants was rare, these variables were not controlled routinely in the multivariate analyses. Instead, their influence was assessed by rerunning all analyses yielding significant alcohol effects, omitting the infants whose mothers reported using these substances at least once per week during pregnancy.

cocaine exposure assessed by maternal self-report alone, but was related to cocaine when assessed on the basis of both self-report and urine assay data. In the Detroit study, urine screens obtained routinely at the first prenatal clinic visit were positive for 6.0% of the women who denied using cocaine, 0.8% of those who denied using opiates, and 12.0% who denied using marijuana. Instead of omitting these subjects from the analysis, the values for the women who had tested positive but denied any use were estimated by assigning them the median values reported by those who tested positive but did not deny use of these drugs. As with alcohol, it is preferable to construct a continuous measure of prenatal drug exposure to facilitate detection of effects that may be evident only at relatively high exposure levels.

Multivariate analysis is used to determine the degree to which effects of exposure are seen after statistically removing the influence of potential confounders. Although some researchers (e.g., Ernhart, in press) have advocated including all control variables in every statistical analysis, that approach has at least two disadvantages. Coefficients estimating the magnitude of effects tend to be unstable unless there are at least 20 subjects for each variable (Tabachnick & Fidell, 1983). In addition, the inclusion of variables unrelated to outcome in a multivariate analysis may increase the size of the error term and consequently the size of the p values. Inflation of the p level for exposure due to the inclusion of extraneous control variables can increase the risk of failure to detect a reliable effect.

Because a control variable cannot be the true cause of an observed effect unless it is related to both exposure and outcome (Schlesselman, 1982), control variables can be selected for inclusion in the statistical analysis based on their relation to either exposure or outcome. In the Detroit alcohol study, control variables were selected on the basis of their relation to outcome. Selection in relation to outcome has the advantage that where a control variable unrelated to exposure increases the amount of variance explained in the outcome, its inclusion reduces the error term, thereby improving the chances of detecting real effects (Kleinbaum, Kupper, & Muller, 1988). In other words, the removal of variance in the outcome unrelated to alcohol can make it easier to detect the real effects of the alcohol exposure. In the alcohol study, we controlled statistically for all control variables related even weakly to the outcome in question (at $p < .10$). Where exposure is assessed by a continuous measure (e.g., oz AA/day), multiple regression is usually the analysis of choice. Analysis of covariance (ANCOVA) is appropriate for dichotomous or grouped exposure measures.

Although relevant potential confounders should be included in all statistical analyses, it is not always appropriate to include mediating or intervening variables. A mediator is a variable that is influenced by exposure and, in turn, influences a subsequent developmental outcome. For example, prenatal cocaine exposure is associated with reduced birth size, which could lead to poorer neurobehavioral outcome. If so, reduced birth size might be the mechanism through which cocaine affects infant behavior. Confusion can arise because confounders and mediators are tested statistically in the same manner. If birth size is added to a regression of neurobehavioral outcome on cocaine, an observed effect of cocaine on that outcome may no longer be significant. If birth size were a confounder, the correct inference would be that the observed cocaine effect is a spurious consequence of the correlation of cocaine with birth size. But, if reduced birth size is a result of the cocaine exposure and causally related to the outcome, the reduction in the cocaine effect suggests that birth size mediates the effect. Potential confounders should be included routinely in all analyses because effects of exposure are of interest only after alternative explanatory variables have been statistically controlled. Because inclusion of a mediating variable causally linking exposure with outcome can make the effect of the exposure appear nonsignificant, mediators should not be entered routinely. Their effects can be understood only if analyses excluding them are compared with analyses that include them.

DOSE–RESPONSE RELATIONSHIPS
AND THRESHOLDS

Although teratogenic effects are often evaluated in linear regression models, there is considerable interest in the degree to which observed effects are dose dependent. Dose–response relationships have typically been investigated in human behavioral teratology studies by grouping subjects by exposure level and looking for progressive decrements in mean group performance as level of exposure increases (e.g., Greene et al., 1991; J. L. Jacobson, S. W. Jacobson, & Humphrey, 1990; Streissguth et al., 1980; see Fig. 7.1). From a toxicological perspective, effects should always be more severe among the more highly exposed. Therefore, even where the regression coefficient is significant, a finding that moderately exposed infants performed markedly poorer than highly exposed infants would raise serious questions regarding the validity of inferring a toxic effect.[4]

In addition to checking for dose dependence, dose–reponse analysis can provide information regarding threshold; that is, the level of exposure required before a reliable effect is seen. Given the body's ability to tolerate low doses of many toxic substances, most effects are seen only when exposure exceeds a minimum threshold dose. Severe effects, such as fetal death, mental retardation, and the craniofacial dysmorphology associated with FAS, have relatively high thresholds, and they occur only in the most heavily exposed infants. Figure 7.1 illustrates two patterns of dose–response relationships. For some behaviors, even

---

[4]This general principle might not hold, however, in a case where infants most highly exposed to cocaine are removed from their biological mothers and raised by another relative or in foster care. In that case, the moderately exposed infants reared by cocaine-using mothers might perform poorer than more highly exposed infants raised in more optimal environments.

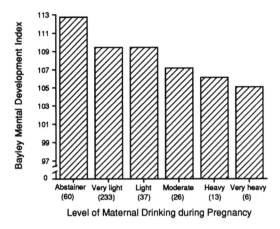

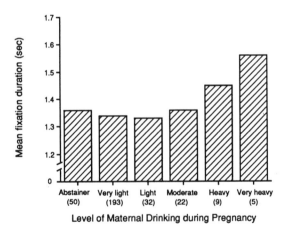

FIG. 7.1. Dose–response relationships between maternal drinking during pregnancy and two infant developmental outcomes. All group means are adjusted for potential confounding influences following the methodology described in J. L. Jacobson et al. (1993).

the smallest dose appears to have some adverse effect, and the severity of the effect increases gradually with increasing levels of exposure (Fig. 7.1a). This pattern can be termed *linear with no apparent threshold.* Most neurobehavioral effects seem to have relatively high thresholds, however, with dose–response patterns typically resembling those in Fig. 7.1b (S. W. Jacobson et al., 1992). No adverse effect is seen at less than 1 oz AA/day during pregnancy, and the effect becomes more severe with increased exposure over that level.

Thresholds can be determined more precisely in laboratory animal experiments than with human subjects. In animal studies, experiments are performed to determine a median lethal dose (LD50), and it is assumed that individual differences in sensitivity to the exposure are normally distributed around that value (Klaassen, 1986). If a large number of doses is used with a large number of animals per dose, a normally distributed sigmoid curve (represented by the embryolethality curve in Fig. 7.2) is observed. This curve reflects individual differences in vulnerability to a substance, because some individuals survive at higher doses than others. Threshold is defined as the lowest dose at which an adverse effect is seen; that is, the dose at which the most vulnerable individuals are affected. As illustrated in Fig. 7.2, certain domains are expected to have lower thresholds than others (see Vorhees, 1986).

By contrast to the sigmoid curves generated in animal studies, the thresholds derived for human studies (Fig. 7.1) represent sample averages and are relatively insensitive to individual differences in vulnerability. Children diagnosed with FAS vary markedly in severity of symptoms (Streissguth, Herman, & Smith, 1978), and not all offspring of women who drink heavily during pregnancy manifest full FAS (Coles et al., 1987; Sokol et al., 1986). This differential susceptibility may be due to genetic variation, the occurrence of exposure during a narrow critical period, synergistic interactions with drug abuse or other risk factors, or protective effects from certain as yet unidentified maternal characteristics. Because the threshold values derived from human studies are based on group averages, it is not appropriate to infer that exposure just below a threshold level is necessarily "safe"; some individuals could be markedly more vulnerable than others.

In evaluating risk associated with exposure to environmental and food contaminants, a margin of safety is usually incorporated to allow for individual differences in sensitivity. Where human data are available, a factor of 10 is used for this purpose (Sette & Levine, 1986). Taking this approach, one might divide a threshold value of 0.5 oz AA/day by 10 and conclude that 0.05 oz/day (one drink every 10 days) during pregnancy is likely to be "safe." On the other hand, even if no functional deficits are associated with a given level of exposure in

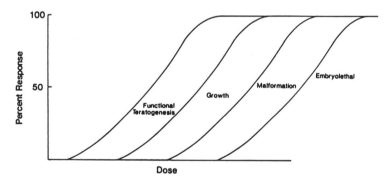

FIG. 7.2. Idealized dose–response curves for four domains of teratogenesis. Neurobehavioral outcomes are included under "functional teratogenesis" in this model. From Vorhees (1986).

infancy and childhood, there can be subclinical neurostructural damage, which could lead to functional deficits when the child is stressed or challenged by a complex task (Riley, 1990) or when the individual reaches old age. For this reason, although there is little evidence of impairment at low levels of prenatal alcohol exposure (J. L. Jacobson & S. W. Jacobson, 1994), many investigators are reluctant to condone even low-level drinking during pregnancy.

CONCLUSION

When compared with research on other teratogens, such as alcohol or heroin, current cocaine studies present unique problems. Combining biological measures of exposure with self-report greatly enhances the determination of whether cocaine was used during pregnancy (Zuckerman et al., 1989), although it does not as yet provide information regarding degree of exposure. If, as with alcohol, the behavioral effects of cocaine occur only in more highly exposed individuals, studies based on dichotomous yes/no exposure measures are likely to yield inconsistent results depending on the exposure level of those studied. When compared with other teratogens studied to date, cocaine appears to have less effect on Bayley Scale performance (e.g., Chasnoff et al., 1992), leading some investigators to hypothesize that deficits will be seen most readily on measures relating to regulation of arousal and affect (e.g., Alessandri, Sullivan, Imaizumi, & Lewis, 1993; Rodning, Beckwith, & Howard, 1991). Given the relative paucity of reliable measures of affective function in infants and children, investigators may need to develop innovative approaches, such as Alessandri et al.'s (1993) use of facial expression to evaluate affective response in the context of a learning paradigm.

Contemporary cocaine research also faces many of the same challenges as the earlier teratological studies, including the need to oversample higher exposed individuals to reduce the risk of failing to detect effects seen only in the offspring of heavier users. As in earlier studies, it is important to use control variables that provide reliable and valid measurement of important potential confounders to limit the risk of erroneously attributing deficits to cocaine exposure. Potential mediating variables, such as birth weight and gestational age, should not be controlled routinely, however, to avoid obscuring true cocaine effects. Because investigators are only beginning to identify the specific domains affected by cocaine exposure, study designs need to incorporate a broad range of developmental outcomes, protecting against Type I error through replication rather than overly conservative Bonferroni corrections. Given that apical cognitive tests, such as the Bayley Scales, may be insensitive to the effects of cocaine, increased attention needs to be devoted to developing more narrow-band tests to assess the specific domains affected by cocaine exposure.

The current interest in prospective, longitudinal studies of the effects of cocaine exposure provides a unique opportunity for developmental psychology and allied fields to evaluate the latest theoretical models regarding the nature of development, including the transactional model (Sameroff & Chandler, 1975) and the role of the environment in protecting against the deleterious consequences of biological risk (e.g, Hans et al., 1992; Rutter, 1987).

REFERENCES

Alessandri, S. M., Sullivan, M. W., Imaizumi, S., & Lewis, M. (1993). Learning and emotional responsivity in cocaine-exposed infants. *Developmental Psychology, 29*, 989–997.

Aronson, M., Kyllerman, M., Sabel, K.-G., Sandin, B., & Olegard, R. (1985). Children of alcoholic mothers: Developmental, perceptual and behavioural characteristics as compared to matched controls. *Acta Paediatrica Scandinavica, 74*, 27–35.

Barnard, K. E., Bee, H. L., & Hammond, M. A. (1984). Home environment and cognitive development in a healthy, low-risk sample: The Seattle study. In A. W. Gottfried (Ed.), *Home environment and early cognitive development: Longitudinal research* (pp. 117–149). New York: Academic Press.

Bayley, N. (1969). *Bayley Scales of Infant Development.* New York: Psychological Corporation.

Beck, A. T., Ward, C. H., Mendelson, M., Mock, F., & Erbaugh, J. (1961). An inventory for measuring depression. *Archives of General Psychiatry, 4*, 561–571.

Bellinger, D. C., Needleman, H. L., Leviton, A., Waternaux, C., Rabinowitz, M. B., & Nichols, M. L. (1984). Early sensory-motor development and prenatal exposure to lead. *Neurobehavioral Toxicology and Teratology, 6*, 387–402.

Bowman, R. S., Stein, L. I., & Newton, J. R. (1975). Measurement and interpretation of drinking behavior. *Quarterly Journal of Studies on Alcohol, 36*, 1154–1172.

Brown, R. T., Coles, C. D., Smith, I. E., Platzman, K. A., Silverstein, J., Erickson, S., & Falek, A. (1991). Effects of prenatal alcohol exposure at school age. II. Attention and behavior. *Neurotoxicology and Teratology, 13*, 369–376.

Caldwell, B. M., & Bradley, R. H. (1979). *Home observation for measurement of the environment.* Little Rock: University of Arkansas Press.

Chasnoff, I. J., Griffith, D. R., Freier, C., & Murray, J. (1992). Cocaine/polydrug use in pregnancy. *Pediatrics, 89*, 284–289.

Coles, C. D., Brown, R. T., Smith, I. E., Platzman, K. A., Erickson, S., & Falek, A. (1991) Effects of prenatal alcohol exposure at school age. I. Physical and cognitive development. *Neurotoxicology and Teratology, 13*, 357–367.

Coles, C. D., Platzman, K. A., Smith, I., James, M. E., & Falek, A. (1992). Effects of cocaine and alcohol use in pregnancy on neonatal growth and neurobehavioral status. *Neurotoxicology and Teratology, 14*, 22–33.

Coles, C. D., Smith, I. E., Lancaster, J. S., & Falek, A. (1987). Persistence over the first month of neurobehavioral differences in infants exposed to alcohol prenatally. *Infant Behavior and Development, 10*, 23–37.

Colombo, J., & Mitchell, D. W. (1990). Individual differences in early visual attention: Fixation time and information processing. In J. Colombo & J. Fagen (Eds.), *Individual differences in infancy: Reliability, stability, prediction* (pp. 193–227). Hillsdale, NJ: Lawrence Erlbaum Associates.

Colombo, J., Mitchell, D. W., Coldren, J. R., & Freeseman, L. J. (1991). Individual differences in infant visual attention: Are short lookers faster processors or feature processors? *Child Development, 62*, 1247–1257.

Day, N., Jasperse, D., Richardson, G., Robles, N., Sambamoorthi, U., Taylor, P., Scher, M., Stoffer, D., & Cornelius, M. (1989). Prenatal exposure to alcohol: Effect on infant growth and morphologic characteristics. *Pediatrics, 84*, 536–541.

Dietrich, K. N., Krafft, K. M., Bornschein, R. L., Hammond, P. B., Berger, O., Succop, P. A., & Bier, M. (1987). Low-level fetal lead exposure effect on neurobehavioral development in in early infancy. *Pediatrics, 80,* 721–730.

Dunn, L. M., & Dunn, L. M. (1981). *PPVT manual for Forms L and M.* Circle Pines, MN: American Guidance Service.

Ernhart, C. B. (in press). Cofactors in observational research: Issues and examples from the lead effects literature. In G. R. Melton, S. R. Schroeder, & T. B. Sonderegger (Eds.), *Behavioral toxicology of childhood.* Lincoln: University of Nebraska Press.

Fagan, J. F., & Singer, L. T. (1983). Infant recognition memory as a measure of intelligence. In L. P. Lipsitt (Ed.), *Advances in infancy research* (Vol. 2, pp. 31–72). Norwood, NJ: Ablex.

Fried, P. A., & Watkinson, A. (1988). 12- and 24-month neurobehavioural follow-up of chldren prenatally exposed to marihuana, cigarettes and alcohol. *Neurotoxicology and Teratology, 10,* 305–313.

Gladen, B. C., Rogan, W. J., Hardy, P., Thullen, J., Tingelstad, J., & Tully, M. (1988). Development after exposure to polychlorinated biphenyls and dichlorodiphenyl dichloroethene transplacentally and through human milk. *Journal of Pediatrics, 113,* 991–995.

Golden, N. L., Sokol, R. J., Kuhnert, B. R., & Bottoms, S. (1982). Maternal alcohol use and infant development. *Pediatrics, 70,* 931–934.

Gottfried, A. W., Rose, S. A., & Bridger, W. H. (1977). Cross-modal transfer in human infants. *Child Development, 48,* 118–123.

Greene, T., Ernhart, C. B., Ager, J., Sokol, R., Martier, S., & Boyd, T. (1991). Prenatal alcohol exposure and cognitive development in the preschool years. *Neurotoxicology and Teratology, 13,* 57–68.

Gunderson, V. M., Grant, K. S., Burbacher, T. M., Fagan, J. F., III, & Mottet, N. K. (1986). The effect of low-level prenatal methylmercury exposure on visual recognition memory in infant crab-eating macaques. *Child Development, 57,* 1076–1083.

Haith, M. M., Hazan, C., & Goodman, G. S. (1988). Expectation and anticipation of dynamic visual events by 3.5-month-old babies. *Child Development, 59,* 467–479.

Hans, S. L., Henson, L. G., & Jeremy, R. J. (1992). The development of infants exposed in utero to opioid drugs. In C. W. Greenbaum & J. G. Auerbach (Eds.), *Longitudinal studies of children at psychological risk: Cross-national perspectives* (pp. 155–173). Norwood, NJ: Ablex.

Hurt, H., Malmud, E., Brodsky, N., & Giannetta, J. (1992). Prenatal exposure to cocaine has no effect on infant performance on Bayley Scales. *Pediatric Research, 31,* 251A.

Jacobson, J. L., & Jacobson, S. W. (1994). Prenatal alcohol exposure and neurobehavioral development: Where is the threshold? *Alcohol Health and Research World, 18,* 30–36.

Jacobson, J. L., Jacobson, S. W., & Humphrey, H. E. B. (1990). Effects of in utero exposure to polychlorinated biphenyls and related contaminants on cognitive functioning in young children. *The Journal of Pediatrics, 116,* 38–45.

Jacobson, J. L., Jacobson, S. W., Sokol, R. J., Martier, S. S., Ager, J. W., & Kaplan-Estrin, M. G. (1993). Teratogenic effects of alcohol on infant development. *Alcoholism: Clinical and Experimental Research, 17,* 174–183.

Jacobson, S. W. (1987). *Protocols for administering the Home Observation for Measurement of the Environment.* Unpublished manuscript, Wayne State University, Detroit, MI.

Jacobson, S. W., Fein, G. G., Jacobson, J. L., Schwartz, P. M., & Dowler, J. K. (1985). The effect of intrauterine PCB exposure on visual recognition memory. *Child Development, 56,* 853–860.

Jacobson, S. W., Jacobson, J. L., & Frye, K. F. (1991). Incidence and correlates of breast-feeding in disadvantaged women. *Pediatrics, 88,* 728–736.

Jacobson, S. W., Jacobson, J. L., O'Neill, J. M., Padgett, R. J., Frankowski, J. J., & Bihun, J. T. (1992). Visual expectation and dimensions of infant information processing. *Child Development, 63,* 711–724.

Jacobson, S. W., Jacobson, J. L., & Sokol, R. J. (1994). Effects of prenatal alcohol exposure on infant reaction time. *Alcoholism: Clinical and Experimental Research, 18,* 1125–1132.

Jacobson, S. W., Jacobson, J. L., Sokol, R. J., Martier, S., & Ager, J. (1993). Prenatal alcohol exposure and infant information processing. *Child Development, 64*, 1706–1721.

Jones, K. L., & Smith, D. W. (1973). Recognition of the fetal alcohol syndrome in early infancy. *Lancet, 2*, 999–1001.

Klaassen, C. D. (1986). Principles of toxicology. In C. D. Klaassen, M. O. Amdur, & J. Doull (Eds.), *Casarett and Doull's toxicology* (3rd ed., pp. 11–32). New York: Macmillan.

Kleinbaum, D. G., Kupper, L. L., & Muller, K. E. (1988). *Applied regression analysis and other mutivariable methods* (2nd ed.). Boston: PWS-Kent.

Loevinger, J., & Wessler, R. (1970). *Measuring ego development* (Vol. 1). San Francisco: Jossey-Bass.

Mayes, L. C., Granger, R. H., Bornstein, M. H., & Zuckerman, B. (1992). The problem of prenatal cocaine exposure: The rush to judgment. *Journal of the American Medical Association, 267*, 406–408.

Mayes, L. C., Granger, R. H., Frank, M. A., Schottenfeld, R., & Bornstein, M. H. (1993). Neurobehavioral profiles of infants exposed to cocaine prenatally. *Journal of Pediatrics, 91*, 778–783.

McCall, R. B., Hogarty, P. S., & Hurlburt, N. (1972). Transitions in infant sensorimotor development and the prediction of childhood IQ. *American Psychologist, 27*, 728–748.

Needleman, H. L., Gunnoe, C., Leviton, A., Reed, R., Peresie, H., Maher, C., & Barrett, P. (1979). Deficits in psychologic and classroom performance of children with elevated dentine lead levels. *New England Journal of Medicine, 300*, 689–695.

O'Connor, M. J., Brill, N. J., & Sigman, M. (1986). Alcohol use in primiparous women older than 30 years of age: Relation to infant development. *Pediatrics, 78*, 444–450.

Richardson, G. A., & Day, N. L. (1991). Maternal and neonatal effects of moderate cocaine use during pregnancy. *Neurotoxicology and Teratology, 13*, 455–460.

Riley, E. P. (1990). The long-term behavioral effects of prenatal alcohol exposure in rats. *Alcoholism: Clinical and Experimental Research, 14*, 670–673.

Rodning, C., Beckwith, L., & Howard, J. (1991). Quality of attachment and home environments in children prenatally exposed to PCP and cocaine. *Development and Psychopathology, 3*, 351–366.

Rogan, W. J., & Gladen, B. C. (1991). PCBs, DDE, and child development at 18 and 24 months. *Annals of Epidemiology, 1*, 407–413.

Rutter, M. (1987). Psychological resilience and protective mechanisms. *American Journal of Orthopsychiatry, 57*, 316–331.

Sameroff, A. J., & Chandler, M. J. (1975). Reproductive risk and the continum of caretaking casualty. In F. D. Horowitz, M. Hetherington, S. Scarrf-Salapatek, & G. Sigel (Eds.), *Review of child development research* (Vol. 4, pp. 187–244). Chicago: University of Chicago Press.

Sampson, P. D., Streissguth, A. P., Barr, H. M., & Bookstein, F. L. (1989). Neurobehavioral effects of prenatal alcohol: Part II. Partial least squares analysis. *Neurotoxicology and Teratology, 11*, 477–491.

Schlesselman, J. (1982). *Case-control studies: Design, conduct, analysis*. New York: Oxford University Press.

Seltzer, M. L. (1971). The Michigan Alcoholism Screening Test: The quest for a new diagnostic instrument. *American Journal of Psychiatry, 127*, 1653–1658.

Sette, W. F., & Levine, T. E. (1986). Behavior as a regulatory endpoint. In Z. Annau (Ed.), *Neurobehavioral toxicology* (pp. 391–403). Baltimore: Johns Hopkins University Press.

Shaywitz, S. E., Cohen, D. J., & Shaywitz, B. A. (1980). Behavior and learning difficulties in children of normal intelligence born to alcoholic mothers. *Journal of Pediatrics, 96*, 978–982.

Siegel, L. S. (1984). Home environmental influences on cognitive development in preterm and full-term children during the first 5 years. In A. W. Gottfried (Ed.), *Home environment and early cognitive development: Longitudinal research* (pp. 197–233). Orlando, FL: Academic Press.

Sigman, M. D., Cohen, S. E., Beckwith, L., Asarnow, R., & Parmelee, A. H. (1991). Continuity in cognitive abilities from infancy to 12 years of age. *Cognitive Development, 6*, 47–57.

Sigman, M. D., Cohen, S. E., Beckwith, L., & Parmelee, A. H. (1985, July). *Infant attention in relation to intellectual abilities in childhood.* Paper presented at the International Society for the Study of Behavioural Development, Tours, France.

Singer, L., Arendt, R., & Yamashita, T. (1992). Development of infants exposed in utero to cocaine. *Pediatric Research, 31,* 260A.

Smith, I. E., Coles, C. D., & Falek, A. (1982). *A prospective study of the effects of alcohol in utero.* Paper presented at the annual meeting of the American Public Health Association, Montreal, Quebec.

Sokol, R. J., Ager, J., Martier, S., Debanne, S., Ernhart, C., Kuzma, J., & Miller, S. I. (1986). Significant determinants of susceptibility to alcohol teratogenicity. *Annals of the New York Academy of Sciences, 477,* 87–100.

Sokol, R. J., Martier, S., & Ernhart, C. (1983). Identification of alcohol abuse in the prenatal clinic. In N. C. Chang & H. M. Chao (Eds.), *Early identification of alcohol abuse* (Research Monograph No. 17, pp. 209–227). Rockville, MD: Alcohol, Drug Abuse, and Mental Health Administration.

Streissguth, A. P., Barr, H. M., Martin, D. C., & Herman, C. S. (1980). Effects of maternal alcohol, nicotine, and caffeine use during pregnancy on infant mental and motor development at 8 months. *Alcoholism: Clinical and Experimental Research, 4,* 152–164.

Streissguth, A. P., Barr, H. M., & Sampson, P. D. (1990). Moderate prenatal alcohol exposure: Effects on child IQ and learning problems at age 7½ years. *Alcoholism: Clinical and Experimental Research, 14,* 662–669.

Streissguth, A. P., Barr, H. M., Sampson, P. D., Parrish-Johnson, J. C., Kirchner, G. L., & Martin, D. C. (1986). Attention, distraction and reaction time at age 7 years and prenatal alcohol exposure. *Neurobehavioral Toxicology and Teratology, 8,* 717–725.

Streissguth, A. P., Bookstein, F. L., Sampson, P. D., & Barr, H. M. (1989). Neurobehavioral effects of prenatal alcohol: Part III. PLS analyses of neuropyschologic tests. *Neurotoxicology and Teratology, 11,* 493–507.

Streissguth, A. P., Herman, C. S., & Smith, D. W. (1978). Intelligence, behavior and dysmorphogenesis in the fetal alcohol syndrome: A report on 20 patients. *The Journal of Pediatrics, 92,* 363–367.

Streissguth, A. P., Martin, D. C., Barr, H. M., Sandman, B. M., Kirchner, G. L., & Darby, B. L. (1984). Intrauterine alcohol and nicotine exposure: Attention and reaction time in 4-year-old children. *Developmental Psychology, 20,* 533–541.

Streissguth, A. P., Martin, D. C., Martin, J. C., & Barr, H. M. (1981). The Seattle longitudinal prospective study on alcohol and pregnancy. *Neurobehavioral Toxicology and Teratology, 3,* 223–233.

Tabachnick, B. G., & Fidell, L. S. (1983). *Using multivariate statistics.* New York: Harper & Row.

Vorhees, C. V. (1986). Principles of behavioral teratology. In E. P. Riley & C. V. Vorhees (Eds.), *Handbook of behavioral teratology* (pp. 23–48). New York: Plenum.

Zuckerman, B., Frank, D. A., Hingson, R., Amaro, H., Levenson, S. M., Kayne, H., Parker, S., Vinci, R., Aboagye, K., Fried, L. E., Cabral, H., Timperi, R., & Bauchner, H. (1989). Effects of maternal marijuana and cocaine use on fetal growth. *New England Journal of Medicine, 320,* 762–768.

8

▼▼▼▼▼▼▼

A Cohort Study of Prenatal Cocaine Exposure: Addressing Methodological Concerns

Heather Carmichael Olson
Therese M. Grant
Joan C. Martin
Ann P. Streissguth
University of Washington School of Medicine

There are common themes in recent discussions of the impact of prenatal cocaine and other drug exposure on child development (Coles & Platzman, 1993; Hutchings, 1993a, 1993b; Lutiger, Graham, Einarson, & Koren, 1991; Myers, Britt, Lodder, Kendall, & Williams-Petersen, 1992; Neuspiel & Hamel, 1991; Richardson, Day, & McGaughey, 1993; Robins & Mills, 1993; Singer, Garber, & Kliegman, 1991; Zuckerman, 1991b). First, in examining whether prenatal exposure to cocaine impairs later function, research on human subjects continues to provide equivocal results, although it is clear that earlier concerns about widespread, serious developmental effects have not been confirmed. Second, there is a lack of human data, particularly studies on neurobehavioral outcome in cocaine-exposed infants and on the long-term consequences of prenatal cocaine exposure. Among the studies that do exist, there are methodologic problems, and recommendations have been made to address these methodologic concerns. Third, it is clear from this recent literature that it is a challenge to distinguish behavioral dysfunction caused by a specific drug, such as cocaine, or to separate drug effects from problems arising from other causes, using either animal models or human study. It is also clear that the developmental toxicity of cocaine is not yet established, and that the mechanism(s) underlying any impact of cocaine on fetal and postnatal development are not yet defined.

The most convincing argument for the developmental toxicity of cocaine requires a confluence of data from solid experimental animal studies, hypothesis-driven clinical investigation of human subjects, and careful prospective epidemiologic research. In epidemiologic studies, one criterion for making a causal argu-

129

ment about prenatal cocaine effects lies in investigating a dose–response relationship between cocaine exposure in utero and later outcome, while exerting the best possible experimental and statistical control of carefully chosen confounding factors. Yet it is a methodological challenge to design and carry out this kind of epidemiologic study and to analyze a possible dose–response relationship.

Four main areas of methodological concern can be identified in the epidemiologic study of prenatal cocaine exposure and child outcome (see reviews cited earlier; also see Volpe, 1992; Zuckerman, 1991b). First is the difficult task of ensuring that sample size and selection, choice and definition of comparison group, and other aspects of research design are not biased, and provide sufficient power and methodological control over confounding variables to discern the developmental toxicity of cocaine. A second concern lies in the problem of sample maintenance when following chemically dependent subjects, who may actively avoid research scrutiny, often have transient and unpredictable lifestyles, and among whom the highest risk subjects are least likely to cooperate. A third concern involves the complexities of measurement and analysis: measuring the timing and extent of prenatal cocaine use (both among the case and comparison groups); assessing (at the appropriate level of accuracy) important intervening pregnancy and postnatal factors; and analyzing transactions between prenatal drug exposure and other influences on child development. Fourth are the difficulties of maintaining a developmental perspective and following the development of drug-exposed offspring over time, including the need to assess the specific physiological and behavioral functions that may be sensitive to prenatal drug exposure using appropriate measures taken at the proper time in the child's life.

Well-designed epidemiologic research on cocaine effects must take into account these areas of methodological concern. This chapter describes the study design and procedures from the epidemiologic Seattle Cocaine and Pregnancy Study, a longitudinal cohort study of cocaine and pregnancy that was designed as an effort to address many of these methodological issues. Sections of this chapter deal with: (a) a description of the Cocaine and Pregnancy Study, and study assumptions about cocaine as a risk factor in child development; (b) sample selection in the study; (c) sample maintenance techniques used in the study; (d) quantification of prenatal substance exposure in the study, including the measurement of cocaine using maternal hair samples; (e) measures used in this cohort study, and data collection and data analysis issues in examining effects of prenatal cocaine exposure on child development; and (f) research and public policy contributions of the Cocaine and Pregnancy Study. In this chapter, prevalence data and information on the parameters of cocaine use among subjects in the Cocaine and Pregnancy Study are presented. Developmental findings are not discussed. Instead, the chapter focuses on how this study addressed methodological concerns current in the field. Strategies used in this study and suggestions for examining drug effects on child development over time may be helpful to other investigators interested in the consequences of prenatal drug exposure.

THE SEATTLE COCAINE AND PREGNANCY STUDY

In 1987, a pilot study in Seattle highlighted an alarming 15-fold increase in cocaine use over the level of use documented 12 years previously among pregnant women at a teaching hospital (Streissguth et al., 1991). Research literature at the time reported neurobehavioral effects of prenatal cocaine exposure on early infant outcome, and there was suggestive evidence that these effects persisted through the infant's first year of development (Chasnoff, Burns, Schnoll, & Burns, 1985; MacGregor et al., 1987; Ryan, Erlich, & Finnegan, 1987). In response to this apparently serious and growing problem, the Seattle Cocaine and Pregnancy Study began in 1988, funded by the National Institute of Drug Abuse, with the primary purpose of examining the potentially adverse effects of prenatal cocaine exposure on early offspring development.

Goals of the Study

The Cocaine and Pregnancy Study screened over 7,000 postpartum women and focused on a carefully constructed cohort of over 500 women and their infants. The cohort was selected with the primary goal of detecting the presence and degree of developmental toxicity of prenatal cocaine exposure on child outcome through the first 2 years of life. Other goals of the study included: (a) assessing the prevalence of cocaine (and other drug) use during pregnancy in a large and varied population of women in the Seattle area, (b) assessing the validity of self-reported cocaine use as verified by a biologic marker (in this case, radioimmunoassay of hair), and (c) delineating the parameters of cocaine use during pregnancy, including dose, pattern, frequency, timing, and duration of use, as well as describing the characteristics of cocaine users in the sample, and the correlates of their drug use.

Cocaine as a Risk Factor in Offspring Development and Study Hypotheses

The Cocaine and Pregnancy Study was built on lessons learned from earlier longitudinal studies of the effects of fetal alcohol exposure on offspring. Also important in designing the study was information from experimental animal research. The animal studies suggested then, and have continued to suggest (although there are mixed findings), that cocaine may have an effect on development apart from that of other drugs (Dow-Edwards, 1993; Dow-Edwards, Freed, & Milhorat, 1988; Fantel, 1993; Foss & Riley, 1991; Goodwin et al., 1992; Riley & Foss, 1991a, 1991b; Spear, 1993; Spear & Heyser, 1992). As much as possible, the Cocaine and Pregnancy Study was built on the principles of behavioral teratology (Vorhees, 1986) and developmental psychopathology (Cicchetti, 1984), recognizing the complex interrelationships of substance exposure, social, and other biological factors in determining difficulties in child outcome (Neuspiel, 1993).

Thus, the Cocaine and Pregnancy Study began in 1988 with the assumption that prenatal exposure to cocaine, like alcohol, places the developing child at risk. The study was based on the idea that cocaine is an agent which, when administered prenatally under appropriate conditions, can potentially disrupt the formation and function of the fetus' developing somatic and central nervous system, and so affect how the child later thinks and behaves. Historically, researchers assumed that cocaine was a structural and functional teratogen (see survey in Koren, Gladstone, Robeson, & Robieux, 1992). This was the viewpoint current when the Cocaine and Pregnancy Study was initiated. More recently, cocaine has been variously described as a "weak" teratogen (Fantel, 1993; Hutchings, 1993a, 1993b), as producing particular functional alterations when administered in sufficiently high doses (Dow-Edwards, 1993), and as a developmental toxicant that affects certain classes of behavior and can alter neural function (Spear, 1993). Recent articles have suggested several direct and indirect mechanisms, at several levels of analysis, to explain different categories of cocaine effects on offspring development, and have suggested that the effects of cocaine may differ according to level of dose and individual susceptibility (Church, 1993; Greenspan, 1991a, 1991b; Hutchings, 1993a; Koren, 1993; Kosofsky, 1991; Neuspiel & Hamel, 1991; Volpe, 1992; Zuckerman, 1991a).

The primary goal of the Cocaine and Pregnancy Study was to ascertain the developmental toxicity of cocaine, with the expectation that prenatal cocaine exposure would show varied but adverse effects on child outcome. Cocaine effects were examined in the presence of other drug use, because essentially all users also ingest other drugs. Two hypotheses were formulated about the developmental impact of cocaine exposure. The first study hypothesis stated that maternal cocaine use in a nonclinical population would contribute to differential offspring development in a dose-dependent fashion. A second study hypothesis stated that neurobehavioral outcomes (rather than growth parameters) would be relatively sensitive indicators of the effects of cocaine exposure in utero, and perhaps of a dose–response relationship between cocaine and offspring effects. To examine these hypotheses, the type and degree of in utero exposure to "doses" of cocaine was quantified, a large number of offspring were enrolled who had been exposed to a broad spectrum of maternal use, mediating and confounding variables were dealt with as much as possible in the study design, and development was examined in varied domains (such as growth, difficulties in neonatal behavior, infant neuromotor skills, toddler behavior problems and representational abilities, etc.). The next section of this chapter presents the study design and procedures of the Cocaine and Pregnancy Study, and describes data on the prevalence and parameters of cocaine use in this cohort study based in the Seattle metropolitan area.

SAMPLE SELECTION, PREVALENCE DATA, AND THE PARAMETERS OF COCAINE USE DURING PREGNANCY

Careful sample selection can help to deal with many confounding variables, making reliance on statistical adjustment during data analysis less necessary. The impact of confounding variables is a major methodological concern in studies of the effects of cocaine use during pregnancy. The Cocaine and Pregnancy Study had several sample selection and stratification features that improved the ability of the study to separate prenatal cocaine exposure from the effects of other important predictors. These included: an initially large screening population drawn from women delivering at local hospitals; a two-phase cocaine self-report system for assessing prenatal exposure, with verification of self-report by a biologic marker (hair analysis); stratification of cocaine (COC) and noncocaine (NO-COC) groups by marijuana, alcohol, and cigarette (MAC) use; exclusion of self-reported users of opiates, amphetamines, barbiturates, and other street drugs except cocaine and MAC; and efforts to balance the COC and NO-COC groups for maternal education.

Recruiting Subjects at Delivery

Subjects were recruited on the day following birth from all women delivering at four study hospitals. Three hospitals at which recruitment took place were urban (one a teaching hospital), and one was suburban. All were in the metropolitan Seattle area. Hospital recruitment provided a community-based sample that was fairly representative of our geographic area. The multiple-hospital strategy was aimed at including the full continuum of users: from middle-income cocaine-using mothers who had experienced few adverse environmental circumstances, to social users, to heavier cocaine users who had not received prenatal care. Other recruitment strategies may select less broad-based samples. Studies using only urban hospitals may fail to include many middle-income women. Studies recruiting during pregnancy, rather than at delivery, may miss the highest risk substance-using mothers who fail to receive prenatal care. Studies relying on recruitment from drug treatment centers, rather than hospitals, do not accrue a very representative sample of all cocaine users.

Hospital Screening Questionnaire and Data on Prevalence and Parameters of Cocaine Use During Pregnancy

A self-administered Hospital Screening Questionnaire (HSQ), shown in Fig. 8.1, was developed for the study to collect prevalence data and identify cocaine users in a cost-efficient manner. The HSQ takes 5 min to complete, is confidential and

HOSPITAL SCREENING STUDY (206) 543-7155
Pregnancy and Health Study II, University of Washington Medical School
Dr. Ann P. Streissguth, Dr. Zane Brown, Dr. Joan C. Martin, Dr. Sharon Landesman,
Ms. Pam Phipps, Ms. Therese Grant, Ms. Joan Sienkiewicz

Dear New Mother:

We are trying to get an idea of the kinds of drugs that women in the Seattle area are taking before and during pregnancy. Please help us by completing this attached brief, confidential questionnaire.

Participation is voluntary; this is not part of your hospital care and you have the right to refuse to answer any question or to refuse to participate at all. Only research staff will have access to the questionnaires and they will be shredded at the end of the study. If you have any questions, please ask any of the above persons. Pam Phipps, Therese Grant, or Joan Sienkiewicz will collect the questionnaires, and may come back to talk with you about participating in other study activities. No information from this questionnaire will be entered into your medical record or discussed with your health care providers.

Your willingness to be honest is appreciated. Please do NOT put your name on the questionnaire.

Have you used these drugs either in the month or so before pregnancy or during this pregnancy? Please circle yes or no in each column:

	MONTH OR SO BEFORE PREGNANCY		DURING THIS PREGNANCY	
1. Marijuana (pot, grass)	yes	no	yes	no
If yes, number of times per month	# _____		# _____	
2. Heroin (smack, horse)	yes	no	yes	no
3. Methadone	yes	no	yes	no
4. Cocaine (crack, rock, coke)	yes	no	yes	no
If yes, number of times per month............................	# _____		# _____	
If yes, what is the most cocaine that you used over a two-day period?	_____		_____	
5. Barbiturates (downers, reds, phenobarb, pentobarb, Seconal)	yes	no	yes	no
6. Amphetamines (uppers, crystal, crank)	yes	no	yes	no
7. Any other street drugs (acid, PCP, angel dust)............................	yes	no	yes	no
If yes, what?_____				
8. Any medications (prescriptions, over counter)............................	yes	no	yes	no
If yes, what?_____				
9. Smoke cigarettes?	yes	no	yes	no
If yes, number per day	# _____		# _____	
10. Any alcohol (wine, beer, liquor)?	yes	no	yes	no
11. Five or more drinks at a time?	yes	no	yes	no
If yes, number of times per month	# _____		# _____	

12. Have you ever used IV street drugs (intravenous)?   yes   no

13. Have you ever used cocaine in any form   yes   no
    If yes, when was the last time you used it?_____

14. What is your age? _____   15.   What is your race? _____

16. How many live-born children have you had counting baby just delivered? _____

17. What is your marital status now? Circle one:
    Married   Divorced   Separated   Single   Living as Married

18. What is the highest grade of regular school you have completed? Circle one:
    Jr. High/High School   University/College   Graduate School
    -7 8 9 10 11 12   13 14 15 16   17 18 19 20+

Please place this form in the attached envelope and seal it. THANKS EVER SO MUCH!
Dr. Ann P. Streissguth

FIG. 8.1.   Hospital Screening Questionnaire (HSQ).

easy to distribute using research nurses or outreach staff, and can be used to screen women who do not receive prenatal care. This questionnaire was a useful research tool, and the critical first step of our cohort selection process. The HSQ was also useful for public health reasons, and provided the community with prevalence information on substance use during pregnancy in the Seattle metropolitan area.

During the 112-week period from March 1, 1989 through April 23, 1991, 7,178 HSQs were collected almost daily from all medically available postpartum women at four Seattle-area hospitals. Of the 7,178 HSQs collected, only 66 were judged to be invalid (two thirds of these due to inconsistency between self-report and urine toxicology screens in the medical record; the remaining one third due to problems on the part of the mother [suspected mental retardation, psychosis, uncooperativeness, or mental confusion]). Final sample size for the Cocaine and Pregnancy Study screening sample was 7,112.

Table 8.1 illustrates the percentages of prenatal drug use reported by women delivering at the four hospitals participating in the study. Analysis of HSQ data showed a decline in self-reported drug use in all categories of illegal drugs during the 2 years of the prevalence study (1989 to 1991). When the Cocaine and Pregnancy Study was conceived, cocaine use still appeared to be fashionable among women of middle or upper income. During study start-up and the study period, intense media coverage of the sorry plight of "crack babies" may have had an effect on either usage patterns or on the willingness of women to self-report. Labeling of substance-abusing pregnant women as criminals, or women's fear and denial of the consequences of drug use to their infants, may also have caused a decrease in maternal self-reported drug use in spite of guarantees of confidentiality. As can be seen in Table 8.1, reported cocaine use at the urban teaching hospital, which had the highest rates of reported use, dropped from 19% at the outset to 9% at the end of the study period. Though not shown in the table, it appeared that the type of cocaine usage shifted toward increased use of crack cocaine and, with greater affordability, toward increased use by those with lower incomes. On the other hand, alcohol use during pregnancy remained fairly stable over the 2-year duration of this study. At the teaching hospital, "any alcohol use" hovered at 43% to 51% of the sample over the course of the study, and "binge alcohol use" (defined as five or more drinks on one occasion) was seen in 9% to 15% of the sample. It is notable that in 1989 to 1991, according to maternal report as shown in Table 8.1, only a little more than one third of the 7,112 babies in the screening sample were *not* exposed to any alcohol, cigarettes, or illegal drugs before birth.

Examination of drug use within demographic subgroups (not presented in table format) revealed that illegal drugs were used more frequently by young mothers, those without a high school education, and single or divorced mothers. Cocaine use was reported four times more often by African-Americans than Whites. Although most demographic groups showed some decline in illegal drug use over this 2-year period, cocaine use among young mothers (19 years and under) showed the most dramatic decrease. Inspection of drug use screening data showed that only 10 of the 7,112 women in the screening sample reported cocaine use without any use of other drugs (including alcohol, marijuana, cigarettes, or other illicit drugs). Twenty-four percent of mothers reporting cocaine use also took illicit drugs other than marijuana.

TABLE 8.1

Percentage (Self-Reported) Prenatal Drug Use by Mothers Delivering at Selected Seattle Area Hospitals by Consecutive 28-Week Periods During 1989 to 1991 ($N = 7,112$)

A. Illegal Drug Use During Pregnancy

Percentage Using Drugs in Consecutive 28-Week Period

Hospital Type	(n)	Any Illegal Drug Use				Use of Marijuana				Use of Cocaine				Use of Other Illegal Drugs[b]			
28-Week Period.[a]		1	2	3	4	1	2	3	4	1	2	3	4	1	2	3	4
Urban teaching	(3,472)	36	27	24	23	27	21	18	16	19	13	11	9	8	4	6	5
Suburban	(2,549)	11	9	9	–	10	8	9	–	3	3	2	–	1	2	1	–
Other urban #1	(887)	–	–	15	16	–	–	13	15	–	–	5	2	–	–	1	2
Other urban #2	(204)	–	–	13	8	–	–	12	7	–	–	2	2	–	–	2	0

B. Use of Alcohol, Cigarettes or No Drug Use

Percentage Using Drugs in Consecutive 28-Week Period

Hospital Type	(n)	Alcohol Use								Use of Cigarettes				No Use of Drugs[c]			
		Any Use				Binge/Massed											
28-Week Period.[a]		1	2	3	4	1	2	3	4	1	2	3	4	1	2	3	4
Urban teaching	(3,472)	51	44	43	47	15	12	9	15	52	45	46	46	27	32	33	36
Suburban	(2,549)	49	43	56	–	8	5	6	–	29	28	26	–	39	43	35	–
Other urban #1	(887)	–	–	45	46	–	–	8	9	–	–	27	31	–	–	45	42
Other urban #2	(204)	–	–	56	57	–	–	5	11	–	–	22	22	–	–	35	34

Notes: $N = 7,112$.
[a]Time Period 1 = March 1, 1989–September 12, 1989   (28 weeks, $n = 2,220$)
Time Period 2 = September 13, 1989–March 27, 1990   (28 weeks, $n = 2,024$)
Time Period 3 = March 28, 1990–October 9, 1990   (28 weeks, $n = 1,380$)
Time Period 4 = October 10, 1990–April 23, 1991   (28 weeks, $n = 1,488$)
[b]Other illegal drugs, e.g., heroin, barbiturates, amphetamines, acid, psychedelic mushrooms, MDMA.
[c]No drugs = No alcohol, no cigarettes, no marijuana, no cocaine, and no other illegal drugs.

Two-Phase Self-Report System: Hospital Screening Questionnaire and the Postpartum Maternal Interview

Mothers from the screening sample who appeared eligible for the Cocaine and Pregnancy Study follow-up cohort, based on their drug use and demographic responses on the HSQ, were told about the study and invited to participate. Signed consents were obtained from 90% of those who appeared to be eligible; these women were then interviewed in detail by a female research assistant in a private setting within the hospital. Postpartum Maternal Interviews (PPMI), given on the day after delivery whenever possible, elicited timing, dose, and pattern of licit and illicit drug use during each trimester, the extent of prenatal care received by the mother, and so on. Specialized interview techniques, including a calendar and reminders of special events, were used to increase the precision of reported timing and quantity of drug use. By using a well-designed maternal interview, conducted in a nonjudgmental setting of patience, confidentiality, and trust, an attempt was made to elicit accurate disclosure of drug use. Hair samples were obtained from mother and baby prior to discharge. Data from these biological samples, along with data from medical records, were analyzed later in the study and used to verify and modify the cocaine exposure scores obtained from our two-phase self-report system of the HSQ and PPMI.

Enrollment and Stratification of the Sample

The follow-up cohort was comprised of a group of cocaine users (COC) and an approximately equal-sized group of non-cocaine users (NO-COC). The COC group included women who reported any level of cocaine use during the 9 months of pregnancy; in both the COC and NO-COC groups women could also have used cigarettes, alcohol, and/or marijuana. There were several a priori exclusionary criteria. Mothers reporting use of street drugs other than cocaine and marijuana were excluded to sharpen the study focus on potential cocaine effects. No mother under 17 years could participate, and residence had to be within the Seattle metropolitan area. The only infant characteristic used in enrollment was the requirement for a singleton birth. Medically fragile infants housed in the Neonatal Intensive Care Unit were unlikely to be included in the study. Remuneration for study participation was ultimately set at $50 for each of four clinical follow-up visits. This was important to ensure subject compliance and reimbursement to the women for their time and effort.

The NO-COC group was matched with the COC users on the basis of the three other prenatal exposures that characterized most cocaine users (namely marijuana, alcohol, and/or cigarette use, referred to here as MAC). As available, additional subjects who used no cocaine and no MAC ("nonusers") were added to the NO-COC group. These nonusers met four criteria: no cocaine exposure, no marijuana exposure, no cigarettes during the second and third trimesters, and never more than 1 to 2 drinks in any month/never more than 10 drinks overall/and no more than 5 oz of absolute alcohol during the gestational period.

Enrollment into the follow-up cohort occurred on a nearly daily basis, based on perusing responses to the screening questionnaires. Adjustments were made in the makeup of the study groups on a regular basis over the course of the investigation in order to keep COC and NO-COC groups as similar as possible with regard to demographic characteristics. About one fourth of the NO-COC group were nonusers of any substance, enrolled with care taken to match the demographic profile of the cocaine users, in an effort to increase the power of the study in untangling the impact of cocaine from the other drugs with which it is customarily used. Efforts were made to balance the COC and NO-COC groups on the potentially confounding variables of maternal education, marital status, parity, and race so that potential cocaine effects were less likely to be obscured by the impact of these factors.

Using such selective criteria for cohort selection meant that many cocaine-using women found in the screening sample (56%) were ineligible for enrollment. Reasons for ineligibility included: use of street drugs other than cocaine and/or marijuana (24%), race recorded as African-American prior to time African-Americans were enrolled in the cohort (16%), early hospital departures (5%), residence out of area (3%), age less than 17 years (2%), and multiple births or other infant issues (< 1%). Only 10% of cocaine-using women asked to be involved in the study actually refused to participate.

Composition of the Cocaine and Pregnancy
Study Follow-Up Cohort

The follow-up cohort was comprised of a sample of 532 women and children. Understanding the substance use and demographic characteristics of this follow-up cohort is critical in considering how research findings from this cohort will fit with those of other cohort studies, an important concern in the study of cocaine, pregnancy, and offspring development (Chasnoff, 1993).

Table 8.2 presents the drug use characteristics of the 7,112 screened mothers, and of the 532 mothers enrolled in the follow-up cohort. As can be seen in Table 8.2, the sample selection process resulted in more frequent maternal cocaine use within the follow-up cohort relative to the Seattle-area hospital population from which the screening sample was drawn. Thus, 49% of the enrolled follow-up cohort used cocaine during pregnancy, in contrast to 8% in the screening sample, so that cocaine use was oversampled. Population-based studies of environmental toxins and teratogens that have not adequately included a sufficient number of users can fail to detect exposure effects that do, in fact, exist. Note that this sampling procedure also stratified for MAC and, compared to the screening sample, resulted in a threefold increase in the rate of marijuana use, a twofold increase in alcohol use and cigarette use, and a fourfold increase in "binge"

TABLE 8.2

Drug Use[a] by Mothers in the Screening Sample (N = 7,112)
Compared to Mothers Enrolled in the Follow-Up Cohort (N = 532)

Drug	Screening Sample (N = 7,112)	Follow-up Cohort (N = 532)
Cocaine use	8%[b]	49%
Marijuana use	15%	47%
Alcohol (any use)	47%	82%
Alcohol ("binge")/Massed drinking[c]	10%	40%
Cigarette use	38%	73%
Illegal drug use (other than cocaine and/or marijuana)	4%	0%

Notes: [a]Drug use includes any use during the first, second, and/or third trimesters, or in the one month "prior to pregnancy recognition."
[b]These percentages should not be interpreted as population drug prevalence figures.
[c]"Binge" or massed drinking is defined as consuming five or more drinks on any drinking occasion.

alcohol use (massed drinking of 5 or more drinks on one occasion) within the follow-up cohort.

The follow-up cohort had the following levels of drug use (not presented in table format). The 259 cocaine users reported a median usage frequency of 10 times during pregnancy and a median use of 5.9 total grams of cocaine during the pregnancy. The 251 marijuana users reported median usage frequency of 25 occasions and total median use of 16 marijuana cigarettes or pipes during pregnancy. There were 434 alcohol users, who reported a median of 14 drinking occasions during the pregnancy and a total of 17.4 ounces of absolute alcohol (35 average drinks) during the pregnancy. The 389 cigarette users in the follow-up cohort all reported daily use, for a median of 174 packs per pregnancy (between ½ and 1 pack per day).

Table 8.3 presents follow-up cohort demographics in the "Total Cohort" column, and demographics by user groups in the COC and NO-COC columns. In the follow-up cohort, there were 259 women in the·COC group, and 273 cocaine abstainers in the follow-up cohort in the NO-COC group (including 202 enrollees who were cocaine abstainers and MAC users, and another 71 enrolled as nonusers of any substance during pregnancy). The "Total Cohort" column shows that 78% of the sample were White or Hispanic and 22% listed were African-American. Sixty-eight percent of the sample were between 20 and 30 years old, 64% had received a high school education or some college, 55% were living without a partner, and 58% were multiparous. Fifty-two percent of the women listed welfare as their primary source of income, and 52% of the children in the follow-up cohort were male. From figures available in Table 8.1, note that 49% of the cohort came from the urban teaching hospital, 15% from the two urban nonteaching hospitals, and 36% from the suburban hospital.

The association of drug use with demographic variables was also considered in sample selection. Table 8.3 compares demographics of the total cohort with

TABLE 8.3
Demographic Characteristics of Follow-Up Cohort
by Presence of Cocaine Use (*N* = 532)

| | | | Cohort by Cocaine Use | | | |
| | Total Cohort (N = 532) | | Any Use (COC) (n = 259) | | No Use (NO-COC) (n = 273) | |
Demographic Characteristic	*n*	*(%)*	*n*	*(%)*	*n*	*(%)*
Maternal Education (years)						
< 12 years	194	(36%)	109	(42%)	85	(31%)
12–15 years	327	(62%)	148	(57%)	179	(66%)
≥ 16 years	11	(2%)	2	(1%)	9	(3%)
Marital Status						
Married	145	(27%)	42	(16%)	103	(38%)
Living as married	95	(18%)	44	(17%)	51	(19%)
Divorced/separated/widowed/single	292	(55%)	173	(67%)	119	(43%)
Maternal Age (years)						
< 20 years	102	(19%)	30	(11%)	72	(26%)
20–30 years	363	(68%)	191	(74%)	172	(63%)
> 30 years	67	(13%)	38	(15%)	29	(11%)
Parity						
Primiparous	222	(42%)	83	(32%)	139	(51%)
Multiparous	309	(58%)	175	(68%)	134	(49%)
Maternal Race						
White/Hispanic	414	(78%)	182	(70%)	232	(85%)
African-American	118	(22%)	77	(30%)	41	(15%)
Source of Income						
Welfare	278	(52%)	179	(69%)	99	(36%)
Other	254	(48%)	80	(31%)	174	(64%)
Sex of Infant						
Girls	253	(48%)	125	(48%)	128	(47%)
Boys	279	(52%)	134	(52%)	145	(53%)

Note: "Cocaine use" includes any use during the first, second, and/or third trimesters, or in the one month prior to the recognition of pregnancy.

the COC and NO-COC groups, revealing how the sample selection helped distribute demographic factors of race, marital status, and maternal age and education across the COC and NO-COC groups. This was done in an effort to minimize the possible attrition of existing cocaine effects in study findings when statistically adjusting for the possible influences of demographic covariates. The two primary sample selection criteria considered in enrollment were maternal race and education, especially important variables in studies of child outcome. The COC and NO-COC groups were balanced on demographic characteristics as much as possible. A reasonably good match was achieved between COC and NO-COC groups in terms of maternal education, and the demographic balance between user groups was vastly improved in the follow-up cohort relative to the screening sample. However, the effort to balance demographic characteristics was not completely successful, as subjects in the COC group were less likely to be White, married, primiparous, less than 20 years old, and were more likely to be welfare recipients. Note that there was deliberately no attempt made to match for infant variables between user groups, on characteristics such as birth weight or gestational age, because those factors may be direct or indirect consequences of prenatal cocaine exposure.

In summary, the Cocaine and Pregnancy Study follow-up cohort appears overall to have the potential to detect cocaine effects, and at the same time to address important demographic confounding factors. The follow-up cohort includes a relatively lower risk group of cocaine-using women than are found in many other studies of the impact of cocaine use during pregnancy. It is useful to follow such a lower risk cohort because it is possible, as Robins and Mills (1993) have suggested, that the subtler effects of drug exposure may be somewhat more visible in a population not simultaneously dealing with a number of other serious disadvantages.

SAMPLE MAINTENANCE

Sample attrition is another significant area of methodological concern in the study of prenatal drug effects. Over the time span of the Cocaine and Pregnancy Study, which followed all target children until the age of 2 years, sample maintenance remained at or above 90% in the four follow-up visits to the research laboratory. This high level of follow-up success is attributed to the use of labor-intensive sample maintenance efforts, based on lessons learned from talking to and working with these cocaine-using subjects, and knowledge gleaned from two decades of following families with fetal alcohol-exposed children.

Details of sample maintenance procedures used in this laboratory are available in Streissguth and Giunta (1992). As is true of most developmental studies, the key to low sample attrition was a dedicated outreach team. At enrollment, female research staff were utilized rather than hospital staff or social services workers (who might unintentionally alter the client's medical services based on information obtained for the purposes of research). For each phase of the study, a female outreach worker was assigned to trace, schedule, transport to child testing, and interview the subjects. Calls to clients were made every 6 to 8 months to schedule a research visit, and more often when necessary. Periodically, Mother's Day cards, personalized communications, and newsletters with child development information were sent out with an address correction requested, to both provide positive feedback and useful information to the women, and to monitor address changes. Frequent follow-up is a key to successful tracing. Our outreach workers and enrollment staff were all college-educated and interested in research, substance abuse, and further study in social services. They were distinguished not by any specific training background, but by their determination, efficiency, straightforward communication style, and ability to problem solve, remain flexible, and be concerned about and bond with our clients. Important aspects of our sample maintenance procedures involved remaining helpful and nonjudgmental, leaving each woman feeling good about her participation in the study, and maintaining an attitude of recognizing clients' strengths and the importance of their personal goals. The outreach workers were not required to be "blind" to drug use status, as were the examiners who tested the infants. Therefore, the outreach workers were able to build a supportive and informed relationship with the subjects.

At the outset of the project, informed consent was obtained from subjects for all procedures in the funded study. A Certificate of Confidentiality was obtained from the Department of Health and Human Services, U.S. Public Health Service, in order to protect research staff from subpoena and subjects from unwarranted use of research information. At each contact, subjects were asked for information helpful in future tracing, such as telephone numbers and the addresses of friends. If a woman was so socially isolated that she could list no friends, or if the outreach worker was concerned about the future success of tracing a particular woman, then the subject was designated as a "special needs mother," and very frequent contact was maintained.

Clearly, positive inducements were also important to high sample maintenance. For each visit, $50 was given to the subject, as an initially lower amount of $10 was not sufficient inducement. Mothers were transported to and from visits. After each testing, general information was given to the mothers about their children's developmental status, positive aspects of the child's performance, and needed referrals for well-child care. If a subject requested a small amount of assistance from the outreach workers, such as brief child-related advice, extra diapers to take home after a research visit, or help with filling out forms or finding safe baby furniture, such assistance was given. Women were not differentially treated based on exposure history. Specific referrals for serious medical problems or well-child care, and the minor amount of assistance already described were given to any family that needed them.

QUANTIFICATION OF PRENATAL
SUBSTANCE EXPOSURE

Information about dose is important in the study of developmental toxicants and teratogens, and precise assessment of prenatal substance exposure has been identified as a major area of methodological concern in the study of cocaine effects. To our knowledge, the Cocaine and Pregnancy Study is the first large investigation to evaluate pregnancy outcomes associated with cocaine exposure ascertained by self-report and verified by hair analysis. This information is discussed by Grant and colleagues (Grant, Brown, Callahan, Barr, & Streissguth, 1994), and is presented in detail in this section of the chapter.

Overview of Cocaine and Pregnancy Study
Measurements of Prenatal Substance Exposure

In the Cocaine and Pregnancy Study, the Hospital Screening Questionnaire (HSQ) and Postpartum Maternal Interview (PPMI) together provided the self-report information on cocaine, marijuana, alcohol, cigarette, and illicit drug use. Care was taken to gather information as detailed as self-report methodology allows, including the use of calendar prompts, precise questioning, and a confidential venue for the maternal interview. Questions about use were asked separately for each trimester, in order to allow for fluctuation in pattern of use over the course of pregnancy. The measurement of cocaine is fully discussed in later sections, and exposure to other substances was assessed as follows. Cigarettes were assessed in terms of self-report of total number of cigarettes smoked per day in each trimester. Marijuana was assessed in terms of self-report of total number of marijuana cigarettes or pipes smoked in each trimester of the gestational period. Alcohol use in each trimester was assessed via self-report, using quantity/frequency/variability indices (Streissguth, Barr, Sampson, Bookstein, & Darby, 1989). Exclusionary data on opiate, amphetamine, and barbiturate exposure were obtained from infant or maternal urine screening, or infant meconium screening, when available.

Differences Between Methods of Measurement
of Prenatal Cocaine Exposure

Correct determination of quantity and timing of intrauterine cocaine exposure is critical in establishing a link with subsequent maternal and infant outcomes. Self-report and urine toxicology are the most commonly used research methods for determining prenatal cocaine (or other drug) exposure, but each has serious drawbacks. The obvious problem with self-report is a tendency for individuals who are chemically dependent to underestimate or deny drug use, particularly if the drug is an illegal one. Among pregnant women, the widely publicized criminalization of drug-using mothers further exacerbates problems with the validity of self-report (Frank et al., 1988; Zuckerman, Amaro, & Cabral, 1989). In addition, long-term drug users may suffer memory impairment, retrospective report of any substance is subject to recall bias, and self-reported cocaine doses are inexact because street cocaine is not subject to standards for purity or weight.

Maternal or infant urine is limited as a chronological marker of drug use, because cocaine and its metabolites have short half-lives and are not detectable in urine 3 to 5 days following the last use (Saxon, Calsyn, Haver, & Delaney, 1988). As a result, outcome studies enrolling subjects based on either maternal or infant positive urine screens at delivery, which are quite common in the literature, are likely to underestimate the number of users. Results may be biased toward overestimation of cocaine effects because identified subjects are likely to be chronic, heavy users (those who use until the time of delivery).

Meconium has shown promise as a more sensitive biologic indicator of prenatal exposure than urine. However, timing of exposure for an individual fetus cannot be established from meconium samples, and the gestational threshold at which cocaine is deposited in meconium has not yet been determined (Ostrea, Brady, Gause, Raymundo, & Stevens, 1992; Ostrea, Brady, Parks, Asensio, & Naluz, 1989). In a small substudy conducted among 59 women drawn from the larger Cocaine and Pregnancy Study follow-up cohort, comparison of the sensitivity of tests of newborn infant hair, meconium, and urine in detecting gestational cocaine exposure was carried out (Callahan et al., 1992). Radioimmunoassay of infant hair and gas chromatography–mass spectrometry of meconium were significantly more sensitive than immunoassay of urine, which failed to identify 60% of cocaine-exposed infants. The quantity of cocaine metabolite in the newborn infant hair correlated best with the segment of maternal hair closest to the scalp, representing the last 12 weeks of antepartum hair growth. Based on these results, the conclusion was drawn that analyses of the newborn infant hair by radioimmunoassay, or of meconium by gas chromatography–mass spectrometry, are more sensitive than analysis of urine by immunoassay and can detect fetal cocaine exposure occurring during the last two trimesters of pregnancy. But it was found that neither urine, meconium, nor infant hair can be expected to reveal gestational exposure during early pregnancy.

In contrast to these methods, radioimmunoassay of postpartum maternal hair (RIAH) provides a biologic marker that records levels of cocaine use during the entire gestational period. Cocaine, and a cocaine metabolite, benzoylecgonine, are incorporated into the hair follicle as it grows (Baumgartner, Hill, & Blahd, 1989). Therefore, maternal hair samples collected postpartum and assayed for these substances in segments at measured distances from the hair root may provide an estimate of quantity and timing of cocaine use during the full course of pregnancy (Forman et al., 1992; Graham, Koren, Klein, Schneiderman, & Greenwald, 1989; Welch, Martier, Ager, Ostrea, & Sokol, 1990).

Use of Radioimmunoassay of Postpartum Maternal Hair (RIAH)

Maternal postpartum hair samples were collected from women enrolled in the follow-up cohort, and analyzed using radioimmunoassay techniques as a biologic and historic measure of cocaine exposure. (RIAH for other illicit drugs was not carried out because of its expense.) RIAH findings for cocaine were then compared with self-report of cocaine use from the structured two-part HSQ/PPMI interview process. This was done to evaluate the concordance of hair and self-report as measures of prenatal cocaine exposure. Specifically, the precision of information on quantity available from self-report data was examined, and the limitations of RIAH were noted. In addition, the characteristics of women for whom there were discrepancies in assessment of cocaine exposure by the two methods were carefully scrutinized.

To gather the hair samples, women were informed that at the end of the PPMI a small sample of maternal hair would be collected, with their consent, for the purpose of determining drug exposure. Maternal hair samples were obtained by cutting approximately 40 full-length hairs with scissors from the back of the head close to the scalp. Samples were packaged individually and sent to Psychemedics Corporation, in Los Angeles, California, for measurement of cocaine-benzoylecgonine by RIAH using a proprietary method. Methodologic details of hair decontamination (washing), extraction, and evaluation of the impact of cosmetic hair damage on findings are described elsewhere (Baumgartner et al., 1989; Marques, Tippetts, & Branch, 1993). Laboratory technicians were blind to the self-reported drug status of the subjects.

Only the proximal 11.7 cm of the hair sample, measured from the scalp, was analyzed because adult hair grows at an average rate of 1.3 cm per month, or approximately 11.7 cm over a 9-month pregnancy (Baumgartner et al., 1989; Saitoh, Uzuka, & Sakamoto, 1969). Each hair sample was analyzed in three sections, representing approximate growth in each trimester. Hair analysis results were reported in nanograms (ng) of cocaine-benzoylecgonine (coc-ben) per 10 mg of hair. Per a decision by the laboratory, the cutoff value used for determining a positive test for each hair section was 2.0 ng of coc-ben/10 mg of hair. If any of the three hair segments was positive, the subject was classified as cocaine exposed. The average reported value of the three segments defined the level of prenatal exposure over three trimesters.

Concordance of Findings from Self-Report and RIAH

Of the 532 women in this follow-up cohort, 478 (90%) provided a hair sample. Fifteen percent were excluded from comparison because their hair was too short or they self-reported cocaine use only during the month prior to conception. The final group of 405 women providing hair samples were primarily White or Hispanic, unmarried, between 20 and 30 years old, with at least a high school education, and were multiparous. Only 56 (14%) of the women in this final hair sample group were African-Americans.

Table 8.4 shows the number of women identified as cocaine users by self-report only ($n = 148$) and by positive RIAH only ($n = 165$). Table 8.4 also shows that there were 129 women who were identified as cocaine positive on both measures. Note that 184 women were identified as cocaine users by a combination of methods (*either* a positive interview *or* a positive hair assay for cocaine), and that relying on either methodology *alone* led to notable misclassification of maternal cocaine exposure status. Taking the combination of methods as the standard, and 184 as the total number of women who were actually cocaine positive, Table 8.4 shows that if RIAH alone had been used to identify cocaine

TABLE 8.4
Radioimmunoassay of Hair for Cocaine-Benzoylecgonine Compared
to Self-Report of Prenatal Cocaine Use (N = 405)

| | Total Hair Sample Group (N = 405) | | Findings from Radioimmunoassay of Hair for Cocaine/Benzoylecgonine | | | |
| | | | Positive (n = 165) | | Negative (n = 240) | |
Findings from Self Report	n	(%)	n	(%)	n	(%)
Cocaine Use Reported First, and/or Second, and/or, Third Trimesters	148	(37%)	129	(87%)	19	(13%)
No Cocaine Use Reported	257	(63%)	36	(14%)	221	(86%)

Note: The total number of cocaine-positive women was comprised of all women with either positive self report for cocaine use (129 + 19) *or* a cocaine-positive hair assay (129 + 36). Thus, there were a total of 129 (70.1%) + 19 (10.3%) + 36 (19.6%), equaling 184 (100%) individuals identified as cocaine-positive by a combination of methods.

exposure, 19 of the infants would have been misclassified as nonexposed (10.3%). If interview alone had been used to classify exposure, 36 infants would have been misclassified (19.6%).

Table 8.4 also shows that 36 women denied cocaine use on interview, but actually had cocaine-positive hair. Several factors characterized this group of women, and this information may help to understand what affects the accuracy of self-report data on cocaine use. First, the mean value of coc-ben in the hair samples of these 36 women was significantly less than that found among the 129 women who both reported cocaine use and had cocaine-positive hair. (Levels were 21.3 ± 34.6 ng/10 mg hair among the women with discrepant reports, vs. 237 ± 477 ng/10 mg among women with congruent reports.) Second, these 36 women showed distinguishing demographic characteristics. Women with discrepant reports were significantly more likely to be unmarried, African-American, and multiparous. Third, 7 of these 36 women reported passive exposure to cocaine smoke during the pregnancy. Because a number of reports have indicated that positive urine toxicology screens have been obtained from infants and adults exposed to recreational levels of crack cocaine smoke, low levels of coc-ben found in the hair could be explained by this passive exposure (Baselt, Yoshikawa, & Chang, 1991; Bateman & Heagarty, 1989; Dinnies, Darr, & Saulys, 1990).

Among the 129 women who were cocaine positive on both measures, there was a significant but moderate correlation between the quantity of cocaine detected in hair and that revealed by self-report (r = .32, p < .001). There are complex factors underlying discrepancies in self-report and biological indicators of drug use. To better understand the demographic characteristics that affected the precision of self-report data, the sample was divided by marital status, parity, and race.

From interview information on the entire sample, unmarried women were found to be six times more likely to deny using any cocaine than married women. However, among the women who did admit use when interviewed, there was a better correlation between hair values and self-report among those who were unmarried ($r = .326$) compared to those who were married ($r = .160$); the married women who reported using the least cocaine had hair values most discrepant with self-report. In speculating on these findings, it is possible that *unmarried* women may have been reticent to report *any* cocaine use because of feelings of vulnerability (perhaps to losing their children), particularly in the presence of other indices placing them at risk, such as low income and poor social support. *Married* women's reticence to reveal the *extent* of their drug use may be related to fear of incriminating a drug-using spouse or fear of spousal reprisal, despite the fact that interviews were confidential.

Multiparous women who used cocaine were both more likely to deny drug use and to underreport admitted use. Their unwillingness to accurately report may have been due to prior intervention by child protective services or medical personnel.

There was a complex impact of race on the relationship between RIAH and self-report data, with lower correlations among African-Americans ($r = .039$) as compared to Whites ($r = .386$). Hair values were lowest among White women who reported the least total cocaine use during pregnancy. Among both African-American and White women, hair values were highest among women reporting the greatest number of grams of cocaine used throughout pregnancy. However, African-American women who reported the least cocaine use throughout pregnancy were "underreporters"; they had median hair values nearly 50 times greater than those of White women who reported using similarly low amounts. Hair values for these African-American underreporters were nearly as high as for those African-American women reporting the greatest amount of use of cocaine. There are several possible explanations for these findings. First, a recent study found differences in the ratio of fibrous protein to hair matrix substances among hair samples from African-Americans, Whites, and Asians (Dekio & Jidoi, 1990). These structural differences could have an influence on drug uptake in the hair, and could lead to a possible racial bias in hair testing (Kidwell, 1992). However, there appear to be no published studies documenting differences due to race in hair growth or differences in results of hair analysis for drugs of abuse. Second, Chasnoff, Landress, and Barrett (1990) found that African-American women were nearly 10 times more likely than White women to be reported to public health authorities for substance abuse during pregnancy, although toxicologic screening showed similar rates of use among African-Americans and Whites. Although this study has methodological flaws, it does highlight a valid concern among African-American women regarding biased attitudes and reporting practices, which could help explain the differential accuracy of cocaine self-report for African-American versus White women found in this study.

Advantages and Limitations of RIAH, and the Combination of RIAH and Self-Reported Drug Use Used in the Cocaine and Pregnancy Study

RIAH is a sensitive, comprehensive, and clinically practical technique that produces a biologic marker of gestational exposure across the duration of pregnancy, but it has several limitations. Certain pharmacological and analytical questions regarding its validity and reliability remain to be answered (Mieczkowski, 1992). Subjects must be willing to comply, RIAH is expensive, and there is a wide biologic variability in metabolizing cocaine. In addition, the chronological record of cocaine use from hair is dependent on hair length, condition, and rate of hair growth. If a woman's hair grows faster than average, a hair sample length representing 9 months of growth might not identify use early in pregnancy. If a woman's hair grows more slowly than average, a 9-month hair sample might detect cocaine use that occurred before conception, and would produce a false positive. Hair analysis does not detect cocaine used in the last few days of the pregnancy because of insufficient time for the drug to enter the hair shaft. Results of hair analysis may also be affected if hair is altered by cosmetic treatments, and there are issues of discerning systemic versus passive exposure (Koren, Klein, Forman, & Graham, 1992). Because of these limitations, and because adjustment was not made for gestational age in the Cocaine and Pregnancy Study RIAH/self-report comparisons, caution should be used in attributing exact quantitative values to levels of cocaine exposure at specific points during pregnancy. However, RIAH of postpartum maternal hair does give a record of exposure across three trimesters, as does no other biological marker. Thus, using RIAH of maternal hair, it is possible to objectively categorize levels of use as high, medium, or low, and as stable or increasing/decreasing across gestation.

The combination of RIAH with self-report may provide a more accurate and thorough measure of gestational cocaine exposure than more commonly used toxicology screening methods, for both research and clinical purposes. Biologic markers of drug exposure can provide more precise exposure information, especially when combined with self-report data that can reveal patterns of use. Prospective studies using these more precise classification methods may yield more accurate information on the impact of in utero cocaine and other drug exposure on child development.

EXAMINING THE EFFECTS OF PRENATAL COCAINE EXPOSURE ON DEVELOPMENT OVER TIME IN THE COCAINE AND PREGNANCY STUDY

In a review of the literature, Robins and Mills (1993) stated: "the question of long-term consequences of in utero drug exposure is undoubtedly the most important of all the questions . . . [that] . . . need answering, and the hardest to get satisfactory answers to" (p. 28). In examining the effects of prenatal cocaine exposure on child development over time, once an adequate sample has been selected and maintained over time, and good measures of "dose" are obtained, the following issues must be considered to adequately address methodological concerns: choice of appropriate and theory-driven child outcome measures and timing of assessment, measuring and handling mediating and confounding variables, and examining individual differences. This section of the chapter discusses the choice of measures and data collection strategy, and ideas about data analysis, used in the Cocaine and Pregnancy Study. The design of the Cocaine and Pregnancy Study, not actual findings, are discussed here.

Data Collection Issues: Timing of Assessment and Choice of Appropriate Infant Measures

Research on alcohol effects has shown that assessing the impact of prenatal substance exposure on child development with the wrong measures, at the wrong point in time, or for too short a period, may lead investigators to the premature and perhaps incorrect conclusion that there are no long-term effects on child outcome (Carmichael Olson, Streissguth, Bookstein, Barr, & Sampson, 1994; Jacobson & Jacobson, 1991). When studying the developmental impact of gestational cocaine exposure, then, it is important to assess outcome very early in life, and continue to follow the child over time. Measures of child outcome should be selected to tap both enduring cognitive, affective, and regulatory processes as well as salient developmental tasks; as much as possible, selected measures should have predictive power. Both global developmental assessments and measures of more specific cognitive functions may be important (Jacobson & Jacobson, 1991). Measures (and variables derived from these measures) should also be chosen to capture hypothesized drug effects, as identified in animal and human data, and to assess development fully. Spear (1993) commented that many of the behavioral endpoints critical to the full assessment of neurobehavioral toxicity have not yet been examined in cocaine-exposed infants beyond a rudimentary level, and certainly have not been investigated in older children. She included five functional categories she believed should be assessed: motivational/arousal, sensory, motor, cognitive, and social. Until all these areas are examined, Spear suggested that it may be premature to conclude, as did Hutchings (1993a), that the effects of prenatal cocaine exposure on child development are marginal and transitory.

Data Collection Strategy Used in the Cocaine and Pregnancy Study

Figure 8.2 presents the data collection strategy used in the Cocaine and Pregnancy Study, which followed infants from the day of delivery through the first 2 years of life. Measures were chosen from a developmental perspective to broadly assess child outcome, and tap most of Spear's five functional categories.

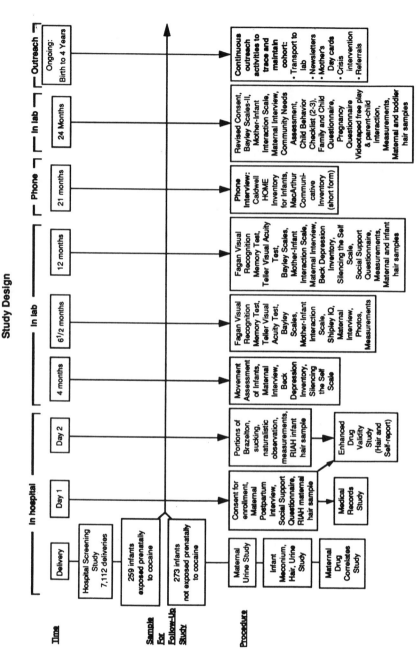

FIG. 8.2. Cocaine and Pregnancy Study: Study design.

The neonatal data collection phase of the study included assessment of growth parameters and review of medical records (e.g., early health and presence of physical anomalies). These data are important, because lowered birth weight and certain physical anomalies have been found to be associated with prenatal cocaine exposure. Newborn movement patterns were videotaped, and a kinematic analysis will be carried out. Neurobehavioral tests were administered to assess as many aspects of newborn functioning as possible within a short time frame, given the logistical constraints of neonatal testing. These tests, which were carried out by highly trained examiners, assessed reflexes, activity level, sucking ability, and state control. These are aspects of neonatal function hypothesized to show effects of prenatal cocaine exposure, depending on individual susceptibility, dosage levels, and so on. Several of these neonatal tests are discussed in Martin, Martin, Streissguth, and Lund (1979). Currently under preparation are discussions of the Cocaine and Pregnancy Study findings from the neonatal neurobehavioral substudy, and the newborn growth data from the entire follow-up cohort.

The Cocaine and Pregnancy follow-up cohort was followed past the neonatal period and through the child's first 2 years. Information was gathered on the relationship between prenatal cocaine exposure and the following domains: neuromotor status at 4 months of age; visual acuity, infant visual recognition memory, and global development status (during structured testing) in the first year of life; and early language skills, developmental status (during structured testing), toddler play (in an unstructured situation), and behavior problems in the second year of life. Systematic, qualitative clinical observations were also made at each data collection point to discern potential effects that health and standardized developmental measures might not pick up, including examiner ratings of unusual behaviors and in vivo and (at 24 months) videotaped mother–infant interaction. No physiological outcome data were collected.

Actual measures used in the Cocaine and Pregnancy Study are listed in Fig. 8.2. The domains assessed in the study were considered important in development and salient to the stage in the infant's life in which they were assessed. Several of these domains have shown predictive validity in relation to later child outcome, and were selected as cocaine sensitive according to leads from animal or human data. For example, there have been suggestions that ocular anomalies may result from teratogen exposure (Stromland, Miller, & Cook, 1991), so that examination of cocaine effects on infant visual acuity and visual recognition memory could be important, especially because the latter skill has been found to predict later cognitive development. As another example, studies of small samples have suggested that toddler play in an unstructured situation may more clearly reveal drug effects in representational abilities, an important developmental arena, than does performance during structured testing (Rodning, Beckwith, & Howard, 1989), so that it is important to have assessments of both.

Data Analysis Issue: Handling Mediating and Confounding Variables

Newborn assessments have advantages in a developmental follow-up study. They are the only evaluations not influenced by the postnatal environment and, as Zuckerman (1991a) stated, "the closer the exposure to the measurement of outcome, the greater the ability to make a causal inference" (p. 352). However, as Kosofsky (1991) and Chasnoff (1993) pointed out, measures taken earlier in a child's life require less complex forms of learning and reasoning, so that evidence of brain insult potentially arising from prenatal drug exposure may not emerge until later in development. Longitudinal assessment should continue through the infant years and beyond.

When following children past the immediate neonatal period, the direct and indirect long-term effects of a potential prenatal toxin like cocaine must be considered within the spectrum of postnatal environmental factors that affect child outcome. Yet the question of how to describe the ongoing, changing, mediating influence of the postnatal environment in a research study of prenatal drug effects is a particular challenge (Neuspiel, 1993). Different strategies have been recommended. Robins and Mills (1993) specified important mediating variables which they believe should be dealt with in research on the long-term consequences of in utero drug exposure, such as maternal IQ, postnatal exposure to drugs, and the quality of the child's postnatal home environment. Coles and Platzman (1993) emphasized that the childrearing environment can have very potent effects on the development of drug-exposed children. Indeed, it is important to identify risk factors as well as "protective factors" (such as good nutrition during pregnancy or a stable home environment) in the lives of drug-exposed children. In studying the developmental effects of prenatal drug exposure, Richardson and Day (1994) suggested focusing on the cumulative effects of substance use and risks of the associated lifestyle. It may also be enlightening to see how differently such risk and protective factors operate in the lives of children who are and are not drug-exposed, as has been done in studying developmental processes among preterm versus full-term children (Carmichael Olson, 1986).

Handling Mediating and Confounding Variables in the Cocaine and Pregnancy Study

The Cocaine and Pregnancy Study has followed a large sample of exposed and nonexposed offspring, and sample attrition has been kept low. As part of the study design, the focus has been on the question of a dose–response relationship between levels of prenatal cocaine exposure and several classes of offspring growth, medical problems, and behavior. Cocaine exposure was oversampled, the sample stratified to control for important biologic confounding factors, and other mediating and confounding factors were described. The Cocaine and Pregnancy Study has attempted to identify the presence and type of developmental toxicity of prenatal cocaine exposure, not to trace the mechanism of action of the drug on development; these fundamentally different research questions were differentiated by Jacobson (1991). The study design and analytic approach taken in the Cocaine and Pregnancy Study has been productive in the study of the effects of prenatal alcohol exposure (Streissguth, Bookstein, Sampson, & Barr, 1993), and has advantages not found in studies of matched comparison groups.

In the Cocaine and Pregnancy Study, the data gathered on mediating variables describe aspects of the postnatal environment at the highest level of detail that was feasible. This included variables such as family structure; presence of foster care; quality of caregiver–child interaction; stresses in the environment over the course of the child's life (including the presence of violence); maternal characteristics such as level of education, a measure of cognitive ability, social support (measured according to both traditional and gender-appropriate terms), presence of an intimate partner or the grandmother in the home; the quality of developmental stimulation and amount of predictability available in the home; postnatal exposure to drug use; and so on.

Analyses of group findings for the newborn outcomes in the Cocaine and Pregnancy Study will center on the question of the dose–response relationship between prenatal cocaine exposure and child growth and neonatal behavior, with competing biological and demographic influences controlled for via study design and regression techniques. The total effects of prenatal cocaine exposure, including both direct and indirect effects, are being examined. Analyses of group findings for outcomes from age 4 months through 2 years will also focus on the dose–response relationship. But these later analyses must deal not only with quantifying dose, and quantifying differences in "response" (effects on growth and several classes of behavior), as did the analysis of neonatal outcomes. They must also take into account the cumulative effects of substance use and the "realities" (characteristics) of the associated lifestyle, which are very diverse within a group of children exposed to cocaine and other drugs in utero (Carmichael Olson, Streissguth, & Barr, 1992). These analyses must contend with the complex notion of direct and indirect effects of prenatal cocaine exposure on development (Neuspiel & Hamel, 1991; Zuckerman, 1991a), as some authors have recently attempted to do (Azuma & Chasnoff, 1993; Lester et al., 1991).

Investigating Individual Differences in the Cocaine and Pregnancy Study

Kosofsky (1991), Volpe (1992), Church (1993), and Koren (1993) have all speculated that there may be individual differences in susceptibility to cocaine effects. Thus, it is critical to understand how and why some individuals may be vulnerable, whereas others are resilient. Beyond considering drug dosage and timing issues such as maternal and fetal genetic factors, observed medical events suffered by a child (such as a stroke), gender differences, and environmental risk and protective factors all eventually need to be examined. Because the Cocaine and Pregnancy Study followed a large group of children over the first 2 years of life, there is an opportunity for "focus studies" to find vulnerable individuals or subgroups, and to identify individuals or subgroups who are particularly unaffected and thus appear to have escaped early exposure unscathed (at least during the infant years). Following the Cocaine and Pregnancy Study cohort through childhood could be important to adequately judge vulnerability and resilience, and the full extent of long-term effects.

Directions for Research Past the Years of Infancy in the Cocaine and Pregnancy Study

In the search to understand whether there are long-term consequences of in utero cocaine exposure in particular areas of function, or consequences for certain exposed individuals vulnerable because of dosage levels, inherent characteristics, and/or environmental circumstance, it is crucial to follow drug-exposed children past infancy and into childhood, through at least the school-age years (Frank & Zuckerman, 1993). The children in the Cocaine and Pregnancy Study cohort, who are now entering kindergarten, could provide a unique opportunity to carry out this type of developmental follow-up. Following the entire cohort, and conducting "focus studies" centering on subgroups of interest, would both be important.

One useful research topic could center on documenting the natural history and "real-life outcomes" of children identified as experiencing prenatal drug exposure, to answer vital questions such as whether a higher proportion of these children really do experience problems in the classroom. Research could target potential drug effects on both physiological (e.g., endocrine function or respiratory control) and behavioral function among cocaine-exposed children, during preschool and beyond. A complete look at behavioral function would involve examining central cognitive, affective, and regulatory processes as well as the performance of stage-salient behavioral tasks and performance under conditions of stress; all five of Spear's (1993) functional domains should be assessed.

An especially productive and intriguing avenue for research on the long-term consequences of prenatal drug exposure could center on regulatory processes, at both the physiologic and behavioral levels, and at the level of the individual or the dyad (Chasnoff, Griffith, Freier, & Murray, 1992; Greenspan, 1991a, 1991b; Zuckerman, 1991a). For example, the potential impact of cocaine on regulatory processes at the neurophysiological level is supported by initial evidence of alterations in neurotransmitter levels and cortisol response to stress among exposed individuals (Magnano, Gardner, & Karmel, 1992; Ward et al., 1991). As another example, Greenspan (1991a, 1991b) suggested a model focusing on regulatory disorders among drug-exposed children, within the context of behaviors and interactions between the infant and his or her caregiver; thus, studies of mutual regulation between caregiver and child are another interesting focus for research. Suggestions have been made by several authors of interactional tasks useful in studying child self-regulation, and mutual regulation in interaction with the caregiver, among drug-exposed toddlers and older children. For example, the Self-Regulatory Play Paradigm is a videotaped situation in which a toddler must transition from free play with a familiar caregiver, to a combination of free play and noncontingent, overly positive, free play with toys with a stranger, and back to play with the familiar caregiver (Tronick, Beeghley, Fetters, & Weinberg, 1991). New tasks from other fields of research may also be useful in the study of self-regulation, and of mutual regulation between child and caregiver. For example, from attachment research has come a videotaped situation called The Waiting Task (Carmichael Olson, 1986). This task is age appropriate in preschool and early childhood, and may be a window on the "transactional process" between caregiver and child. The Waiting Task can provide insight on a child's self-regulatory processes, and on the quality of mutual regulation and goal-corrected partnership during a frustrating task within a drug-exposed child–caregiver dyad.

A related research focus in the developmental study of drug effects could center on the neuropsychological constructs of attention, executive control functioning, and efficient information processing. (Executive control functioning has been defined by some writers as how well a person can organize, plan, resist distraction, and execute responses [West, Goodlett, & Brandt, 1990].) Deficits in these areas may be final common pathways through which drug effects and other biological insults are expressed in child behavior. Enduring alcohol-related deficits have been found in these domains (Carmichael Olson, Feldman, Streissguth, & Gonzalez, 1992; Don, Kerns, Mateer, & Streissguth, 1992; Kodituwakku et al., 1992; Jacobson, Jacobson, Sokol, Martier, & Ager, 1993; Kopera-Frye, Carmichael Olson, & Streissguth, in press; Streissguth et al., in press). Cocaine-related deficits in these areas are at least of theoretical concern. For example, Zuckerman (1991a) stated that the potential central nervous system (CNS) impact of cocaine, as seen in neurotransmitter alterations or small localized hemorrhages, suggests the use of specific outcome measures that tap such constructs as the regulation of attentional states, deficits in information processing, or the ability to regulate affect or anxiety.

CONTRIBUTIONS OF THE COCAINE AND PREGNANCY STUDY TO PUBLIC HEALTH RESEARCH AND POLICY

In work on the Cocaine and Pregnancy Study, it has been clear that fetal alcohol and drug effects are only one aspect of the many problems faced by exposed children and their families. Prenatal drug exposure exacts its toll, but parental drug use is part of a larger set of social concerns that have profound personal and social costs for both the child and the family. Our staff has recognized these as serious public health issues. In response, work on the Cocaine and Pregnancy Study has resulted in several contributions to public health research, community service, and public policy.

Generating Data on Prevalence and Correlates of Substance Use, and on Methods for Quantifying Prenatal Substance Exposure

The Hospital Screening Questionnaire (HSQ) developed for the Cocaine and Pregnancy Study is a methodology that can be used to generate hospital prevalence data on drug and alcohol use during pregnancy. Prevalence data can be used to target appropriate services. In addition, prevalence data can set the context for understanding how the results of a developmental follow-up study of drug effects in a particular geographic area, such as Seattle, will fit with data from follow-up studies in other locations, such as New York or Detroit. The two-phase Hospital Screening Questionnaire/Postpartum Maternal Interview (HSQ/PPMI) self-report process can go beyond prevalence data based on anonymous screening, to generate more thorough self-report of substance use and the correlates of maternal use. Combining information from the HSQ/PPMI self-report process with data from radioimmunoassay of postpartum maternal hair may provide a more accurate and thorough measure of gestational cocaine exposure than more commonly used toxicology screening methods, for both research and clinical purposes. Prospective studies using these more precise classification methods may yield more accurate information on the impact of in utero cocaine and other drug exposure on child development.

Generating Suggestions for Effective Work With Chemically Dependent Pregnant Women

Work on the Cocaine and Pregnancy Study, funded by the National Institute of Drug Abuse (NIDA), was used to inform research on the Seattle-based multidisciplinary, multiagency "MOMS Project." The MOMS Project is a NIDA-funded research and demonstration project designed to provide state-of-the-art, comprehensive services to over 300 chemically dependent pregnant women and their children, to understand who enters and stays in treatment, and to examine the effectiveness of intervention on maternal, child, and interactional outcomes. Sample maintenance techniques, measurement ideas and, most importantly, data on the needs of this population drawn from work on the Cocaine and Pregnancy Study have assisted work in the MOMS Project. Even more broadly, information on the characteristics and needs of these high-risk, chemically dependent women and children from the Cocaine and Pregnancy Study have been disseminated throughout Washington state to assist in treatment and family support services for chemically dependent women and their children.

In addition, a special research demonstration and intervention program for chemically dependent pregnant and parenting women was created, based directly on lessons learned from working with research subjects in the Cocaine and Pregnancy Study. Funded by the Center for Substance Abuse Prevention, the "Birth to Three Project" was designed to intervene for 3 years postpartum with a group of the highest risk drug-using women (who had minimal or no prenatal care). These women were recruited at delivery through the HSQ/PPMI process and community referral. The intervention involves consistent, one-on-one advocacy with a woman and her family. Attention is paid to the complex interplay of drug treatment, housing needs, health care, child custody, poverty, depression, loss of confidence, violence, and other social factors that can accompany drug use and fetal alcohol or drug exposure. The Birth to Three Project draws to a close in 1996, and evidence so far suggests it has been cost effective. It has clearly been positively received both by the community and by the women themselves.

Addressing Methodological Concerns in the Study of Prenatal Cocaine Exposure

As discussed at the outset of this chapter, strategies used in the Cocaine and Pregnancy Study address areas of methodologic concern in the study of the long-term effects of in utero drug exposure. These include sample selection and stratification strategies, sample maintenance techniques, methods of quantifying prenatal substance exposure, a developmental perspective on following the development of drug-exposed offspring over time (including the complexities of measuring child outcome), and ideas about data collection and analysis.

Yet the methodological concerns addressed in the chapter are not the only difficulties facing those carrying out research on prenatal polydrug exposure. Concerns have also been raised about unbalanced interpretation of results in the popular media (Frank & Zuckerman, 1993), publication bias toward studies reporting positive cocaine effects (Koren, Graham, Shear, & Einarson, 1989), possible overgeneralization of results based on proband cases to the full population of drug-exposed children (Day & Richardson, 1993), searching for effects when none may exist or when the social concerns accompanying drug use may actually be the major concern (Coles, 1993; Day & Richardson, 1993; Frank & Zuckerman, 1993), and other issues. To contend with these problems, recent peer consensus suggests careful adherence to the scientific method, and drawing conclusions based on an accumulation of results from well-designed animal and controlled prospective human study (Hutchings, 1993a, 1993b). We believe that the Cocaine and Pregnancy Study will be a significant contribution to the growing body of evidence on prenatal cocaine and polydrug effects on child development, and findings from the study will continue to point toward fruitful directions for public health research and policy.

ACKNOWLEDGMENTS

This project was funded by the U.S. Department of Health and Human Services: National Institute on Drug Abuse, Grant # 5R01 DA05365-01-05 to A. P. Streissguth. We acknowledge the contributions of Sharon Landesman Ramey, and Zane A. Brown, research co-investigators who were crucial to the design and implementation of the Seattle Cocaine and Pregnancy Study. We are grateful for the invaluable statistical assistance of Helen Barr. The contributions of Charles Callahan to the content of this manuscript are also sincerely acknowledged. This study would not have been possible without the dedication and concern for women and children of the following members of the research team (in alphabetical order): Laura Atkins, Kim Carson, Nancy Heller, Denise Anderson Kitikas, Bev LaVeck, Claudia Meadows, Lea Ann Miyagawa, Heidi Myers, Arlett Neumarker, Linda Peters, Pam Richardson, Joan Sienkiewicz, Teresa Stevens, Pamela Swanborne, Mary Tatarka, Alison Voinot, and Gretchen Weiss. Research team members Pam Phipps and Nancy Larson are especially acknowledged for their careful work on the study, and insightful comments on this manuscript. We also wish to thank the nursing staffs in the newborn nurseries of participating hospitals for their cooperation. Finally, and most important, was the energy, willingness, and commitment of the women and children who participated in the study.

REFERENCES

Azuma, S. D., & Chasnoff, I. J. (1993). Outcome of children prenatally exposed to cocaine and other drugs: A path analysis of three-year data. *Pediatrics, 92*(3), 306–402.

Baselt, R., Yoshikawa, D., & Chang, J. (1991). Passive inhalation of cocaine. *Clinical Chemistry, 37*, 2160–2161.

Bateman, D., & Heagarty, M. (1989). Passive freebase cocaine ("crack") inhalation by infants and toddlers. *American Journal of Diseases of Children, 143*, 25–27.

Baumgartner, W. A., Hill, V. A., & Blahd, W. H. (1989). Hair analysis for drug abuse. *Journal of Forensic Sciences, 34*, 1433–1453.

Callahan, C. M., Grant, T. M., Phipps, P., Clark, G., Novack, A. H., Streissguth, A. P., & Raisys, V. A. (1992). Measurement of gestational cocaine exposure: Sensitivity of infants' hair, meconium, and urine. *Journal of Pediatrics, 120*(5), 763–768.

Carmichael Olson, H. (1986). *Developmental process and outcome in preterm children: A transactional study.* Unpublished doctoral dissertation.

Carmichael Olson, H., Feldman, J., Streissguth, A., & Gonzalez, R. (1992). Neuropsychological deficits and life adjustment in adolescents and adults with fetal alcohol syndrome. *Alcoholism: Clinical and Experimental Research, 16*(2), p. 380.

Carmichael Olson, H., Streissguth, A., & Barr, H. (1992). Behavior problems in substance-exposed toddlers. *Society for Research in Child Development, 1993 Abstracts*, p. 37.

Carmichael Olson, H., Streissguth, A., Bookstein, G., Barr, H., & Sampson, P. (1994). Developmental research in behavioral teratology: The impact of prenatal alcohol exposure on child development. In S. L. Friedman & H. C. Haywood (Eds.), *Developmental follow-up: Concepts, genres, domains, and methods* (pp. 67–112). Orlando, FL: Academic Press.

Chasnoff, I. J. (1993). Missing pieces of the puzzle (commentary). *Neurotoxicology and Teratology, 15*, 287–288.

Chasnoff, I. J., Burns, W. J., Schnoll, S. H., & Burns, K. A. (1985). Cocaine use in pregnancy. *New England Journal of Medicine, 313*(11), 666–669.

Chasnoff, I. J., Griffith, D. R., Freier, C., & Murray, J. (1992). Cocaine/polydrug use in pregnancy: Two-year follow-up. *Pediatrics, 89*(2), 284–289.

Chasnoff, I. J., Landress, H. J., & Barrett, M. E. (1990). The prevalence of illicit-drug or alcohol use during pregnancy and discrepancies in mandatory reporting in Pinellas County, Florida. *New England Journal of Medicine, 322*(17), 1202–1206.

Church, M. W. (1993). Does cocaine cause birth defects? (commentary). *Neurotoxicology and Teratology, 15*, 289.

Cicchetti, D. (1984). The emergence of developmental psychopathology. *Child Development, 55*(1), 1–7.

Coles, C. D. (1993). Saying "goodbye" to the "crack baby." (commentary). *Neurotoxicology and Teratology, 15*, 290–292.

Coles, C. D., & Platzman, K. A. (1993). Behavioral development in children prenatally exposed to drugs and alcohol. *The International Journal of Addictions, 28*(13), 1393–1433.

Day, N. L., & Richardson, G. A. (1993). Cocaine use and crack babies: Science, the media, and miscommunication (commentary). *Neurotoxicology and Teratology, 15*, 293–294.

Dekio, S., & Jidoi, J. (1990). Amounts of fibrous proteins and matrix substances in hairs of different races. *Journal of Dermatology, 17*(1), 62–64.

Dinnies, J., Darr, C., & Saulys, A. (1990). Cocaine toxicity in toddlers. *American Journal of Diseases of Children, 144*, 743–744.

Don, A., Kerns, K., Mateer, C., & Streissguth, A. (1992, June). *Cognitive deficits in non-retarded adults with fetal alcohol syndrome*. Paper presented at the meeting of the Research Society for Alcoholism, San Diego, CA.

Dow-Edwards, D. (1993). The puzzle of cocaine's effects following maternal use during pregnancy: Still unsolved (commentary). *Neurotoxicology and Teratology, 15*, 295–296.

Dow-Edwards, D., Freed, L., & Milhorat, T. (1988). Stimulation of brain metabolism by perinatal cocaine exposure. *Developmental Brain Research, 42*, 137–141.

Fantel, A. G. (1993). Puzzle of cocaine's effects following maternal use during pregnancy: Are there reconcilable differences? (commentary). *Neurotoxicology and Teratology, 15*, 297.

Forman, R., Schneiderman, J., Klein, J., Graham, K., Greenwald, M., & Koren, G. (1992). Accumulation of cocaine in maternal and fetal hair; The dose response curve. *Life Sciences, 50*(18), 1333–1341.

Foss, J. A., & Riley, E. P. (1991). Failure of acute cocaine administration to differentially affect acoustic startle and activity in rats prenatally exposed to cocaine. *Neurotoxicology and Teratology, 13*(5), 547–551.

Frank, D., & Zuckerman, B. (1993). Children exposed to cocaine prenatally: Pieces of the puzzle. (commentary). *Neurotoxicology and Teratology, 15*, 298–300.

Frank, D. A., Zuckerman, B. S., Amaro, H., Aboagye, K., Bauchner, H., Cabral, H., Fried, L., Hingson, R., Kayne, H., & Levenson, S. M. (1988). Cocaine use during pregnancy: Prevalence and correlates. *Pediatrics, 82*(6), 888–895.

Goodwin, G. A., Heyser, C. J., Moody, C. A., Rajachandran, L., Molina, V. A., Arnold, H. M., McKinzie, D. L., Spear, N. E., & Spear, L. P. (1992). A fostering study of effects of prenatal cocaine exposure: II. Offspring behavioral measures. *Neurotoxicology and Teratology, 14*, 423–432.

Graham, K., Koren, G., Klein, J., Schneiderman, J., & Greenwald, M. (1989). Determination of gestational cocaine exposure by hair analysis. *Journal of the American Medical Association, 262,* 3328–3330.

Grant, T., Brown, Z., Callahan, C., Barr, H., & Streissguth, A. (1994). Cocaine exposure during pregnancy: Improving assessment with radioimmunoassay of maternal hair. *Obstetrics & Gynecology, 83,* 524–531.

Greenspan, S. (1991a). Regulatory disorders I: Clinical perspectives. In M. M. Kilbey & K. Asghar (Eds.), *Methodological issues in controlled studies on effects of prenatal exposure to drug abuse* (NIDA Research Monograph), *114,* 165–172.

Greenspan, S. (1991b). Regulatory disorders II: Psychophysiologic perspectives. In M. M. Kilbey & K. Asghar (Eds.), *Methodological issues in controlled studies on effects of prenatal exposure to drug abuse* (NIDA Research Monograph), *114,* 173–181.

Hutchings, D. E. (1993a). The puzzle of cocaine's effects following maternal use during pregnancy: Are there reconcilable differences? (Open peer commentary: Perspective). *Neurotoxicology and Teratology, 15,* 281–286.

Hutchings, D. E. (1993b). Response to commentaries. *Neurotoxicology and Teratology, 15,* 311–312.

Jacobson, J. L. (1991). Discussion: Measurement of drug-induced physical and behavioral delays and abnormalities—A general framework. In M. M. Kilbey & K. Asghar (Eds.), *Methodological issues in controlled studies on effects of prenatal exposure to drug abuse* (NIDA Research Monograph), *114,* 182–186.

Jacobson, J. L., & Jacobson, S. W. (1991). Assessment of teratogenic effects on cognitive and behavioral development in infancy and childhood. In M. M. Kilbey & K. Asghar (Eds.), *Methodological issues in controlled studies on effects of prenatal exposure to drug abuse* (NIDA Research Monograph), *114,* 248–261.

Jacobson, S., Jacobson, J., Sokol, R., Martier, S., & Ager, J. (1993). Prenatal alcohol exposure and infant information processing ability. *Child Development, 64,* 1706–1721.

Kidwell, D. A. (1992). Discussion: Caveats in testing for drugs of abuse. In M. M. Kilbey & K. Asghar (Eds.), *Methodological issues in epidemiological, prevention, and treatment research on drug-exposed women & their children* (NIDA Research Monograph), *117,* 98–120.

Kodituwakku, P., Handmaker, N., Cutler, S., Weathersby, E., Handmaker, S., & Aase, J. (1992, June). *Specific impairments of self-regulation in FAS/FAE: A pilot study.* Paper presented at the meeting of the Research Society for Alcoholism, San Diego, CA.

Kopera-Frye, K., Carmichael Olson, H., & Streissguth, A. (in press). Teratogenic effects of alcohol exposure on attention. In J. Burack & J. Enns (Eds.), *Development, attention, and psychopathology.* New York: Guilford Press.

Koren, G. (1993). Cocaine and the human fetus: The concept of teratophilia (commentary). *Neurotoxicology and Teratology, 15,* 301–304.

Koren, G., Gladstone, D., Robeson, D., & Robieux, I. (1992). The perception of teratogenic risk of cocaine. *Teratology, 46,* 567–571.

Koren, G., Graham, K., Shear, H., & Einarson, T. (1989). Bias against the null hypothesis: The reproductive hazards of cocaine. *Lancet, 2,* 1440–1442.

Koren, G., Klein, J., Forman, R., & Graham, K. (1992). Hair analysis of cocaine: Differentiation between systemic exposure and external contamination. *Journal of Clinical Pharmacology, 32*(7), 671–675.

Kosofsky, B. E. (1991). The effect of cocaine on developing human brain. In M. M. Kilbey & K. Asghar (Eds.), *Methodological issues in controlled studies on effects of prenatal exposure to drug abuse* (NIDA Research Monograph), *114,* 128–143.

Lester, B., Corwin, M. J., Sepkoski, C., Seifer, R., Peucker, M., McLaughlin, S., & Golub, H. L. (1991). Neurobehavioral syndromes in cocaine-exposed infants. *Child Development, 62,* 694–705.

Lutiger, B., Graham, K., Einarson, T. R., & Koren, G. (1991). Relationship between gestational cocaine use and pregnancy outcome: A meta-analysis. *Teratology, 44,* 405–414.

MacGregor, S. N., Keith, L. G., Chasnoff, I. J., Rosner, M. A., Chisum, G. M., Shaw, P., & Minogue, J. P. (1987). Cocaine use during pregnancy: Adverse perinatal outcome. *American Journal of Obstetrics & Gynecology, 157*(3), 686–690.

Magnano, C., Gardner, J., & Karmel, B. (1992). Differences in salivary cortisol levels in cocaine exposed and noncocaine exposed NICU infants. *Developmental Psychobiology, 25,* 92–103.

Marques, P. R., Tippetts, A. S., & Branch, D. G. (1993). Cocaine in the hair of mother–infant pairs: Quantitative analysis and correlations with urine measures and self report. *American Journal of Drug & Alcohol Abuse, 19*(2), 159–175.

Martin, D. C., Martin, J. C., Streissguth, A. P., & Lund, C. A. (1979). Sucking frequency and amplitude in newborns as a function of maternal drinking and smoking. In M. Galanter (Ed.), *Currents in alcoholism* (Vol. 5, pp. 359–366). New York: Grune & Stratton.

Mieczkowski, T. (1992). New approaches in drug testing: A review of hair analysis. *Annals of the American Academy of Social Sciences, 521,* 132–150.

Myers, B. A., Britt, G. C., Lodder, D. E., Kendall, K. A., & Williams-Petersen, M. G. (1992). Effects of cocaine exposure on infant development: A review. *Journal of Child and Family Studies, 1*(4), 393–415.

Neuspiel, D. R. (1993). Cocaine and the fetus: Mythology of severe risk (commentary). *Neurotoxicology and Teratology, 15,* 305–306.

Neuspiel, D. R., & Hamel, S. C. (1991). Cocaine and infant behavior. *Journal of Development and Behavioral Pediatrics, 12*(1), 55–61.

Ostrea, E. M., Jr., Brady, M., Gause, S., Raymundo, A. L., & Stevens, M. (1992). Drug screening of newborns by meconium analysis: A large-scale, prospective, epidemiologic study. *Pediatrics, 89*(1), 107–113.

Ostrea, E. M., Jr., Brady, M. J., Parks, P. M., Asensio, D. C., & Naluz, A. (1989). Drug screening of meconium in infants of drug-dependent mothers: An alternative to urine testing. *Journal of Pediatrics, 115*(3), 474–477.

Richardson, G. A., & Day, N. L. (1994). Detrimental effects of prenatal cocaine exposure: Illusion or reality? *Journal of the American Academy of Child and Adolescent Psychiatry, 33*(1), 28–34.

Richardson, G. A., Day, N. L., & McGaughey, P. J. (1993). The impact of prenatal marijuana and cocaine use on the infant and child. *Clinical Obstetrics and Gynecology, 36*(2), 302–318.

Riley, E. P., & Foss, J. A. (1991a). The acquisition of passive avoidance, active avoidance, and spatial navigation tasks by animals prenatally exposed to cocaine. *Neurotoxicology and Teratology, 13,* 559–564.

Riley, E. P., & Foss, J. A. (1991b). Exploratory behavior and locomotor activity: A failure to find effects in animals prenatally exposed to cocaine. *Neurotoxicology and Teratology, 13,* 553–558.

Robins, L. N., & Mills, J. L. (Eds.). (1993). Effects of in utero exposure to street drugs. *American Journal of Public Health, 83*(Supplement).

Rodning, C., Beckwith, L., & Howard, J. (1989). Characteristics of attachment organization and play organization in prenatally drug-exposed toddlers. *Development and Psychopathology, 1,* 277–289.

Ryan, L., Erlich, S., & Finnegan, L. (1987). Outcome of infants born to cocaine using drug dependent women. *Pediatric Research, 20,* 209A.

Saitoh, M., Uzuka, M., & Sakamoto, M. (1969). Rate of hair growth. *Advances in the Biology of the Skin, 9,* 183–201.

Saxon, A. J., Calsyn, D. A., Haver, V. M., & Delaney, C. J. (1988). Clinical evaluation and use of urine screening for drug abuse. *Western Journal of Medicine, 149*(3), 296–303.

Singer, L. T., Garber, R., & Kliegman, R. (1991). Neurobehavioral sequelae of fetal cocaine exposure. *Journal of Pediatrics, 119*(4), 667–672.

Spear, L. P. (1993). Missing pieces of the puzzle complicate conclusions about cocaine's neurobehavioral toxicity in clinical populations: Importance of animal models (commentary). *Neurotoxicology and Teratology, 15,* 307–309.

Spear, L. P., & Heyser, C. J. (1992). Cocaine and the developing nervous system: Laboratory findings. In I. S. Zagon & T. A. Slotkin (Eds.), *Maternal substance abuse and the developing nervous system* (pp. 155–175). Orlando, FL: Academic Press.

Streissguth, A. P., Barr, H. M., Sampson, P. D., Bookstein, F. L., & Darby, B. L. (1989). Neurobehavioral effects of prenatal alcohol: Part I. Research strategy. *Neurotoxicology and Teratology, 11*, 461–476.

Streissguth, A., Bookstein, F., Sampson, P., & Barr, H. (1993). *The enduring effects of prenatal alcohol exposure on child development: Birth through seven years, a partial least squares solution.* Ann Arbor: University of Michigan Press.

Streissguth, A. P., Grant, T. M., Barr, H. M., Brown, Z. A., Martin, J. C., Mayock, D. E., Ramey, S. L., & Moore, L. (1991). Cocaine and the use of alcohol and other drugs during pregnancy. *American Journal of Obstetrics & Gynecology, 164*(5, Pt. 1), 1239–1243.

Streissguth, A. P., & Giunta, C. T. (1992). Subject recruitment and retention for longitudinal research: Practical considerations for a nonintervention model. In M. M. Kilbey & K. Asghar (Eds.), *Methodological issues in epidemiological, prevention, and treatment research on drug-exposed women and their children* (NIDA Research Monograph), *117*, 137–154.

Streissguth, A. P., Sampson, P. D., Carmichael Olson, H., Bookstein, F. L., Barr, H. M., Scott, M., Feldman, J., & Mirsky, A. (in press). Maternal drinking during pregnancy: Attention and short-term memory in 14-year-old offspring: A longitudinal prospective study. *Alcoholism: Clinical and Experimental Research.*

Stromland, K., Miller, M., & Cook, C. (1991). Ocular teratology. *Surveys in Ophthalmology, 35*(6), 429–446.

Tronick, E., Beeghly, M., Fetters, L., & Weinberg, M. K. (1991). New methodologies for evaluating residual brain damage in infants exposed to drugs of abuse: Objective methods for describing movements, facial expressions, and communicative behaviors. In M. M. Kilbey & K. Asghar (Eds.), *Methodological issues in controlled studies on effects of prenatal exposure to drug abuse* (NIDA Research Monograph), *114*, 262–290.

Volpe, J. J. (1992). Effect of cocaine use on the fetus. *New England Journal of Medicine, 327*(6), 399–407.

Vorhees, C. V. (1986). Principles of behavioral teratogenicity. In E. P. Riley & C. V. Vorhees (Eds.), *Handbook of behavioral teratology.* New York: Plenum.

Ward, S., Schuetz, S., Wachsman, L., Bean, X., Bautista, D., Buckley, S., Sehgal, S., & Warburton, D. (1991). Elevated plasma norepinephrine levels in infants of substance-abusing mothers. *American Journal of Diseases of Children, 145*, 44–48.

Welch, R., Martier, S., Ager, J., Ostrea, E., & Sokol, R. (1990). Radioimmunoassay of hair: A valid technique for determining maternal cocaine abuse. *Substance Abuse, 11*, 214–217.

West, J., Goodlett, C., & Brandt, C. (1990). New approaches to research on the long-term consequences of prenatal exposure to alcohol. *Alcoholism: Clinical and Experimental Research, 14*(5), 684–689.

Zuckerman, B. (1991a). Discussion: Drug effects—A search for mechanisms. In M. M. Kilbey & K. Asghar (Eds.), *Methodological issues in controlled studies on effects of prenatal exposure to drug abuse* (NIDA Research Monograph), *114*, 352–362.

Zuckerman, B. (1991b). Selected methodologic issues in investigations of prenatal effect of cocaine: Lessons from the past. In M. M. Kilbey & K. Asghar (Eds.), *Methodological issues in controlled studies on effects of prenatal exposure to drug abuse* [NIDA Research Monograph], *114*, 45–54.

Zuckerman, B., Amaro, H., & Cabral, H. (1989). Validity of self-reporting of marijuana and cocaine use among pregnant adolescents. *Journal of Pediatrics, 115*(5, Pt. 1), 812–815.

9

▼▼▼▼▼▼▼

Measuring the Effects of Prenatal Cocaine Exposure

Margaret Bendersky
Robert Wood Johnson Medical School

Steven M. Alessandri
Medical College of Pennsylvania

Margaret Wolan Sullivan
Michael Lewis
Robert Wood Johnson Medical School

The effects of prenatal exposure to cocaine are of great interest to the research, clinical, and educational communities. As Vorhees and Neuspiel report in this volume, there have been few striking, consistent findings reported thus far in either animal or human studies. It is our belief that the failure to find robust results, particularly in human follow-up studies, is related to three problems inherent in this type of research: identification and quantification of drug use, confounding variables, and insensitive and limited outcome measures.

IDENTIFICATION AND QUANTIFICATION OF DRUG USE

Identifying the specifics of maternal drug use presents a methodological problem for studies of prenatal exposure. It is evident that amount, timing over the course of gestation, pattern of use, and use of other substances that might potentiate the effects of cocaine, are impossible to ascertain reliably for every drug user given the current state of technology. (See Ostrea, chap. 10, this volume, for a more detailed presentation of these issues.) Moreover, animal models cannot adequately address all of the issues of timing, route of administration, and drug use pattern. These problems are discussed more fully in other chapters of this volume.

CONFOUNDING VARIABLES

The effects of the multitude of variables other than substance use that tend to covary with a drug-using lifestyle, and that are related to developmental outcome presents another difficulty. The offspring of drug users are at high risk of developmental problems from such prenatal factors as poor maternal nutrition, high maternal stress levels, and poor maternal health, to list but a few. There are similarly numerous postnatal variables, known to impact a child's development, which may not be optimal for the children of drug users. These include obvious extreme conditions, such as neglect or exposure to violence as victim or witness. There may be inconsistent and numerous caregivers, and the child may have no one with whom to engage in sensitive, responsive, and appropriately stimulating interactions. Most of the children we study live in materially impoverished conditions, and are thus at risk due to suboptimal environments even without being exposed to toxins. Studies have not always considered confounding variables or have controlled for very few. The Jacobsons, Neuspiel, and other contributors to this volume, discuss this issue further.

MEASURING OUTCOMES

The third problem is the relative scarcity of studies that have considered sufficiently sensitive and wide-ranging outcome measures. The majority of human studies of prenatal cocaine exposure to date have examined only two measures—the Brazelton Neonatal Behavioral Assessment Scale, and the Bayley Scales of Infant Development. Studies examining performance on the Brazelton have failed to replicate a pattern of significant findings (e.g., Chasnoff, Burns, Schnoll, & Burns, 1985; Coles, Platzman, Smith, James, & Falek, 1992; Eisen et al., 1991; Mayes, Granger, Frank, Schottenfeld, & Bornstein, 1993; Neuspiel & Hamel, 1991). Moreover, the stability and long-term significance of a single Brazelton score obtained soon after birth have been questioned (Brazelton, 1987). Similarly, Bayley scores in the average range have poor predictive validity (Bornstein & Sigman, 1986; Lewis & McGurk, 1972; McCall, Hogarty, & Hurlburt, 1972). In addition, global or aggregate measures of functioning, such as those derived from the Bayley, often mask more specific deficits, for example language or fine motor problems. The issue of measuring outcome has not been addressed extensively and is the focus of this chapter.

MEASURE OR MEASURES: THE VALUE
OF MULTIPLE, SENSITIVE, AND PREDICTIVE
OUTCOMES

Single global measures of ability, such as IQ, generally assess skill across a variety of functional domains. These usually include language, perception, fine motor, visual-motor integration, memory, and abstract reasoning. Whereas a massive, early insult to the brain may result in general deficits of cognitive and motor functioning, most insults affect much more circumscribed regions or systems of the brain. In addition, central nervous system (CNS) development is relatively lengthy and the timing of a perturbation is an important determinant of impact. Therefore, the majority of insults would be expected to have relatively specific developmental sequelae. An IQ score is analogous to pureeing potatoes, zucchini, onions, and turnips. Various felicitous combinations will produce a decent tasting soup, but will make individual flavors indistinguishable. If perturbation X causes a deficit in Skill A but not Skill B, and the subject is unusually good at Skill B, it would appear that X had no effect at all on the total A + B ability. Thus, limiting our outcome measure to IQ may mask specific effects of particular perturbations.

Another problem of the IQ score is that the tests rely on motor ability in the first 18 months of life, but at older ages, depend on language competence for adequate performance. Thus, an IQ score for an infant informs us mostly about fine motor ability, and for an older child, about language competence. This is one of the reasons that infant IQ scores are not predictive of later ones; that is, early motor ability may be unrelated to language skill (Lewis, Jaskir, & Enright, 1986; Lewis & McGurk, 1972; McCall, Eichorn, & Hogarty, 1977).

It seems clear that we must measure many different functions to begin to study the specific impact of a particular insult such as prenatal cocaine exposure. The region or system of the brain affected by a perturbation, whether the impact is discrete or global, and its timing during CNS development are all likely to affect whether and what specific functional deficits may result. In addition, the young brain is inherently plastic and may have the capacity to compensate for damage, especially if the external environment provides appropriate stimulation (Lee & Barratt, 1993).

In a study of the effects of intraventricular hemorrhage (IVH) on the development of preterm infants, we have taken an approach that underscores the value of using multiple outcomes and accounting for the effect of several confounding variables. As IVH is, like prenatal cocaine exposure, an early CNS insult associated with both specific and diffuse effects on the CNS, this model may be applicable to drug exposure follow-up studies.

Although IVH appears to be a well-defined insult, like prenatal cocaine exposure, it does not usually occur in isolation. Neonates who develop IVH tend to have many other complications of prematurity, especially developmental breathing problems such as respiratory distress syndrome and apnea. These problems may independently affect brain development. Therefore, we have included another measure of biological insult, the number of other common complications of prematurity, along with IVH severity, in our analytic model. As developmental outcome clearly is associated with environmental conditions, and as IVH covaries somewhat with socioeconomic status (SES) due to the mutual association of these variables with low birth weight, measures of environmental risk also have been included in our model (Bendersky & Lewis, 1994; Lewis & Bendersky, 1989).

Thus, we have embraced a model of development of these high-risk infants, applicable to the cocaine-exposed infant, which acknowledges the potential impact of other biological and environmental risk factors even in the face of a relatively specific medical complication. Moreover, our use of a variety of developmental outcomes at different ages allows us to see what outcomes may be related to IVH alone, those related to other biological insults, poor parenting or low SES, and those related to the interaction of these factors. Analyses of attentional, motoric, sensorimotor, language, and abstract visual reasoning abilities over the age span 3 months to 3 years, have produced a fairly cohesive picture of the specific effects of IVH (Bendersky & Lewis, 1991, 1994; Lewis & Bendersky, 1989). It appears that by 3 years of age, IVH itself has sequelae limited to the motor system when the effects of more general medical condition at birth and the family environment are controlled. It is primarily children who had associated white matter lesions who continue to have motor problems.

Figure 9.1 illustrates the amount of variance explained by each of the three types of predictor variables—IVH, general medical condition, and environmental risk—on language, abstract and visual reasoning, and quantitative and motor skill at 3 years of age. IVH primarily explained some of the variance in the motor and language abilities, and the number of other medical complications suffered during the neonatal period (Medical Complications Score; MCS) explained variance in motor, language, and abstract and visual reasoning skills. The environment explained the most variance in language and quantitative ability. It is clear that the independent effects of IVH are very circumscribed. The cumulative impact of other medical complications of prematurity and environmental risk surpass the specific effect of IVH on developmental consequences.

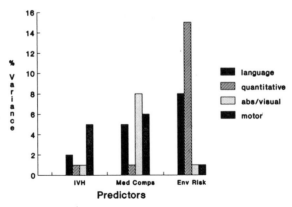

FIG. 9.1. Variance explained in 3-year outcome measures by IVH, general medical condition, and environmental risk.

These findings have several implications generalizable to the study of effects of prenatal drug exposure. First, it is important to have measures of other prenatal or neonatal conditions that may have similar developmental effects. In the case of substance abuse, such variables as exposure to nicotine, prenatal nutrition, exposure to disease organisms, or medical complications of prematurity should be controlled when looking for specific drug exposure effects. Second, postnatal environmental factors must be controlled, lest they become hidden, confounding variables that themselves alone explain the variability in developmental outcome. In this case, outcome differences may be falsely attributed to prenatal drug exposure because drug use is associated with suboptimal environmental conditions. Third, multiple, specific outcomes, related if possible to theoretically predicted functional deficits, must be assessed in order to understand the specific effects of drug exposure, as well as to shed light on the mechanisms of effect.

Having rejected IQ, what kinds of measures of functioning of cocaine-exposed children should we use? Ideally, they should measure specific functions, have a theoretical connection with prenatal cocaine exposure, have long-term functional significance, and have a reliable test procedure. Such capacities as attention, learning, memory, emotional responsivity, and regulation appear to be appropriate areas of inquiry.

Our laboratory has used contingency learning and its emotional concomitants to study early cognitive development in normal samples of infants. We have begun to apply this methodology to the study of the effects of prenatal cocaine exposure as an appropriate alternative to more global measures of function.

LEARNING AND EMOTION AS MEASURES OF INFANT FUNCTIONING

Unlike standardized infant development assessment instruments that measure attainment of developmental milestones and show very poor predictive validity, contingency learning is a measure of the fundamental ability to associate a voluntary behavior with its consequence. Our procedure is language free, requires minimal motor control, and is self-motivating. Moreover, studies of learning in rats have suggested that there is a specific effect of cocaine exposure on brain mechanisms for learning and reward (Heyser, Chen, Miller, Spear, & Spear, 1990; Heyser, Spear, & Spear, 1992; Spear, Kirstein, & Frambes, 1989; Spear et al., 1989). These studies suggest that early learning and accompanying affective responses may be critical functions on which prenatal cocaine exposure has specific effects.

Learning procedures are particularly appealing as measures of infant information processing. They not only tap the subject's ability to form expected associations, but also can be readily employed to study the development and maintenance of motivational systems. They have been used for this purpose in the animal literature for decades. Some of the classic animal paradigms have served as models for human motivational systems. For example, the phenomenon of learned helplessness originated in the animal literature and has found application as a model of depression in the human clinical literature.

Apart from a few early studies of conditioned fear (Watson & Rayner, 1920) and smiling (Brackbill, 1958), the study of learning and emotion proceeded independently in infant research. With the advent of video technology and the development of coding systems for emotion based on facial musculature, more objective coding of infant facial expression is possible (Ekman & Oster, 1979; Izard, 1983). We now have the opportunity to combine traditional learning methods with a very untraditional and uniquely human measure, human facial expression. Before describing our work with cocaine-exposed infants we review the procedures and data on learning and emotion developed in our laboratory.

To study learning in young infants, we use pulling or arm retraction as the target response. Infants between the ages of 2 and 8 months are seated in an infant seat in the apparatus and a ribbon connected to a microswitch is attached to their wrists (see Fig. 9.2). Infants typically do not reach toward and grasp objects until the fourth to fifth month of life. Before this time, however, gross movements of the arm are frequent during infant play activity. Sensitive microswitches, mounted so as to register movement toward the infant's body, record pulls automatically. The need to grasp is avoided by having infants wear an elastic wristlet, which fits snugly and allows the ribbon to be quickly and easily connected to the baby's wrist. Ribbon tension is set so that hand-to-mouth activity alone will not trigger stimulus onset.

Pulling the ribbon produces a colored slide of a smiling infant and a few bars of the Sesame Street theme for 3 sec. The stimulus comes on every time the

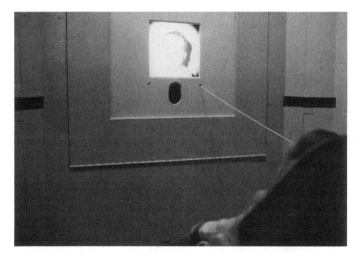

FIG. 9.2. An infant seated in the contingency apparatus, pulling to trigger a burst of slides and music.

string is pulled. Multiple responses occurring within the 3-sec reinforcement window do not prolong the period of stimulation but are registered. (Further details about the test apparatus can be found in Lewis, Sullivan, & Brooks-Gunn, 1985.)

In our initial investigations, we reported that infants found the procedure interesting and were willing to remain in the experimental apparatus for a considerable length of time provided they controlled the stimulus. Figure 9.3 tracks subject loss during testing over time. Subjects were removed from the apparatus if they cried continuously for 60 sec, dozed for 60 sec, or were inactive for 2.5 min. The graph contrasts time remaining in the experiment for a group of infants who received the contingency (contingent) and a group of control infants who received matched rates of the slide–music presentation independent of their pulling (noncontingent). The figure shows that in the noncontingent group subjects began to drop out of the experiment quite dramatically after 4 min, whereas loss from the contingent group was more gradual and exceeded 10% only after 10 min. The longest time logged by a noncontingent subject was 20 min; the longest time recorded by a contingent subject who remained active and awake throughout this time was 36 min. Presumably, this difference in motivation occurs because infants in the contingent group have learned to control the outcome, whereas the noncontingent group has not.

The major age-related difference in responding, replicated now in several studies, is that older infants pull at greater rates because they are stronger, better

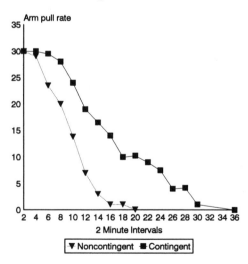

FIG. 9.3. Subject loss under conditions of either contingent or noncontingent presentation of slides and music. The graph shows the number of subjects completing 2-minute intervals in the apparatus without fussing.

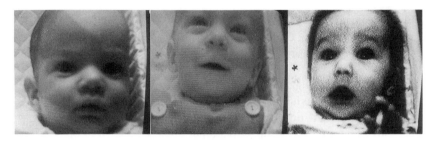

FIG. 9.4. Three positive facial expressions (MAX-coded): Excited Interest
(24/33/51); Enjoyment (0/33/52); and Surprise (20/30/50).

coordinated and more active. It is also the case that the response curves of
contingent and noncontingent infants diverge later in the procedure for the
2-month-old infants than for the older age groups. However, it appears that the
infants learn that they control the stimulus within 3 to 4 min at all ages studied
(Lewis et al., 1985).

In order to study the motivational system as well as learning ability, we
simultaneously videotape full-face close-ups of the infants as they respond in the
procedure. These tapes are subsequently coded using the Maximally Discriminative Facial Coding System for Infants and Young Children (MAX; Izard, 1983).
In brief, the system allows for independent coding of changes in facial musculature in each of three regions of the face (brows, eye/cheek, and mouth). MAX
formulas are then used to objectively determine which distinctive facial expression or blend has occurred.

Figure 9.4 shows the different positive facial expressions commonly observed
in our work. Each of these expressions is usually observed during learning. They
are from left to right: excited interest, enjoyment, and surprise.

Because we are interested in points of change during learning, we initially
examined individual learning curves to determine how to best sample emotion.
Figure 9.5 shows a learning curve produced by a 6-month-old infant in our
procedure. The response curve of an infant of the same age and gender is also
shown. This infant received the same amount of stimulation, but it was not related
to his arm movements. Despite individual differences in response rate, the
learning curves of infants in our study shared several characteristics that are
nicely illustrated in the contingent subject's curve. First, infants typically show
a period early in the learning session (Point 2) when responding is at, or may
fall below, baseline (designated Point 1), as shown by Point 2. This is followed
by a rapid acceleration of response (Points 3 and 4), a period of maximally
elevated responding (Points 5, 6, and 7) and a period of decline (Point 8). Finally,
the baby's level of response typically returns to baseline levels (Point 9). The
operational definitions for each of these points are provided in the figure legend.
Each of these points could be identified in learning curves across all infant age
groups. These points during the procedure were then coded for infant facial

Pulling Over Minutes

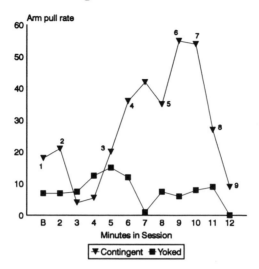

FIG. 9.5. Typical response curves of a matched contingent/noncontingent pair of infants showing transition points of interest during learning: 1—baseline (1 minute in apparatus with no consequences); 2—first minute of contingency; 3—one minute prior to acceleration (point at which responding first exceeds and remains above base); 4—first minute of acceleration; 5—1 minute prior to attainment of peak rate; 6—first minute at peak; 7—1 minute prior to sustained decline in response rate; 8—first minute of decline; 9—last minute of the session.

expression. Our hypothesis was that emotions would vary across these selected points because response rates, and presumably attendant cognitions, were changing, and that maximum enjoyment was likely to co-occur with the peak response—a sign of contingency mastery. The data for 4- and 6-month-olds, described by Sullivan and Lewis (1989) are summarized briefly here. All expressions observed (interest, surprise, enjoyment, sadness, fear, and anger) showed significant changes across the phases of the learning curves. The patterns, with the exception of one expression (anger), were similar.

For purposes of discussion, the 6-month data are presented in Fig. 9.6. Interest and surprise are greatest before the peak response and decline gradually thereafter. Enjoyment occurs at its greatest levels at the point of peak responding. All positive expressions have declined by the final minute when pull responses have also declined. Negative expressions occur rarely across all minutes when the infant is engaged in the task, but increase as pulling declines, presumably because of fatigue or boredom. Fear, expressed predominantly as fear/interest blends, and some sadness, occur at low levels prior to or early in the acceleration phase. The infant may not as yet understand the contingency at this early stage in learning and may be startled by its onset, hence the expression of some negative emotion.

A. Positive Expressions over Selected   B. Negative Expressions over Selected
   Points in the Learning Curve   Points in the Learning Curve

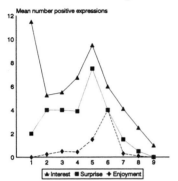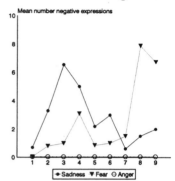

FIG. 9.6. Positive and negative facial expressions (MAX-coded) of 24-week-olds
($n = 10$) observed during particular phases of the learning curve.

In more recent work, we have examined negative expressions in greater detail by studying infants' emotional responses when the expected contingency between pull response and interesting outcome is stopped (Alessandri, Sullivan, & Lewis, 1990; Lewis, Alessandri, & Sullivan, 1990; Sullivan, Lewis, & Alessandri, 1992). After a short training period in which infants meet a learning criterion, the contingency is interrupted for 2 minutes. The slide and music will not turn on during this period (extinction). Thereafter the contingency is reinstated. The data from several investigations have consistently shown that pull responses increase during this period, as the infant initially attempts to reinstate the contingency. Figure 9.7 shows data for a group of subjects who persisted through two extinction and two relearning periods. Pull responses increase in rate during extinction, return to the level of the initial contingent phase with the restoration of the contingency, and increase again during the second extinction phase.

The emotional responsivity of infants during extinction is also of interest. Frustration in response to the inability to turn on the stimulus can be expected to produce an increase in negative affect. But the pattern of facial expressions is telling. Anger, but not other negative expressions, increases significantly (Lewis et al., 1990; Sullivan et al., 1992). Figure 9.8 shows this effect for the contingent and the noncontingent control groups. Noncontingent subjects show little anger as can be seen in the figure. For contingent subjects, the increase in anger during extinction is seen at every age, although the number of anger expressions is greater in older subjects. Joy, as measured by infant smiling, shows exactly the opposite pattern. It is high during periods of contingency, and absent during extinction (see Lewis et al., 1990, for further discussion of these data).

Our work shows that contingency learning procedures offer a window not only on the information processing abilities of the young infant, but also on

Pulling Over Learning Phases

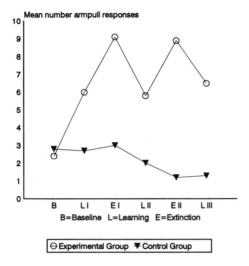

Mean number armpull responses

B=Baseline L=Learning E=Extinction

⊖ Experimental Group ▼ Control Group

FIG. 9.7.   Increases in pulling observed in 4–8-month-old subjects exposed to multiple alternating blocks of either contingent or noncontingent stimulation (LI, LII, LIII) and extinction (EI, EII)

Anger Expressions During Learning and Extinction

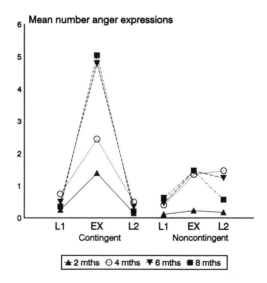

Mean number anger expressions

Contingent   Noncontingent

▲ 2 mths ⊖ 4 mths ▼ 6 mths ■ 8 mths

FIG. 9.8.   Expressions of anger observed during learning and extinction at each of four ages.

173

emerging motivational systems. Responses to frustration are readily studied during periods of extinction or whenever a learned expectancy is violated.

LEARNING AND EMOTION IN COCAINE-EXPOSED INFANTS: A PILOT STUDY

The extensive experience of our laboratory using this contingency learning method with samples of normal infants permitted us to apply it to the question of whether in utero cocaine exposure has an impact on early learning and its emotional concomitants in humans. A sample of 72 4- to 8-month-old infants, half of whom had been prenatally exposed to cocaine, were studied. The procedure was identical to that used in our previous studies. The rates of pulling, frequency of each emotional expression, and amount of fretting during Baseline, Learning 1, Extinction, and Learning 2 were compared for the two groups of infants—exposed and unexposed. (For a complete description of method and results see Alessandri, Sullivan, Imaizumi, & Lewis, 1993.)

Figure 9.9 displays the pull responses for each phase as a function of cocaine exposure group. There were three major differences in the contingency learning of the infants exposed to cocaine compared with their unexposed counterparts. First, the infants exposed to cocaine showed less overall activity, as evidenced by a lower rate of pulling over the entire procedure. Second, although the groups did not differ in pulling during Baseline and Learning 1, the exposed infants did not show the expected increase in pulling during the Extinction period. Finally, the unexposed subjects decreased their response rate when the contingency was reinstated (Learning 2) to a level similar to that during Learning 1. The exposed subjects, however, decreased their pulling to the baseline level. This last finding suggests that cocaine-exposed infants were unmotivated to continue exploring the contingent outcome. After mild frustration, they simply gave up.

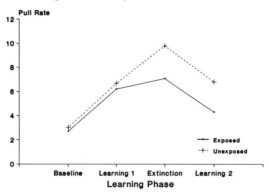

FIG. 9.9. Rates of pulling by cocaine-exposed and unexposed infants during learning and extinction.

The emotion results parallel the learning findings. Figure 9.10 presents the frequencies of positive emotional expressions (i.e., interest and enjoyment) and anger expressions for each phase as a function of exposure group. There were fewer positive and negative expressions overall in the cocaine-exposed group. Exposed infants showed significantly less interest and joy during the initial learning phase compared with the nonexposed subjects. Moreover, there were fewer negative emotional behaviors when the machine stopped "paying off" (extinction). The predominant negative expression observed during extinction was anger. Sad expressions occurred with low frequency during extinction in the unexposed group, replicating our earlier results for normal infants (Lewis et al., 1990). Sad expressions were virtually absent in the exposed group, which in addition, showed significantly less fussing than the control group over the entire procedure.

A. Positive Expressions

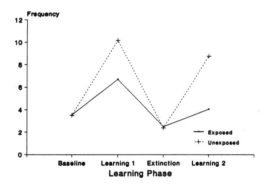

B. Anger Expressions

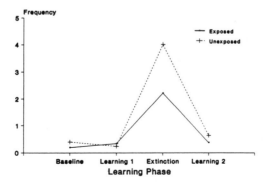

FIG. 9.10.   Frequencies of total positive expressions and anger by cocaine-exposed and unexposed infants during learning and extinction.

Given the possible confounding effects of compromised infant health status and exposure to other potentially harmful substances in utero on learning behavior, analyses were conducted to control for newborn growth characteristics and maternal use of alcohol and cigarettes during pregnancy. The results indicated that cocaine exposure group was the *only* significant predictor of pull rate and frequency of positive or negative expressions during the different phases of the procedure.

Taken together, the findings for the pulling, facial expressions, and fussing suggest that the cocaine-exposed infants were less engaged by the contingency task. Although their pattern of responses paralleled those of the unexposed subjects, the cocaine-exposed infants were much less aroused. Problems with arousal may represent an underlying difficulty with sustained sensory processing and may be related to childhood hyperactivity or learning disabilities at school age (Doyle, 1975). Moreover, an increase in expressions of joy when a problem is mastered is thought to reflect an infant's active cognitive engagement and a sense of efficacy (Lewis et al., 1990; Lewis & Goldberg, 1969; Piaget, 1952; Sullivan & Lewis, 1989; Watson, 1972; White, 1959). Its absence in the exposed group suggests that these infants are unchallenged or unrewarded by the contingency. Finally, the lack of a vigorous reaction to the discontinuation of the contingency, and the failure to respond when the contingency is reinstated, corroborates this lack of motivation to persevere in the face of obstacles. This may be a pattern that places children at risk of failing to develop feelings of competency and mastery motivation (Lewis & Goldberg, 1969; White, 1959).

The lack of emotional responsivity in cocaine-exposed infants has implications for social development as well. Mother–infant interactions are generally characterized by synchronous behavior that results in mutually optimal stimulation levels (Brazelton, Koslowski, & Main, 1974; Stern, 1974). Our results suggest this contingency, reciprocity, and synchrony may be problematic for cocaine-exposed infants. Given the low level of arousal and lack of emotional responsivity seen in response to a contingency that normally is quite enjoyable for young infants, we think that exposed infants may respond with similarly flat affect to the social contingencies present in parent–child interactions. If so, the caregiving relationship may be unsatisfying for the parent. Caregivers of cocaine-exposed infants may be less successful in maintaining the infants' attention and arousal. They also may have difficulty eliciting affective behaviors such as smiles and coos that are necessary for continued engagement (Osofsky, 1976; Osofsky & Danzger, 1974). Furthermore, the feelings of frustration and inadequacy that parents may experience in dealing with apparently unresponsive infants may predispose them to child maltreatment, as has been seen in other high-risk infant groups (Garbarino & Gilliam, 1981).

The results of this preliminary study indicate that cocaine exposure during gestation may specifically influence arousal, engagement in a contingency task, and emotional responsivity in the first year of life. Further study of discrete domains of infant functioning, such as attention, learning, memory, emotional responsivity, and regulation, may be the most fruitful approach to understanding specific problems associated with in utero cocaine exposure.

ACKNOWLEDGMENT

This work was supported by a grant from the National Institute on Drug Abuse, #R01DA07109, to Michael Lewis.

REFERENCES

Alessandri, S. M., Sullivan, M. W., Imaizumi, S., & Lewis, M. (1993). Learning and emotional responsivity in cocaine exposed infants. *Developmental Psychology, 29*, 989–997.

Alessandri, S. M., Sullivan, M. W., & Lewis, M. (1990). Violation of expectancy and frustration in early infancy. *Developmental Psychology, 26*, 738–744.

Bendersky, M., & Lewis, M. (1991, April). *Effects of IVH, other medical complications, and environmental risk on development at age three.* Paper presented at the Society for Research in Child Development, Seattle, WA.

Bendersky, M., & Lewis, M. (1994). Environmental risk, medical risk, and cognition. *Developmental Psychology, 30*, 484–494.

Bornstein, M. H., & Sigman, M. D. (1986). Continuity in mental development from infancy. *Child Development, 57*, 251–274.

Brackbill, Y. (1958). Extinction of smiling responses in infants as a function of reinforcement schedule. *Child Development, 29*, 115–124.

Brazelton, T. B. (1987). Neonatal behavioral assessment scale. In J. D. Osofsky (Ed.), *Handbook of infant development* (pp. 780–817). New York: Wiley.

Brazelton, T. B., Koslowski, B., & Main, M. (1974). The origins of reciprocity: The early mother–infant interaction. In M. Lewis & L. Rosenblum (Eds.), *The effect of the infant on its caretaker: The origins of behavior* (Vol. 1, pp. 49–76). New York: Wiley.

Chasnoff, I., Burns, W., Schnoll, S., & Burns, K. (1985). Cocaine use in pregnancy. *New England Journal of Medicine, 313*, 666–669.

Coles, C., Platzman, K., Smith, I., James, M., & Falek, A. (1992). Effects of cocaine and alcohol use in pregnancy on neonatal growth and neurobehavioral status. *Neurotoxicology and Teratology, 14*, 23–33.

Doyle, A. (1975). Infant development in daycare. *Developmental Psychology, 11*, 655–656.

Ekman, P., & Oster, H. (1979). Facial expressions of emotion. *Annual Review of Psychology, 30*, 527–554.

Eisen, L., Field, T., Bandstra, E., Roberts, J., Morrow, C., Larson, S., & Steele, B. (1991). Perinatal cocaine effects on neonatal stress behavior and performance on the Brazelton scale. *Pediatrics, 88*, 477–480.

Garbarino, J., & Gilliam, G. (1981). *Understanding abusive families.* Lexington, MA: Lexington Press.

Heyser, C., Chen, W., Miller, J., Spear, N., & Spear, L. (1990). Prenatal cocaine exposure induces deficits in Pavlovian conditioning and sensory preconditioning among infant rat pups. *Behavioral Neuroscience, 104*, 955–963.

Heyser, C., Spear, N., & Spear, L. (1992). Effects of prenatal exposure to cocaine on conditional discrimination learning in adult rats. *Behavioral Neuroscience, 106*, 837–845.

Izard, C. E. (1983). *The maximally discriminative facial coding system (MAX), (Revised)*. Newark: University of Delaware, Instructional Resources Center.

Lee, H., & Barratt, M. S. (1993). Cognitive development of preterm low birthweight children at 5 to 8 years old. *Journal of Developmental and Behavioral Pediatrics, 14*, 242–249.

Lewis, M., Alessandri, S. M., & Sullivan, M. W. (1990). Violation of expectancy, loss of control, and anger expressions in young infants. *Developmental Psychology, 26*, 745–751.

Lewis, M., & Bendersky, M. (1989). Cognitive and motor differences among low birth weight infants: The impact of IVH, medical risk, and social class. *Pediatrics, 83*, 187–192.

Lewis, M., & Goldberg, S. (1969). Perceptual-cognitive development in infancy: A generalized expectancy model as a function of the mother–infant interaction. *Merrill-Palmer Quarterly, 15*, 81–100.

Lewis, M., Jaskir, J., & Enright, M. (1986). Development of mental abilities in infancy. *Intelligence, 10*, 331–354.

Lewis, M., & McGurk, H. (1972). Evaluation of infant intelligence: Infant intelligence scores—true or false? *Science, 178*, 1174–1177.

Lewis, M., Sullivan, M. W., & Brooks-Gunn, J. (1985). Emotional behavior during the learning of a contingency in early infancy. *British Journal of Development, 4*, 307–316.

Mayes, L., Granger, R., Frank, M. A., Schottenfeld, R., & Bornstein, M. (1993). Neurobehavioral profiles of neonates exposed to cocaine prenatally. *Pediatrics, 91*, 778–783.

McCall, R. B., Eichorn, D. H., & Hogarty, P. S. (1977). Transitions in early mental development. *Monographs of the Society for Research in Child Development, 42*.

McCall, R. B., Hogarty, P. S., & Hurlburt, N. (1972). Transitions in infant sensori-motor development and the prediction of childhood IQ. *American Psychologist, 27*, 728–748.

Neuspiel, D., & Hamel, S. (1991). Cocaine and infant behavior. *Journal of Developmental and Behavioral Pediatrics, 12*, 55–64.

Osofsky, J. D. (1976). Neonatal characteristics and mother–infant interaction in two observational situations. *Child Development, 47*, 1138–1147.

Osofsky, J. D., & Danzger, B. (1974). Relationships between neonatal characteristics and mother–infant interaction. *Developmental Psychology, 10*, 124–130.

Piaget, J. (1952). *The origins of intelligence in children*. New York: International Universities Press.

Spear, L., Kirstein, C., Bell, J., Yoottanasumpun, V., Greenbaum, R., O'Shea, J., Hoffmann, H., & Spear, N. (1989). Effects of prenatal cocaine exposure on behavior during the early postnatal period. *Neurotoxicology and Teratology, 11*, 57–63.

Spear, L., Kirstein, C., & Frambes, N. (1989). Cocaine effects on the developing nervous system: Behavioral, psychopharmacological, and neurochemical studies. *Annals of the New York Academy of Science, 562*, 290–307.

Stern, D. N. (1974). The goal and structure of mother–infant play. *Journal of the American Academy of Child Psychiatry, 13*, 402–421.

Sullivan, M. W., & Lewis, M. (1989). Emotion and cognition in infancy: Facial expressions during contingency learning. *Journal of Behavioral Development, 12*, 221–237.

Sullivan, M. W., Lewis, M., & Alessandri, S. M. (1992). Cross-age stability in emotional expressions during learning and extinction. *Developmental Psychology, 28*, 58–63.

Watson, J. B., & Rayner, R. (1920). Conditioned emotional reactions. *Journal of Experimental Psychology, 3*, 1–14.

Watson, T. (1972). Smiling, cooing, and the game. *Merrill-Palmer Quarterly, 18*, 323–339.

White, R. W. (1959). Motivation reconsidered: The concept of competence. *Psychological Review, 66*, 297–333.

10
▼▼▼▼▼▼▼

Meconium Drug Analysis

Enrique M. Ostrea, Jr.
Wayne State University

According to a national survey in 1990, about 4.8 million women used some form of illicit drugs (Khalsa & Gfroerer, 1991). A sizable portion of this population are women of childbearing age or pregnant women. It has been reported that the prevalence of drug abuse among pregnant women ranges between 0.4% to 27% (Chasnoff, 1989). These figures are probably underestimated, because recently, we found in a large survey of infants delivered at our hospital, that 42% of the infants were exposed to cocaine, heroin, or cannabinoids in contrast to the 10.5% rate of illicit drug use in the same population obtained by maternal self report (Ostrea, Brady, Gause, Raymundo, & Stevens, 1992).

Drug abuse during pregnancy is a major health problem because the associated perinatal complications are high. These include a high incidence of stillbirths, meconium-stained fluid, premature rupture of the membranes, maternal hemorrhage (abruptio placenta or placenta praevia), and fetal distress (Chasnoff, Burns, Schnoll, & Burns, 1985; McGregor et al., 1987; Oro & Dixon, 1987; Ostrea & Chavez, 1979). For the newborn infant, the mortality rate, as well as morbidity (e.g., asphyxia, prematurity, low birth weight, hyaline membrane disease, infections, aspiration pneumonia, congenital malformations, cerebral infarction, abnormal heart rate and breathing patterns, drug withdrawal, and risk to acquired immunodeficiency disease) are also increased (Chasnoff, Hunt, Kletter, & Kaplan, 1989; Chasnoff, Bussy, Savich, & Stack, 1986; Fulroth, Phillips, & Durand, 1989; Oleske et al., 1983; Ostrea, Chavez, & Strauss, 1976; Ostrea, Kresbach, Knapp, & Simkowski, 1987; Ryan, Ehrlich, & Finnegan, 1987; Zelson, Rubio, & Wasserman, 1971; Zuckerman et al., 1989). Long-term sequelae are not uncommon and include delays in physical growth and mental development, sudden infant death syndrome, and learning disabilities (Chasnoff, Hatcher, & Burns, 1982; Chavez, Ostrea, Stryker, & Smialek, 1979; Chavez, Ostrea, Stryker, & Strauss, 1979; Wilson, 1989; Wilson, McCreary, Kean, & Baxter, 1979). Because of these immediate and long-term problems, infants born to women who have abused drugs during pregnancy should be identified soon after birth so that appropriate intervention and follow-up with the infants can be done. For other reasons, an accurate identification of neonates exposed to drugs, in utero, is important. For instance, the data is vital for epidemiologic surveys, for the identification of women who need postnatal support, to assess the effectiveness of programs designed to reduce the incidence of drug abuse among pregnant women, and so on.

Unfortunately, the identification of the drug-exposed neonate is not easy. Many of the drugs to which the fetus is exposed, in utero, do not produce immediate or recognizable effects in the neonates (Kandall & Gartner, 1974) Maternal admission of drug use is often inaccurate because of fear of the consequences stemming from such admission. Even with maternal cooperation, such information regarding the type and extent of drug use is often inaccurate (Ostrea et al., 1992). One alternative is to test the infant's urine for drugs, but this procedure has its limitations, because successful detection of drug metabolites in the infant's urine is dependent on time of the last drug intake by the mother, or if obtained after birth, when the infant's urine was collected (Halstead, Godolphin, Lockitch, & Segal, 1988). The high rate of false negative results in neonatal urine tests often arise from the mother's abstention from the use of the drug a few days before she delivers or to the inability to obtain a sample of the infant's urine soon after birth. Recently, analysis of the infant's hair for drugs has been used (Graham, Koren, Klein, Schneiderman, & Greenwald, 1989). Technical problems in analysis and sample collection make this method impractical at the moment (Bailey, 1989).

In the last 2 years, we have successfully developed a new method for identifying the exposure of infants to drugs during pregnancy by the detection of drug metabolites in their meconium. Meconium is the green stool of the newborn formed in utero and excreted within a few days after birth. This narrative highlights the chronology of the studies that have demonstrated the usefulness and sensitivity of the meconium drug test.

ANIMAL STUDIES

The concept behind meconium drug testing was based on our initial studies in animals, which showed that a high concentration of the metabolites of drugs that the pregnant animal was exposed to during pregnancy were found in the gastrointestinal tract of their fetuses. The index study (Ostrea, Lynn, Wayne, & Stryker,

TABLE 10.1
Distribution of Morphine in the Tissues of Addicted Newborn Monkeys

	Monkey Fetus					
	#1	#2	#3	#4	#5	#6
Gestational age (days)	118	125	135	147	155	161
Total maternal morphine (g)	11.9	14.8	13.6	17.9	19.4	15.7
Fetal Tissue Concentration of Morphine (µg/g tissue)						
Intestines	15.8	128.9	108.4	53.7	68.4	42.1
Liver	0	0	0	47.6	169.5	0
Cerebellum	–	–	–	17.2	46.2	–
Heart	15.7	37.9	–	73.9	9.8	6.8
Spleen	16.2	72.5	–	0	0	53.3
Thymus	0	0	69.7	0	31.9	16.2
Lungs	0	0	35.5	0	13.2	0
Kidneys	0	0	0	0	24.5	3.0
Cerebrum	0	0	15.4	0	0	0
Brain stem	–	–	–	0	0	–

Note. (−) = Tissue not available for determination of morphine content.

1980) was designed to determine the distribution of morphine in the various organs of the fetuses of pregnant Rhesus monkeys made addicted to morphine. Unexpectedly, the highest concentrations of morphine and its metabolites were found in the fetal gastrointestines (see Table 10.1).

The high concentration of morphine metabolites in the gastrointestines of the fetus was postulated to occur as a consequence of the excretion of the morphine metabolites through the bile or through the urine, the latter swallowed by the fetus via the amniotic fluid (the morphine concentration of amniotic fluid was found to be 1.9 ± 1.0 µg/dl).

Subsequent studies were conducted in rat models. In four, timed pregnant Wistar rats, three were given daily doses of cocaine, morphine, or cannabinoid at the schedule shown in Table 10.2. On the 20th day of gestation, the pups were delivered by cesarean section and their meconium (intestines) was collected, pooled, and analyzed for drugs. The drugs the dams received during pregnancy

TABLE 10.2
Recovery of Drug Metabolites in the Intestines of Rat Pups Whose Dams
Received Drugs During Pregnancy

Drug	Dose per day	Rat weight	No. of Pups	Drugs in Pups (µg/gm)
Control	0	212	15	0.00
Cocaine HCl	50 mg/kg × 10 d	198	11	0.47
Morphine sulfate	50 mg/kg × 12 d	216	13	1.36
Cannabinoid	25 mg/kg × 12 d	223	12	2.50

TABLE 10.3
Cocaine Concentration in the Intestines of Rat Pups Based on Dose and Time
of Cocaine Administration to the Mother

	Mean Cocaine Concentration (μg/gm intestine)					
Group Dose Gestation	Group A Control Day 7–20	Group B 20 mg/kg Day 7–20	Group C 40 mg/kg Day 7–20	Group D 40 mg/kg Day 1–6	Group E 40 mg/kg Day 7–13	Group F 40 mg/kg Day 14–20
x	0.362	6.064	20.040	0.942	0.416	18.177
s.d.	0.227	5.750	9.956	0.985	0.370	11.842

Note. A vs. B,C,F ($p < .001$); B vs. C ($p < .001$); D,E, vs. F ($p < .001$) by t test with
Bonferroni correction.

were found in the intestines of their pups (E. M. Ostrea, Brady, Parks, Asensio,
& Naluz, 1989).

The relationship of the dose and timing of cocaine administration to the
pregnant animal and the concentration of cocaine in meconium was further studied
(Lucena, Silvestre, Raymundo, Roxas, & Ostrea, 1991). Cocaine was injected
daily to timed, pregnant Wistar rats (five per group) at doses and gestational
periods shown in Table 10.3. On Day 20, the meconium (intestines) of the pups
was analyzed for cocaine by radioimmunoassay. The amount of cocaine in
meconium was related to the cocaine dose given to the dams (B vs. C) and the
period in gestation when cocaine was administered (F vs. D and E).

Another subgroup of pregnant rats ($N = 5$ per group) were given cocaine (40
mg/kg) on Days 12–14, 15–17, or 18–20 to further characterize the third-week
gestation of the fetus. Cocaine concentration in meconium was significantly
higher than control only on Days 18–20 ($p < .001$). Thus, the amount of cocaine
in rat meconium is influenced by the gestational age of the fetus.

Similarly, the relationship of the dose and timing of morphine administration
to the pregnant animal and the concentration of morphine in meconium was
studied (Silvestre, Lucena, & Ostrea, 1991). Morphine was injected daily to timed
pregnant Wistar rats (five per group) at doses and gestational periods shown in
Table 10.4. On Day 20, the meconium (intestines) of the pups was analyzed for

TABLE 10.4
Morphine Concentration in the Intestines of Rat Pups Based on Dose and Time
of Morphine Administration to the Mother

	Mean Morphine Concentration (μg/gm intestine)					
Group Dose Gestation	Group A Control Day 7–20	Group B 5 mg/kg Day 7–20	Group C 10 mg/kg Day 7–20	Group D 10 mg/kg Day 1–6	Group E 10 mg/kg Day 7–13	Group F 10 mg/kg Day 14–20
x	0.400	0.900	1.578	0.435	0.602	2.263
s.d.	0.172	0.342	1.022	0.371	0.467	1.198

Note. A vs. B,C,F ($p < .01$); B vs. C ($p < .04$); F vs. D,E ($p < .001$).

morphine by radioimmunoassay. The amount of morphine in meconium was related to the morphine dose given to the dams (B vs. C) and the time during gestation when morphine was administered (F vs. D and E). A subgroup of pregnant rats ($N = 5$ per group) were given morphine (10 mg/kg) but only on Days 12–14, 15–17, or 18–20 of pregnancy. Morphine in meconium was higher than control only on Days 18–20 ($p < .001$). Thus, gestational age of the fetus significantly affects the amount of morphine in meconium.

From these observations evolved the hypothesis that meconium contains the metabolites of drugs the fetus was exposed to during gestation and the amount of drugs in meconium was related to the dose and period in gestation when the drug was administered during pregnancy.

DEVELOPMENT OF THE MECONIUM ASSAY

Meconium drug testing has been adapted to various analytical methods, including radioimmunoassay (Ostrea, Parks, & Brady, 1988), enzyme immunoassay (Ostrea, Romero, & Yee, 1993), fluorescence polarization immunoassay (Ostrea, Romero, & Yee, 1993), and gas chromatography/mass spectroscopy (Bandstra, Steele, & Chitwood, 1992; Callahan et al., 1992; Clark, Rosenweig, & Raisys, 1990; Montes, Romero, Ostrea, & Ostrea, 1993; Ostrea, Yee, & Thrasher, 1991).

Radioimmunoassay

The initial assay of meconium for drugs was by radioimmunoassay and was reported in 1988 (Ostrea et al., 1988). The percentage recovery of morphine and cocaine from meconium was determined by spiking meconium with known amounts of morphine glucuronide and benzoylecgonine and having it analyzed by Abuscreen radioimmunoassay. Recovery of drugs was 84% to 97% for morphine and 70% to 100% for benzoylecgonine.

A comparison of two commercially available radioimmunoassays (DPC Coat-a-Count and Roche Abuscreen) was also done to determine which assay was best suited for meconium analysis. Twenty meconium samples from control and drug-dependent infants were tested for cocaine, opiate, and cannabinoid. For cocaine, a high correlation ($r = 0.9$) between the two methods was observed. However, the amount of cocaine detected by DPC was substantially higher than by Abuscreen, because DPC detects both cocaine and its metabolites. All meconium samples except one tested negative for opiate and cannabinoid by both methods. The one sample was positive for opiate by DPC but negative by Abuscreen. The results demonstrate the advantage of DPC radioimmunoassay for total drug analysis in meconium.

We also analyzed meconium for methamphetamine by radioimmunoassay (Gervasio & Ostrea, 1991). Drug-free meconium was spiked with methamphetamine to achieve concentrations from 250 to 1000 ng/ml. Methamphetamine was analyzed by Abuscreen radioimmunoassay. Meconium from 21 infants of drug-dependent mothers was also analyzed for cocaine, opiate, and methamphetamine. The recovery of methamphetamine from spiked meconium samples was high (96.8%). Meconium from 21 infants of drug-dependent mothers was 90% positive for cocaine, 10% positive for opiate, and 5% positive for methamphetamine.

Studies were also conducted to determine the sensitivity, specificity, precision, and drug cross-reactivity of the radioimmunoassay analysis of drugs in meconium (Romero, Mac, Knapp, & Ostrea, 1993).

Sensitivity/Specificity. Eight drug-free meconium samples were spiked with known amounts of morphine 3 glucuronide, benzoylecgonine, and 11-nor, delta-9-tetrahydrocannabinol-9-carboxylic acid to achieve drug concentrations ranging from 0 to 500 ng/ml. These were analyzed by DPC radioimmunoassay. As shown in Table 10.5, radioimmunoassay showed 100% sensitivity and specificity for cocaine, opiate, and cannabinoid detection and a high recovery rate for the three drugs: 122.2% for cocaine, 114.5% for morphine, and 73.4% for cannabinoid.

Intra-assay Precision. Eight meconium samples from drug-dependent infants were analyzed in triplicate for cocaine, cannabinoid, and morphine by DPC radioimmunoassay. The mean coefficient of variation for the triplicate analysis was 12.6% for cocaine, 4.8% for morphine, and 11.9% for cannabinoid.

Drug Interference. Meconium contains significant amounts of bilirubin, blood, and some protein. These endogenous compounds were not found to interfere with the recovery of cocaine, morphine, and cannabinoid in meconium. Some common drugs were also tested for drug interference. The following drugs, added at high concentrations (100,000 ng/ml) to meconium, only had 0% to 0.2% cross-reactivity with the radioimmunoassay for cocaine, opiate, or cannabinoid: acetaminophen, phenobarbital, acetylsalicylic acid, propoxyphene, pentazocine, chlorpromazine, ibuprofen, meperidine, diazepam, lidocaine, and caffeine.

TABLE 10.5
Recovery of Cocaine, Morphine, and Cannabinoid from Spiked Meconium
by DPC Radioimmunoassay

	Sensitivity	Specificity	Positive Predictive Value	Negative Predictive Value	Recovery Rate
Cocaine	100% (8/8)	100% (3/3)	100% (3/3)	100% (8/8)	122.2 ± 31.5%
Morphine	100% (10/10)	100% (3/3)	100% (10/10)	100% (3/3)	114.5 ± 21.9%
Cannabinoid	100% (7/7)	100% (3/3)	100% (7/7)	100% (3/3)	73.5 ± 13.0%

Studies were further conducted to determine the appropriate method of collection and storage of meconium. The stability of cocaine, morphine, and cannabinoid in meconium were studied under three storage conditions: (a) at room temperature for 24 hrs, (b) emulsified in meconium solvent for 72 hrs at room temperature, and (c) frozen at −15° C for 12 weeks.

Meconium kept at room temperature without refrigeration for 24 hrs resulted in a 25% decrease in cocaine concentration, a 62% increase in morphine concentration, and a 30% decrease in cannabinoid concentration. The increase in morphine concentration represents the hydrolysis of morphine glucuronide into morphine due to the action of beta glucuronidase in meconium and the 40 times higher sensitivity of DPC radioimmunoassay for morphine compared to its glucuronide. Meconium should therefore be sampled and processed within 12 hrs after its excretion by the infant to avoid loss of drugs, specifically cocaine and cannabinoid.

Meconium emulsified in the meconium solvent (buffered methanol) and kept at room temperature for 72 hrs did not show a significant decrease in cocaine, morphine, or cannabinoid concentration. Drugs are therefore stable in meconium solvent for at least 72 hrs at room temperature. For transport purposes, meconium in buffered methanol can be transported, without the need for refrigeration, for at least 72 hrs.

Freezing of meconium for at least 16 weeks (109 days) at −15° C did not cause a significant change in the concentration of cocaine, opiate, and cannabinoid.

Enzyme Immunoassay/Fluorescence Polarization Immunoassay

The original analysis of drugs in meconium was by radioimmunoassay. For wide-scale clinical application, meconium analysis was adapted to enzyme immunoassay (EIA) or fluorescence polarization immunoassay, two methods commonly used in clinical laboratories (Gervasio & Ostrea, 1991; Ostrea et al., 1993). Drug-free meconium was spiked with cocaine, morphine, or cannabinoid at concentrations ranging from 0 to 450 ng/ml and analyzed by enzyme immunoassay (enzyme multiplied immunoassay technique; EMIT), fluorescence polarization immunoassay (ADx), and DPC radioimmunoassay (Table 10.6). By radioimmunoassay, the sensitivity and specificity of cocaine, morphine, and cannabinoid analyses were 100%. By EMIT and ADx, the sensitivity for cocaine, morphine, and cannabinoid detection was 75%, 40%, and 100%, respectively; however, the specificity for the three drugs was 100%. The lower sensitivity of EMIT versus radioimmunoassay was due to nondetection of drugs at low concentrations. Thus, cutoff concentrations are 50 ng/ml for cocaine, 100 ng/ml for morphine, and 25 ng/ml for cannabinoid (Romero, Mac, Knapp, & Ostrea, 1993).

Using the previously given cutoff concentrations, meconium was obtained from 61 newborn infants and analyzed for cocaine, opiate (morphine), and

TABLE 10.6
Sensitivity/Specificity of RIA, EIA, and FPI for the Detection of Cocaine,
Opiate, and Cannabinoid in Spiked Meconium

	RIA	EIA	FPI
1. Cocaine			
Sensitivity (%)	100 (8/8)	75 (6/8)	75 (6/8)
Specificity (%)	100 (3/3)	100 (3/3)	100 (3/3)
Recovery rate (%)	104.5 ± 14.1		
Cutoff conc (ng/ml)	25	50	50
2. Opiate			
Sensitivity (%)	100 (10/10)	40 (4/10)	40 (4/10)
Specificity (%)	100 (3/3)	100 (3/3)	100 (3/3)
Recovery rate (%)	135.6 ± 9.6		
Cutoff conc (ng/ml)	25	100	100
3. Cannabinoid			
Sensitivity (%)	100 (7/7)	100 (8/8)	100 (8/8)
Specificity (%)	100 (3/3)	100 (3/3)	100 (3/3)
Recovery rate (%)	96.6 ± 6.2		
Cutoff conc (ng/ml)	15	25	25

cannabinoid by radioimmunoassay and enzyme immunoassay (EMIT). Opiate
was detected in eight infants (13%) by radioimmunoassay and in nine (15%) by
EMIT; cocaine was detected in 39 infants (64%) by radioimmunoassay and in
39 (64%) by EMIT. The concordance between the negative or positive results
of the radioimmunoassay versus EMIT were 95% and 98%, respectively, for
cocaine, and 98% and 100%, respectively, for opiate.

Gas Chromatography/Mass Spectroscopy (GC/MS)

GC/MS analysis has been successfully applied to meconium drug testing (Bandstra et al., 1992; Callahan et al., 1992; Clark et al., 1990; Montes et al., 1993;
Ostrea et al., 1991). The mass spectrum (M/Z = 98, 119, and 176) of cotinine
(metabolite of nicotine) in meconium and deuterated cotinine (M/Z = 101, 122,
179) as internal standard are shown in Fig. 10.1.

However, analysis by GC/MS is difficult because each drug requires a separate
method for analysis, and analysis for opiate or cannabinoids requires preliminary
hydrolysis of their metabolites prior to GC/MS analyses. We recently developed
an improved method of GC/MS analysis of meconium that features the simulta-
neous detection of cocaine, morphine, and cannabinoid and the omission of
preliminary hydrolysis of drug metabolites of morphine and cannabinoid (Montes
et al., 1993). Twenty meconium samples from drug-exposed and control infants

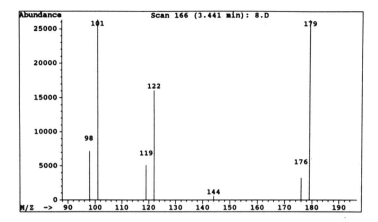

FIG. 10.1. Mass spectrum of cotinine (M/Z = 98, 119 + 176) and deuterated cotinine M/Z = 101, 122, 179) in meconium.

were analyzed for cocaine, opiate, and cannabinoid by RIA, EMIT, ADx and the improved GC/MS method. Table 10.7 shows the total number of samples positive for the drugs using the four methods of analysis.

The GC/MS method confirmed 100% of cocaine and 78% of morphine positive samples. GC/MS was more sensitive for cannabinoid detection than the three immunoassays.

CLINICAL STUDIES

We conducted a number of clinical studies with the meconium drug test. Meconium from 20 infants of drug-dependent mothers and 5 control infants was analyzed by radioimmunoassay for morphine, cocaine, and cannabinoid.

As shown in Table 10.8, control stools showed no drug. Meconium from the infants of drug-dependent mothers showed the presence of at least one drug metabolite: 80% of the infants of drug-dependent mothers showed cocaine (range 0.14 to 19.91 µg/g stool), 55% showed morphine (range 0.41 to 14.97 µg/g stool), and 60% showed cannabinoid (range 0.05 to 0.67 µg/g stool). The con-

TABLE 10.7
Analysis of Meconium for Cocaine, Opiate, and Cannabinoid by
GC/MS ADx, Radioimmunoassay (RIA), Enzyme Immunoasay (EMIT),
and Fluorescence Polarization Immunoassay (ADx)

	GC/MS	RIA	EMIT	ADx
Cocaine (+)	18/20	18/20	18/20	18/20
Opiate (+)	7/20	9/20	6/20	6/20
Cannabinoid (+)	5/20	3/20	1/20	1/20

TABLE 10.8
Recovery of Drug Metabolites in Meconium of Drug-Dependent Infants

Cocaine (µg/gm stool)			Morphine (µg/gm stool)			Cannabinoid (µg/gm stool)			Urine Screen[a]
Day 1	Day 2	Day 3	Day 1	Day 2	Day 3	Day 1	Day 2	Day 3	
6.35	3.23	(-)	3.28	1.72	0.56	(-)	(-)	(-)	(-)
2.34	2.17	1.17	1.19	1.17	(-)	(-)	(-)	(-)	(-)
1.77	9.68	3.67	(-)	(-)	(-)	(-)	(-)	(-)	(-)
10.86	11.29	(-)	(-)	(-)	(-)	0.13	0.29	(-)	(-)
(-)	(-)	(-)	5.38	12.11	(-)	0.05	(-)	(-)	Opiates
4.54	17.78	1.03	(-)	(-)	(-)	0.34	0.66	(-)	Cocaine
(-)	(-)	(-)	0.69	0.97	0.54	(-)	(-)	(-)	(-)
2.39	2.16	1.07	3.75	2.43	2.31	(-)	(-)	(-)	(-)
5.40	8.41	0.41	(-)	(-)	(-)	(-)	0.09	(-)	Cocaine
(-)	(-)	NS	11.74	14.97	NS	(-)	(-)	NS	Opiates
(-)	(-)	(-)	(-)	(-)	(-)	0.06	0.09	(-)	(-)
11.48	0.41	(-)	(-)	(-)	(-)	0.13	(-)	(-)	Cocaine
7.40	6.70	NS	5.36	5.73	NS	0.48	0.37	NS	Cocaine
11.42	0.29	NS	6.95	0.73	NS	0.67	(-)	NS	(-)
3.29	19.91	6.10	(-)	(-)	(-)	(-)	(-)	(-)	NS
0.26	(-)	NS	2.26	0.77	NS	0.14	(-)	NS	(-)
1.76	3.52	2.42	1.24	1.21	1.24	(-)	(-)	0.12	(-)
NS	16.23	13.15	NS	0.41	(-)	NS	0.22	0.09	Cocaine
0.95	0.14	(-)	(-)	(-)	(-)	0.07	(-)	(-)	(-)
0.06	0.03	(-)	(-)	(-)	(-)	0.19	0.17	0.05	(-)

Note. (-) = negative for drug tested; NS, no sample.
[a]urine drug screen by the TDX immunosasay system.

centrations of metabolites were highest during the first 2 days; some stools tested positive up to the third day. In contrast, only 37% of the infants had a positive urine drug screen by fluorescence polarization immunoassay (Ostrea et al., 1989).

With the successful adaptation of the meconium analysis to EMIT and ADx analyses, mass drug screening of newborn infants was initiated (Ostrea et al., 1993). A total of 4409 infants from our institution (Hutzel Hospital) and from three other neonatal centers were tested (see Table 10.9). Hutzel Hospital showed the highest percentage of positive tests among the four centers; 38% positive samples, of which 90% were positive for cocaine. The high prevalence of drug use in the pregnant population at Hutzel Hospital corroborates the findings of an earlier report on the same population. In the remaining three centers, the prevalence of drug abuse was low and ranged between 1% to 4%. These centers represent low-risk rural or middle-class communities. Furthermore, in Center C, which represents a rural community, the principal drug found was cannabinoid, which contrasts sharply to the predominance of cocaine at Hutzel Hospital, which serves an urban population. The disparate results in the prevalence and types of drug abuse between the four centers are consistent with the low- or high-risk characteristics of the population tested.

TABLE 10.9
Meconium Drug Analysis in Four Neonatal Centers

Center	No. Tested	No. Positive	Cocaine +	Opiate +	Cannabinoid +
1. Hutzel	2,032	773 (38%)	693 (90%)	117 (15%)	31 (4%)
2. Center A	269	10 (3.7%)	4 (40%)	4 (40%)	3 (30%)
3. Center B	1,329	39 (2.9%)	22 (56%)	6 (15%)	15 (39%)
4. Center C	779	14 (1.8%)	1 (7%)	4 (29%)	10 (71%)

Routine meconium drug screening of all newborn infants is not practical because of cost, even in high drug prevalence areas. Thus, criteria were established to select the appropriate infants for testing (Ostrea & Romero, 1992). An infant was tested if (a) the mother admitted to the use of illicit drugs during the current (i) or past (ii) (denies current) pregnancy, (b) the mother admitted only to the use of marijuana or alcohol (iii), (c) the mother was a "walk-in" mother with some prenatal care elsewhere (iv), (d) the mother was a "walk-in" mother without prenatal care (v), (e) the infant manifested withdrawal and the mother denied drug use (vi), or (f) there was a social service request (e.g., infant for adoption/home placement, etc.) (vii). A total of 1,036 infants at Hutzel Hospital were tested using these screening criteria (Table 10.10).

Of 1,036 infants screened, 46% were positive for drugs, principally cocaine (90%); 83% of infants in Group 1 tested positive for drugs, which confirmed the high sensitivity of the meconium test; 38% to 47% in Groups 2 and 3 were drug positive, indicative of the high denial rate and the high illicit drug use associated with alcohol or marijuana; 16% to 20% in Groups 4 and 5 were drug positive, which indicates that women with poor prenatal care are at high risk for illicit drug use. Finally, 75% of the drug-positive infants were clinically normal at birth; thus drug screening was the only method to identify these high-risk infants. We conclude that selection criteria for routine drug screening of newborns can be established to efficiently identify the drug-exposed group.

A large-scale, prospective drug screening of newborn infants by meconium analysis was done to determine the prevalence and epidemiologic characteristics of drug use in a high-risk urban obstetric population (Ostrea, Brady, et al., 1992). Every other infant that was delivered in our high-risk perinatal center was enrolled

TABLE 10.10
Drug Screening of Infants Based on Selection Criteria

Groups	i	ii	iii	iv	v	vi	vii
# of cases	416	39	78	120	253	20	110
+ any drug	83%	38%	47%	16%	20%	10%	8%
Cocaine +	79%	28%	33%	12%	18%	10%	4%
Opiate +	12%	8%	5%	4%	2%	0%	4%
Cannabin +	2%	5%	14%	2%	1%	0%	1%

TABLE 10.11
Meconium Drug Screen of 3,010 Infants for the Metabolites of
Cocaine, Opiate, and Cannabinoid

Total stools (meconium) analyzed	3,010 (100.0%)
Positive for drugs	1,333 (44.3%)[a]
1. Positive for cocaine	923 (30.7%)
2. Positive for opiate	617 (20.5%)
3. Positive for cannabinoid	346 (11.5%)
Negative for drug	1,677 (55.7%)

Note. [a]Prevalence of drug exposure based on maternal self-report = 335/3,010 (11.1%).

from November 1988 to September 1989 and their meconium was analyzed for the metabolites of the three commonly abused drugs (cocaine, morphine [opiates], and cannabinoid) by radioimmunoassay. Of 3,010 subjects studied (Table 10.11), 44% were positive for cocaine, morphine, or cannabinoid: 31% positive for cocaine, 21% positive for morphine, and 12% for cannabinoid. Only 11% of the mothers admitted to illicit drug use: 52% of their infants had a positive urine drug screen, whereas 88% had a positive meconium drug screen. Prevalence of drug use among the pregnant women varied per month. A profile of the pregnant addict in the population studied was noted ($p < .001$): service patient, single, multigravid (> 3) and little or no prenatal care. The major problems associated with drug use during pregnancy were principally noted in the group that was exposed to cocaine and opiates and in the group where the mothers admitted to the use of illicit drugs. On the other hand, a large number of infants who have been exposed to drugs in utero, but whose mothers denied the use of drugs, may appear normal at birth and go unrecognized. Improved detection of these infants at risk can be achieved with a high index of suspicion and meconium drug analysis.

In the same population, the prevalence of illicit drug exposure among infants admitted to the neonatal intensive care unit was also determined. Fifty percent of the infants were positive for drugs: 44% positive for cocaine, 11% for opiates, and none for cannabinoids (Ostrea, Brady, et al., 1992).

RECENT DEVELOPMENTS
IN MECONIUM DRUG TESTING

Serial meconium drug analysis can estimate the chronology and degree of the infant's in utero drug exposure (Ostrea, Knapp, Ostrea, Tannenbaum, & Saleri, 1994). We enrolled 58 pregnant drug users early in gestation (18–20 weeks) and prospectively monitored their drug use by: (a) in-depth maternal interview every 2 weeks; (b) maternal hair analysis of samples obtained at enrollment, midgestation, and delivery; and (c) serial meconium analysis by examination of every

TABLE 10.12
Incidence of Cocaine, Opiate, and Cannabinoid Use as Determined
by Maternal Interview, Hair Analysis, and Meconium Analysis

Drug Use Determined By	Cocaine +	Opiate +	Cannabinoid +
Maternal interview	30 (50.8%)	16 (27.1%)	18 (30.5%)
Meconium analysis	40 (67.8%)	19 (32.2%)	7 (11.8%)
Hair analysis	46 (78%)	21 (35.6%)	10 (16.9%)

stool passed by the infant after birth for 3 days. Hair and meconium were quan-titated by RIA and GC/MS for cocaine, opiate, and cannabinoid. Sensitivity, specificity, and correlations between interview, hair, and meconium analyses for type, amount, and timing of drug use were made.

The incidence of cocaine, opiate, and cannabinoid use in the study population as determined by comprehensive maternal interview (excludes drug use during the periconception period), maternal hair analysis, and meconium analysis are shown in Table 10.12. For each method, a positive specific drug use was defined as the presence of a single positive test for that drug within the study period. Hair analysis showed the highest incidence of cocaine (78%) and opiate (35.6%) use, whereas maternal history showed the highest incidence of cannabinoid use (30.5%). Drugs were detected mostly in the drug-abusing group.

The sensitivity and specificity of each method of drug detection was analyzed in the following manner: For each subject, the result of the test for a drug by one method (e.g., meconium analysis), whether positive or negative, was com-pared to the combined test results of the other two methods (i.e., history and hair analysis). Concordance in test results between the combined methods was re-quired to allow for a valid comparison. The reason for this is that the concordance in the test results of the two tests increased the reliability of their results and the validity of serving as the "gold standard" for comparison. As shown in Table 10.13, meconium analysis had the highest sensitivity and specificity for cocaine and opiate detection (97%–100%), followed by hair analysis, which also had high sensitivity but lower specificity (87%). For cannabinoid detection, maternal

TABLE 10.13
Sensitivity and Specificity of Maternal Interview, Meconium Analysis, and
Hair Analysis in Detecting Gestational Use of Cocaine, Opiate, or Cannabinoid

	Cocaine Detection			Opiate Detection			Cannabinoid Detection		
	N^a	Sens	Spec	N^a	Sens	Spec	N^a	Sens	Spec
Maternal interview	54	75%	100%	50	94%	97%	39	100%	75%
Meconium analysis	44	97%	100%	52	100%	97%	40	60%	94%
Hair analysis	43	100%	87%	54	100%	87%	42	38%	91%

Note. [a]Indicates number of valid comparisons (see text for definition).

interview had the highest sensitivity (100%) compared to meconium (60%) and hair (38%) analyses.

By calculating the positive and negative predictive values (p, in percent) of each test, their rates of false positive and false negative tests were determined ($100 - p$), and these are shown in Table 10.14. Maternal interview had the highest false negative rate for cocaine detection (42%) and hair analysis had the highest false positive rates for cocaine (13%) and opiate (24%) detection. Due to the low sensitivity of meconium and hair analysis for cannabinoid detection, each showed a 6% and 14% false negative rate, respectively, for the detection of that drug.

The comparatively low specificity of hair analysis that resulted in a high rate of false positive tests for cocaine (13%) and opiate (24%) was probably due to hair contamination as a result of passive exposure of hair to drugs in the environment. Human hair can be passively exposed to cocaine either from vaporized cocaine freebase (smoking of "crack" cocaine) or from cocaine hydrochloride dust particles in the air or clothes. In the former, it has been shown that even with prewashing of contaminated hair prior to drug analysis, cocaine cannot completely be removed from the hair and enough cocaine residue is left to produce false positive results.

Both meconium and hair analyses showed lower sensitivity to cannabinoid detection (60% and 38%, respectively) than maternal interview. This is because in 54% of the mothers who admitted to cannabinoid use, use of cannabinoid during pregnancy was sparse and episodic, which resulted in mild exposure of the fetus to the drug and drug levels below the detection limits of the two tests. For its clinical relevance, however, this small amount of exposure of the fetus to cannabinoid probably has little or no consequence on ultimate outcome (Fried & Watkinson, 1990). Meconium analysis, like hair analysis, had a high false positive rate for cannabinoid detection (40%). This value may be artificially high, because the calculation was based on a very small sample size of positive results ($n = 5$). Furthermore, in one case, the cannabinoid concentration in meconium was high and the drug was also confirmed by GC/MS; thus, the false positive rate of meconium analysis for cannabinoid could be further adjusted down to 20%.

Safeguards were instituted to ensure the accuracy of the maternal interview, which was the most subjective of the methods used. These included a prospective design in the study, with the maternal interview starting at early gestation and at bimonthly intervals, plus the institution of use of a "bogus pipeline" technique. This technique consisted of informing the patient prior to the interview that their drug use would be confirmed by a sensitive laboratory test. Despite these safeguards, the false negative rate of maternal interview for cocaine use was high (42%). Thus, even under ideal conditions, maternal interview is subject to significant denial by the mother, particularly for cocaine use. On the other hand, if a mother admits to the use of a drug, there seems to be no valid reason to doubt it. Thus, the high false positive rate (75%) of maternal interview for cannabinoid use (Table 10.14) is erroneous and is the result of its comparison to meconium and hair analyses, both of which are not sensitive methods to detect small amounts of cannabinoid use by the mother.

In summary, a comparison of the sensitivity and specificity of maternal interview, meconium analysis, and hair analysis for detecting gestational exposure to cocaine, opiate, and cannabinoid reveal that comprehensive maternal interview is a tedious and time-consuming process, impractical for clinical use. Even in research settings, one may question its overall usefulness because of its high false negative rate for detecting cocaine use. Meconium and hair analyses are drug detection methods more applicable for clinical use. However, meconium analysis shows a clear advantage over hair analysis because the former is non-invasive and it is more sensitive and specific. In particular, the high false positive rates of hair analysis for cocaine and opiate detection due to passive exposure, pose a serious limitation to the use of the test.

One of the objectives in meconium drug testing was to determine whether serial, quantitative analysis of meconium for drugs can estimate the amount and the period(s) in gestation when the fetus was exposed to the drug(s). The assumption is that as meconium is deposited in the fetal intestines throughout gestation, the earliest formed meconium would be located in the most distal portion of the colon, whereas the most recently formed meconium would be in the proximal segments. Thus, as the infant excretes meconium after birth, the order in which meconium is passed should correspond to the time order of its formation in utero, and the quantity of drugs in meconium will also reflect the degree of fetal drug exposure during that period. Unfortunately, no data exist that establish this specific time sequence. Thus, for the purpose of the study, we set the following approximations: (a) meconium excreted between 0 and 10 hrs after birth represents early gestation meconium, (b) meconium excreted between 11 and 20 hrs after birth represents midgestation meconium, and (c) meconium excreted at more than 21 hrs after birth represents late gestation meconium. Our reason for choosing this time sequence stems from our observation that by 36 hrs after birth, the majority of the infant's stools have become transitional, which

TABLE 10.14
Rates of False Positive and False Negative for Maternal Interview,
Meconium Analysis, and Maternal Hair Analysis in Detecting Gestational
Exposure to Cocaine, Opiate, and Cannabinoid

	Cocaine Detection		Opiate Detection		Cannabinoid Detection	
	False +	False −	False +	False −	False +	False −
Maternal interview	0%	42%	6%	3%	75%	0%
Meconium analysis	0%	7%	6%	0%	40%	6%
Hair analysis	13%	0%	24%	0%	50%	14%

indicates mixture of meconium with milk stools. For the purpose of correlating meconium data with hair analysis and maternal interview data, the periods we outlined for meconium were set to correspond to the following gestation: early gestation = less than 20 weeks, midgestation = 21 to 30 weeks, and late gestation = more than 30 weeks. The mean concentrations of cocaine, opiate, and cannabinoid in meconium and hair, and the amount of drug use by maternal history correponding to these time periods were determined. By multiple regression analysis, the correlations between the concentration of drugs in meconium and hair and drug use by maternal interview are shown in Table 10.15.

The concentrations of cocaine and cannabinoid in meconium correlated well to the amount of cocaine and cannabinoid found in maternal hair, and drug use based on maternal interview. For opiate use, however, the correlation was only significant between hair analysis and interview. The reason for the latter is probably overestimation of opiate in meconium by radioimmunoassay. There is a almost a 40-fold greater sensitivity of the radioimmunoassay to morphine compared to morphine glucuronide. The conversion of morphine glucuronide to morphine can occur in meconium due to the presence in meconium of intestinal beta glucuronidase; thus the presence of morphine will substantially increase the opiate concentration in meconium by a factor of 40.

Since the advent of meconium drug testing, one of the frequent questions asked is how early in gestation drugs are detected in meconium. We studied three pregnant women who had early interruptions of their pregnancies (Ostrea, Knapp, Romero, & A. R. Ostrea, 1994). Autopsies were done on their fetuses: two delivered by spontaneous abortions at 16 and 20 weeks of gestation and 1 stillborn delivered at 32 weeks who had jejunal atresia (Case 3). Meconium was obtained from the fetal small (SI) and large (LI) intestines and analyzed for cocaine, opiate, and cannabinoid by DPC radioimmunoassay. The mothers of all three fetuses used cocaine during pregnancy. The three fetuses were all positive for cocaine but negative for opiate and cannabinoid. Cocaine concentration in maternal hair and meconium are shown in Table 10.16.

Cocaine was detected in meconium as early as the 16th week of gestation. The amount of cocaine in meconium was proportional to the cocaine concentration in maternal hair. Drugs are deposited in meconium either from bile secretion or from swallowed amniotic fluid (fetal urine); thus, intestinal obstruction in the

TABLE 10.15
Correlation Between the Amount of Drug Use by the Mother Based on
Maternal Interview, Meconium Analysis, and Hair Analysis

Correlation Coefficient	Cocaine	Opiate	Cannabinoid
Meconium vs. Hair	0.471*	0.150	0.446*
Meconium vs. Interview	0.530*	0.132	0.386*
Hair vs. Interview	0.452*	0.418*	0.561*

*p < .01.

TABLE 10.16
Concentration of Cocaine in the Meconum of Three Preterm Fetuses

Fetus			Cocaine (ng/ml)		
#	Gest Age	Weight	Meconium (SI)	Meconium (LI)	Hair
1	16 wks	110 g	84	33	480
2	21 wks	400 g	2,665	3,426	570
3	32 wks	2,029 g	0	21	128

fetus can affect the deposition of drugs in meconium due to the interruption of flow of the intestinal contents. This was demonstrated in Case 3. High jejunal obstruction in this fetus prevented the passage of cocaine through the intestines. Because cocaine was detected only in the distal segment of the large intestine and not in the small intestine, jejunal obstruction in the fetus must have occurred early in gestation.

We studied fetal exposure to nicotine in passive and active maternal smoking by meconium analysis and for the first time provided evidence that nicotine metabolites (cotinine and trans 3′-hydroxycotinine) can be detected in meconium (Ostrea, Knapp, Romero, Montes, & Ostrea, 1994). There is also a correlation between the concentration of nicotine metabolites in meconium and degree of maternal active and passive smoking. Meconium was collected from 55 infants whose mothers were nonsmokers ($N = 10$), passive smokers ($N = 25$), light (< 1 pack per day) active smokers ($N = 13$), and heavy ($\geq$ 1 pack per day) active smokers ($N = 7$). Meconium was analyzed for nicotine metabolites (cotinine and 3-OH cotinine) by radioimmunoassay (see Table 10.17).

The mean concentration of nicotine metabolites in meconium in the passive and active smokers was significantly higher compared to nonsmokers ($p < .05$, ANOVA). However, the nicotine concentrations in meconium from passive smokers were *not* significantly different from the light active smokers ($t = 0.65$, $p > .05$). The correlation coefficient between nicotine metabolites in meconium and the degree of maternal smoking graded as 1 for control, 2 for passive, 3 for light active, and 4 for heavy active smoking was 0.54 ($p < .001$). Thus, gestational

TABLE 10.17
Mean (SD) Meconium Concentration of Nicotine Metabolites in Infants of
Control, Passive, and Active Smokers, as Analyzed by Radioimmunoassay

Category	N	Concentration (ng/ml)
Nonsmoker	10	10.9 ± 7.6
Passive smoker	25	31.6 ± 17.2*
Light, active smoker (< 1 pack per day)	13	34.7 ± 22.3*
Heavy, active smoker (≥ 1 pack per day)	7	54.6 ± 19.9**

*$p < .05$ compared to nonsmoker (one way ANOVA).
**$p < .05$ compared to light, active smoker, passive smoker and nonsmoker (one way ANOVA).

exposure of the fetus to nicotine in both active and passive maternal smoking can be quantitatively measured in the fetus by analysis of meconium for nicotine metabolites. Of significance, in utero exposure to tobacco smoke in infants of passive smokers was as high as among infants whose mothers actively smoked less than 1 pack per day during pregnancy.

We previously reported on the analysis of meconium for cocaine and its metabolites by GC/MS in drug-dependent infants (Ostrea et al., 1991). In nine infants studied, we found that 67% of the cocaine in meconium was present as the parent compound, cocaine. This was unusual, because most of the cocaine excreted in the fetal urine is in the form of its water-soluble metabolite, benzoylecgonine. To study this observation, we analyzed, by GC/MS, cocaine and benzoylecgonine in meconium, gastric aspirate, and urine of 10 infants (Garcia, Romero, Garcia, & Ostrea, 1994). We observed that benzoylecgonine was the principal form of cocaine in both urine and gastric aspirate with little or no cocaine (Table 10.18). Yet in meconium, cocaine was present in 50% of the specimens analyzed. The explanation for this difference is yet unknown, although the observation is clinically significant because cocaine is lipid soluble and can therefore be absorbed back into fetal circulation. Thus, this implies endogenous and repeated exposure of the fetus to cocaine.

The prevalence of illicit drug exposure in infants in the intensive care unit was studied (Ostrea, Lizardo, & Tanafranca, 1992). The meconium drug test was used to prospectively screen for drugs (opiates, cocaine, and cannabinoids) every infant admitted to a neonatal intensive care unit (NICU) at a high-risk perinatal center from June 10 to August 15, 1991. The morbidity, mortality, and cost of care for the infants were determined. A total of 122 infants were enrolled but 40 were not tested because of insufficient or no meconium samples collected. Of the 82 infants tested, 41 (50%) were positive for drugs, 36 (44%) positive for cocaine, 9 (11%) positive for opiates, and none for cannabinoid. The maternal

TABLE 10.18

Concentrations (ng/mL) of Cocaine (COC) and Benzoylecgonine (BE)
in Meconium, Gastric Aspirate, and Urine of 10 Infants

	Meconium		Gastric Aspirate		Urine	
	Coc	BE	Coc	BE	Coc	BE
1	56.74	63.83	0	199.37	0	86.85
2	0	0	0	0	0	0
3	0	10.75	144.08	18.57	0	0
4	0	7.47	0	24.74	0	0
5	27.31	25.85	0	11.08	0	34.90
6	0	0	0	0	0	10.80
7	22.62	22.23	0	0	43.70	0
8	0	67.32	0	0	0	25.88
9	16.71	14.04	0	7.47	0	7.04
10	0	16.10	0	24.46	0	131.64

profile or complications in the drug-positive group was: 83% Medicaid, 90% African American, 90% unmarried, 75% no prenatal care, 54% Cesarean section, 8% meconium-stained fluid, and 30% prolonged rupture of membranes. The neonatal profile was: premature (78%), small for gestational age (6%), weight less than 1,500g (48%), length less than 35 cm (3%), head circumference less than 28 cm (30%), and Apgar less than 6 at 1 min (29%). The total length of hospital stay of the drug-positive infants was 979 days, or an average of 26 days per infant. At an average NICU cost (excluding physician's fee) per day of $1,250, this amounted to a total cost of $1,223,750. Thus, the prevalence of drug exposure in infants admitted to the NICU is very high. Fifty percent of the morbidity, the mortality, and the high cost of care of infants in the NICU is associated with illicit drugs.

We also studied whether the recent upsurge in the incidence of congenital syphilis was a drug-related event (Sison, Ostrea, & Saleri, 1992). Although reports have shown that the resurgence of congenital syphilis is related to illicit drug use, these reports were based on a restricted population of pregnant women who have openly admitted to the use of drugs. Thus, the true relationship of congenital syphilis to drug use is not known because a large number of pregnant women deny their use of drugs. Infants in a high-risk nursery were screened for drugs by the meconium drug screen test, if (a) the mother admitted to the use of illicit drug during the current or past (denies current) pregnancy, (b) the mother admitted only to the use of marijuana or alcohol, (c) the mother was a "walk-in" mother with some prenatal care elsewhere, (d) the mother was a "walk-in" mother without prenatal care, (e) the infant manifested "withdrawal" and the mother denied drug use, and (f) social service request (e.g., infant for adoption/home placement, etc). Similarly, all parturients in the obstetric service were routinely screened on admission for syphilis by the RPR and FTA-ABS (if RPR is positive) tests. Thus, in this large and more encompassing population of drug- and syphilis-screened maternal infant dyads ($N = 1,012$), the relationship between congenital syphilis and drug abuse in pregnancy was studied.

Meconium drug screen (MDS) was positive for one or more drugs in 449 infants (44.4%). Seventy-two mothers (7%) had positive RPR/FTA-ABS tests. Forty-six of their infants (4.5%) had congenital syphilis based on current definitions. Of 449 infants with positive MDS, 47 mothers (10.5%) were RPR positive and 32 (7%) infants had congenital syphilis, whereas of 563 infants with negative MDS, 25 (4.4%) mothers were RPR reactive and 14 (2.5%) infants had congenital syphilis ($x = 13.7$, $p < .001$). The incidence of positive RPR and congenital syphilis in the MDS positive group was not significantly different ($p > .10$) whether mother admitted to illicit drug use (11% and 8%, respectively) or not (8.8% and 4.4%, respectively). We conclude that maternal drug abuse is truly a significant factor that is related to the resurgence of congenital syphilis.

A study was also conducted to determine if meconium analysis can detect acute, intrapartum drug exposure. We therefore studied 12 infants, 2 control and

TABLE 10.19
Detection of Meperidine in Meconium

Meperidine (ng/ml)	Day 1 Meconium	Day 2 Meconium
Mean	282.9 ± 821.4	145.2 ± 178.2
Range	0–3,450	0–3,590

10 whose mothers were given meperidine during labor (Morales, Knapp, Utarnachitt, Utarnachitt, & Ostrea, 1994). The infants' meconium was collected for 2 days and individually tested for meperidine and normeperidine by GC/MS. Two infants whose mothers were given codeine just before labor were included. Meconium from the control group was negative for meperidine or normeperidine. In the treated group, meperidine was the predominant drug found in meconium and was identified in samples collected on Days 1 and 2 (Table 10.19). In one third of the samples, normeperidine was also isolated at concentrations approximately half those of meperidine. In two infants whose mothers received codeine before labor, the MDS by radioimmunoassay was positive for "opiates" and by GC/MS was positive for codeine.

We conclude that MDS can detect both *acute* and *chronic* fetal exposure to drugs. This demonstrates that a wide range of gestational drug exposure, from early midgestation to labor, can be detected by the meconium drug test. Analgesics, which contain codeine, are easily available and are used before or during labor. This may result in a positive, nonspecific meconium drug screen for opiates and underscores the need for specific drug identification, if exposure to illicit opiates is sought.

Lastly, although the fetal effects of alcohol are known, no reliable marker of fetal exposure to alcohol has yet been identified. Fatty acid ethyl esters (FAEE) are enzymatic, nonoxidative products of in vivo ethanol metabolism, with a long half-life, and they are markers of ethanol consumption in the adult. We reported on the identification of FAEE in meconium of alcohol-exposed infants at concentrations proportional to the amount of maternal alcohol use (Mac, Pacis, Garcia, & Ostrea, 1994). Preliminary studies to determine the optimum method for extraction and isolation of FAEE in meconium were done. FAEE standards (ethyl palmitate and stearate) were spiked into meconium and extracted by acetone or hexane:water and isolated by thin layer chromatography or bonded phase column. Detection was by GC/MS. Optimum FAEE extraction and chromatogram were achieved using the hexane:water/bonded phase column combination. With this method, meconium was analyzed for FAEE in 10 control and 15 alcohol-exposed infants. In the latter, FAEE concentrations in meconium were multifold higher than control, with a wide range proportional to the amount of maternal alcohol use (Table 10.20).

We concluded that FAEE in meconium may serve as an important biologic marker of fetal exposure to ethanol and provide an important, objective tool for the precise study of alcohol exposure and its fetal effects.

TABLE 10.20
Fatty Acid Ethyl Esters in Meconium of Control and Alcohol-Exposed Infants

Mean FAEE (ng/ml)	Ethyl Laurate	Ethyl Palmitate	Ethyl Stearate
Control	32.0	67.2	32.3
(range)	(0–29.6)	(2–367)	(0.4–54)
Alcohol exposed	4,799	1,082	338.2
(range)	(76–36,106)	(57–8,290)	(28–1,908)

STUDIES BY OTHERS

Meconium drug analysis has also been studied by other workers and their data confirm the sensitivity, specificity and usefulness of the test.

Drug-free meconium was spiked with benzoylecgonine and cocaine for extraction efficiencies (Clark et al., 1990). The determination was sensitive for spiked samples to 0.3 µg each of cocaine and benzolecgonine per gram of meconium. The assay was linear for cocaine to 10 µg/g and to 3.5 µg/gm for benzoylecgonine. Prechromatographic extraction efficiencies were 100% for cocaine and 30% for benzoylecgonine. Cocaine and benzoylecgonine were analyzed by GC/MS in meconium of three infants of cocaine-dependent mothers: Cocaine was found in one infant whose mother used cocaine heavily in the first two trimesters; cocaine and benzoylecgonine were found in another infant, and none in the third infant who had limited in utero exposure to cocaine.

Meconium from 28 neonates born to women suspected of drug abuse were tested for cocaine, morphine, codeine, and marijuana (Maynard, Amuroso, & Oh, 1991). In each case, testing of urine from the mother, the infant, or both were done because of suspected maternal drug abuse. Seventeen of 28 (61%) meconium samples tested positive; 28 of 47 (60%) urine samples were positive. Meconium test results were concordant with the results of maternal or newborn urine testing in 24 of the 28 (86%) cases. In three cases, meconium was positive for cocaine when newborn urine was negative; in one case, meconium was negative when maternal urine was positive for cocaine. Compared with the combination of maternal and newborn urine testing, meconium testing had an 82% positive predictive value (14 of 17) and a 91% negative predictive value. The authors further added that the collection of meconium was simpler and more reliable than collection of urine and that the testing of meconium was easily incorporated into routine procedures at a busy commercial laboratory.

The sensitivity of newborn hair, meconium, and urine analyses for drugs in detecting gestational exposure to cocaine was studied (Callahan et al., 1992). Infants were born to 59 women who were interviewed to determine their use of cocaine during pregnancy and whose hair was analyzed for the presence of cocaine. Regression analysis was used to evaluate the relationship between cocaine in newborn hair and in maternal hair. Radioimmunoassay of newborn hair and gas chromatography of meconium were more sensitive than immunoassay of urine ($p < .02$). Urine immunoassay failed to identify 60% of cocaine-exposed infants.

A comparative methodologic study was done to detect in utero cocaine exposure (Bandstra, et al., 1992). Maternal history was compared with various assays in meconium, maternal urine, and infant's urine, using GC/MS, EMIT, ADx, and DPC radioimmunoassay. The authors found meconium to be superior to either maternal or infant urine in detecting in utero cocaine exposure, although the need for concomitant maternal histories in some cases was emphasized.

SUMMARY

Drug abuse in pregnancy is an important health-care problem in the United States and globally, as well. In 1990, it was estimated that 4.8 million women in the United States used illicit drugs and 0.4% to 32% used illicit drugs during pregnancy. The impact of illicit drug use during pregnancy on the mother and infant are far reaching. Thus, for the appropriate management and care of the mother and infant, identification of the drug-exposed infant is vital. The meconium drug test has become an important test to detect these infants. For several reasons, meconium drug analysis is ideal for this purpose: (a) the test is sensitive and specific, (b) the test can be performed using common laboratory techniques for purposes of mass screening and with capabilities for GC/MS confirmation, (c) collection of meconium is easy and noninvasive, (d) meconium can be analyzed for a number of illicit and licit drugs, the latter including nicotine, (e) analysis of serial meconium can reflect the type, chronology, and amount of in utero drug exposure of the infant, and, (f) drugs in meconium are present up to the third day after birth; thus late testing of the infant for drugs is possible, if necessary. Meconium drug testing has therefore become an important diagnostic tool for clinical and research purposes.

REFERENCES

Bailey, D. N. (1989). Drug screening in an unconventional matrix: Hair analysis. *Journal of the American Medical Association, 262,* 3331.

Bandstra, E., Steele, B., & Chitwood, D. (1992). Detection of in utero cocaine exposure: A comparative methodologic study. *Pediatric Research 31,* 58A.

Callahan, C. M., Grant, T. M., Phipps, B. S., Clark, G., Novack, A. H., Streissguth, A. P., & Raisys, V. A. (1992). Measurement of gestational cocaine exposure: Sensitivity of newborn hair, meconium and urine. *Journal of Pediatrics, 120,* 763–768.

Chasnoff, I. J. (1989). Drug use and women. Establishing a standard of care. *Annals of New York Academy of Science, 562,* 208–210.

Chasnoff, I. J., Burns, W. J., Schnoll, S. H., & Burns, K. A. (1985). Cocaine use in pregnancy. *New England Journal of Medicine, 313,* 666–669.

Chasnoff, I. J., Bussy, M. E., Savich, R., & Stack, C. M. (1986). Perinatal cerebral infarction and maternal cocaine use. *Journal of Pediatrics, 108*, 456–459.

Chasnoff, I. J., Hatcher, R., & Burns, W. J. (1982). Polydrug and methadone addicted newborns: A continuum of impairment. *Pediatrics, 70*, 210–213.

Chasnoff, I. J., Hunt, C. E., Kletter, R., & Kaplan, D. (1989). Prenatal cocaine exposure is associated with respirating pattern abnormalities. *American Journal of Diseases of Children, 143*, 583–587.

Chavez, C. J., Ostrea, E. M., Stryker, J. C., & Smialek, T. (1979). Sudden infant death syndrome among infants of drug dependent mothers. *Journal of Pediatrics, 95*, 407–409.

Chavez, C. J., Ostrea, E. M., Stryker, J. C., & Strauss, M. E. (1979). Ocular abnormalities in infants as sequalae of prenatal drug addiction. *Pediatric Research, 12*, 367A.

Clark, G. D., Rosenweig, B., & Raisys, V. A. (1990). Analysis of cocaine and benzoylecgonine in meconium of infants born to cocaine dependent mothers. *Clinical Chemistry, 36*, 1022A.

Fried, P. A., & Watkinson, B. (1990). 36 and 48 month neurobehavioral follow up of children prenatally exposed to marijuana, cigarettes, alcohol. *Journal of Development and Behavior, 11*, 49–58.

Fulroth, R., Phillips, B., & Durand, D. (1989). Perinatal outcome of infants exposed to cocaine and/or heroin in utero. *American Journal of Diseases of Children, 43*, 905–910.

Garcia, D., Romero, A., Garcia, G., & Ostrea E. M. (1994). Gastric juice analysis for drugs. *Pediatric Research, 35*, 225A.

Gervasio, C., & Ostrea, E. M. (1991). Bedside meconium drug testing using latex agglutination inhibition test. *Pediatric Research, 29*, 215A.

Graham, K., Koren, G., Klein, J., Schneiderman, & J. Greenwald, M. (1989). Determination of gestational cocaine exposure by hair analysis. *Journal of the American Medical Association, 262*, 3328–3330.

Halstead, A. C., Godolphin, W., Lockitch, G., & Segal, S. (1988). Timing of specimens is crucial in urine screening of drug dependent mothers and infants. *Clinical Biochemistry 21*, 59–61.

Kandall, S. R., & Gartner, L. M. (1974). Late presentation of drug withdrawal symptoms in newborns. *American Journal of Diseases of Children, 127*, 58–61.

Khalsa, J. H., & Gfroerer, J. (1991). Epidemiology and health consequences of drug abuse among pregnant women. *Seminars in Perinatology, 15*, 265–270.

Lucena, J., Silvestre, M. A., Raymundo, A. L., Roxas, R., Jr., & Ostrea, E. M., Jr. (1991). The effect of timing, dosage duration of cocaine intake during pregnancy on the amount of cocaine in meconium in a rat model. *Pediatric Research, 29*, 62A.

Mac, E., Pacis, M., Garcia, G., & Ostrea, E. M. (1994). A marker of fetal exposure to alcohol by meconium analysis. *Pediatric Research, 35*, 238A.

MacGregor, S. N., Keith, L. G., Chasnoff, I. J., Rosner, M. A., Chisum, G. M., Shaw, P., & Minogue, J. P. (1987). Cocaine use during pregnancy. Adverse perinatal outcome. *American Journal of Obstetrics and Gynecology, 157*, 686–690.

Maynard, E. C., Amuroso, L. P., & Oh, W. (1991). Meconium for drug testing. *American Journal of Diseases of Children, 145*, 650–652.

Montes, N., Romero, A., Ostrea, E. M., & Ostrea, A. R. (1993). Improved method of GC/MS analysis of meconium for opiate, cocaine and cannabinoid. *Pediatric Research, 33*, 66A.

Morales, V., Knapp, D. K., Utarnachitt, R., Utarnachitt, D., & Ostrea, E. M. (1994). Meconium analysis will detect intrapartum drug use: Clinical implications. *Pediatric Research, 35*, 87A.

Oleske, J., Minnefor, A., Cooper, R., Thomas, K., Cruz, A. D., Ahdieh, H., Guerrero, I., Joshi, V., & Deposito, F. (1983). Immune deficiency syndrome in children. *Journal of the American Medical Association, 249*, 2345–2349.

Oro, A. S., & Dixon, S. D. (1987). Perinatal cocaine and methamphetamine exposure: Maternal and neonatal correlates. *Journal of Pediatrics, 111*, 571–578.

Ostrea, E. M., Brady, M., Gause, S., Raymundo, A. L., & Stevens, M. (1992). Drug screening of newborns by meconium analysis: A large scale, prospective, epidemiologic study. *Pediatrics, 89*, 107–113.

Ostrea, E. M., Brady, M. J., Parks, P. M., Asensio, D. C., & Naluz, A. (1989). Drug screening of meconium in infants of drug dependent mothers. An alternative to urine screening. *Journal of Pediatrics, 115*, 474–477.

Ostrea. E. M., & Chavez, C. J. (1979). Perinatal problems (excluding neonatal withdrawal) in maternal drug addiction: A study of 830 cases. *Journal of Pediatrics, 94*, 292–295.

Ostrea, E. M., Jr., Chavez, C. J., & Strauss, M. E. (1976). A study of factors that influence the severity of neonatal narcotic withdrawal. *Journal of Pediatrics, 88*, 642–645.

Ostrea, E. M., Knapp, D. K., Romero, A., Montes, M., & Ostrea, A. R. (1994). Meconium analysis to assess fetal exposure to active and passive maternal smoking. *Journal of Pediatrics, 124*, 471–476.

Ostrea, E. M., Knapp, D. K., Romero, A., & Ostrea, A. R. (1994). Postmortem analysis of meconium in early gestation human fetuses exposed to cocaine: Clinical implications. *Journal of Pediatrics, 124*, 477–479.

Ostrea, E. M., Knapp, D. K., Ostrea, A.R., Tannenbaum, L., & Saleri, V. (1994). A prospective study comparing systematic interview and analysis of maternal hair and meconium to determine illicit drug use during pregnancy. *Pediatric Research, 35*, 245A.

Ostrea, E. M., Jr., Kresbach. P., Knapp, D. K., & Simkowski, K. (1987). Abnormal heart rate tracings and serum creatine phosphokinase in addicted neonates. *Neurotoxicology and Teratology, 9*, 305–309.

Ostrea, E. M., Lizardo, E., & Tanafranca, M. (1992). The prevalence of illicit drug exposure in infants in the NICU as determined by meconium drug screen. *Pediatric Research, 31*, 215A.

Ostrea, E. M., Lynn, S. N., Wayne, R. H., & Stryker, J. C. (1980). Tissue distribution of morphine in the newborns of addicted monkeys and humans. *Developmental Pharmacology and Therapy, 1*, 163–170.

Ostrea, E. M., Parks, P., & Brady, M. (1988). Rapid isolation and detection of drugs in meconium of infants of drug dependent mothers. *Clinical Chemistry, 34*, 2372–2373.

Ostrea, E. M., & Romero, A. (1992). Selection criteria for routine drug screening of infants by meconium analysis. *Pediatric Research 31*, 215A.

Ostrea, E. M., Romero, A., & Yee, H. (1993). Adaptation of the meconium drug test for mass screening. *Journal of Pediatrics, 122*, 152–154.

Ostrea, E. M., Yee, H., & Thrasher, S. (1991). GC/MS analysis of meconium for cocaine: Clinical implications. *Pediatric Research, 29*, 63A.

Romero, A., Mac, E., Knapp, D. K., & Ostrea, E. M. (1993). Evaluation of a rapid, meconium drug testing system for clinical use. *Pediatric Research, 33*, 68A.

Ryan, L., Ehrlich, S., & Finnegan, L. (1987). Cocaine abuse in pregnancy: Effects on the fetus and newborn. *Neurotoxicology and Teratology, 9*, 295–299.

Silvestre, M. A, Lucena, J., & Ostrea, E. M., Jr. (1991). The effect of timing, dosage and duration of morphine intake during pregnancy on the amount of morphine in meconium in a rat model. *Pediatric Research, 29*, 66A.

Sison, C., Ostrea, E. M., & Saleri, V. (1992). Resurgence of congenital syphilis is a drug related problem. *Pediatric Research, 31*, 261A.

Wilson, G. S. (1989). Clinical studies of infants and children exposed prenatally to heroin. *Annals of the New York Academy of Science, 562*, 183–194.

Wilson, G. S., McCreary, R., Kean, J., & Baxter, J. (1979). The development of preschool children of heroin addicted mothers: A controlled study. *Pediatrics, 63*, 135–141.

Zelson, C., Rubio, E., & Wasserman, E. (1971). Neonatal narcotic addiction: 10 year observation. *Journal of Pediatrics, 48*, 178–182.

Zuckerman, B., Frank, D. A., Hingson, R., Amaro, H., Levenson, S. M., Kayne, H., Parker, S., Vinci, R., Aboagye, K., Fried, L. E., Cabral, H., Timperi, R., & Bauchner, H. (1989). Effects of maternal marijuana and cocaine use on fetal growth. *New England Journal of Medicine, 320*, 762–768.

III

OUTCOMES

This section presents a comprehensive overview of the functional impact of prenatal cocaine exposure. Results from animal and human studies on basic neural effects through complex cognitive, emotional, and social outcomes are reviewed and evaluated. There are several themes to be found here. One is the preliminary nature of findings reported to date. The methodological hurdles that researchers must overcome have been described already (see the Methods section of this volume). Although presented as caveats in the Outcomes chapters, there is nonetheless an accumulating body of evidence suggesting several specific, direct effects on fetal brain development of cocaine exposure. These are particularly well documented by the exquisite rodent model described by Spear. Her laboratory has found evidence of neural alterations of the dopaminergic, opiate, and serotonergic systems. These effects seem to extend to the behavioral realm. Cocaine-exposed offspring show less adaptability to stress, as well as changes in play behavior. They also exhibit fundamental alterations in cognitive processing, indicated by a host of conditioning studies performed at different developmental stages.

Needlman and colleagues extend the scope of possible early neuropsychological effects by comparing animal and human investigations. They present the evidence for effects of prenatal cocaine exposure on brain growth and injury, neurochemical changes, brain electrical activity, brain stem function, autonomic and endocrine effects, neurobehavioral organization, and learning, cognition, and aggression.

Mayes and Bornstein review what are known and suspected to be the direct and indirect effects of cocaine on the developing CNS. They propose a mechanism by which brain areas involved in the control of reactivity, arousal, and attention are especially vulnerable to these effects. A review of the few existing studies provides support for a specific impact of cocaine exposure on attentional measures, including information processing, novelty responsiveness, arousal, and reactivity to novel stimuli.

Mayes and Bornstein then develop another major theme: the critical importance of the postnatal environment to the developmental outcome of these children. Longitudinal studies of children at high risk by virtue of early medical complications, particularly low birth weight preterm infants, have increasingly emphasized the need to adopt the dynamic perspective that outcome is a function of the interaction between organismic and environmental factors that change over time. Mayes and Bornstein remind us of the myriad problems of parenting associated with cocaine use, including psychosocial and genetic problems that may predispose a woman to abuse drugs. In addition, they point to the chronic uncertainty, despair, and fear that characterize cocaine use. The remainder of the chapters in this section focus specifically on potential behavioral difficulties resulting from gestational cocaine exposure and parenting problems, that have profound implications for the development of cognitive ability, social competence, and interpersonal relationships.

Alessandri and colleagues discuss the impact of prenatal cocaine exposure on a behavioral characteristic with tremendous implications for learning ability, emotional responsivity, and social functioning. Temperamental characteristics such as persistence, fear of novelty, and low frustration tolerance have been associated with cognitive delays. The mechanism is probably indirect, through behavioral disorganization and the negative impact of a difficult temperament on parent–child interactions. As unusual emotional behavior has been associated with cocaine exposure, these authors have begun to examine whether these children exhibit a consistent pattern of temperamental characteristics that might interfere with optimal development. Evidence for decreases in both positive and negative reactivity is presented. Such findings have distinct implications for interventions with caregivers and educators of cocaine-exposed children.

Studies of Beckwith and co-workers report on preschool-age children exposed to PCP and cocaine in utero and provide reason for concern about the development of social competence in these children. A series of innovative studies of children from 15 months through 4½ years indicates that prenatal exposure and a drug-using environment are likely to result in insecure, disorganized attachments to caregivers in the second year of life; to restless, aggressive, and immature play in toddlers; and inattentive, disorganized preschoolers with poor peer interaction skills.

Finally, Woods and colleagues turn the spotlight on the mothers. Using a rural sample free of many of the confounding problems of polydrug use and chaotic urban life, these authors document significant difficulties of psychosocial functioning and parenting skills of these mothers. The authors present preliminary findings that cocaine-using women are more depressed, believe they have less control of their lives, have lower self-esteem, and feel more impact from life events than women who do not use this drug. These characteristics clearly place these women at an increased risk of parenting problems, with all of the implications for child outcome, including intergenerational substance abuse.

This section provides a unique and comprehensive compilation of effects of prenatal cocaine exposure. Although many of the reported findings are preliminary, it seems clear that these children are at increased risk of developing cognitive and social problems. That this is the result of long-term specific effects of cocaine may be debated; however, our belief in the validity of the impact of environmental conditions, particularly in interaction with infant vulnerabilities, convinces us that research must continue to elucidate particular deficits in these critical functional domains. It is only through such efforts that the most effective mechanism for optimizing the outcome of these children will become apparent.

11

▼▼▼▼▼▼▼

Alterations in Cognitive Function Following Prenatal Cocaine Exposure: Studies in an Animal Model

Linda Patia Spear
Binghamton University

With the increase seen since the early 1980s in the incidence of cocaine use during pregnancy (e.g., Neerhof, MacGregor, Retzky, & Sullivan, 1989; Streissguth et al., 1991), it has become increasingly important to examine the consequences of such early exposure on later offspring functioning. Two basic research strategies have been used in this work. Obviously the most direct approach is the use of clinical studies to examine offspring exposed gestationally to cocaine. Numerous such clinical studies have been conducted, although conclusions across these studies regarding infant outcome are rather controversial (e.g., see Hutchings, 1993, and associated commentaries, for discussion), in part due to concerns regarding appropriateness of control groups and validity of experimental designs used in some of this work (e.g., see Koren, Shear, Graham, & Einarson, 1989). Indeed, it is difficult to design well-controlled clinical studies, given methodological challenges such as the accurate detection and quantification of maternal cocaine use and adequate experimental or statistical control of potentially confounding variables (e.g., see Jacobson & Jacobson, 1990; Neuspiel & Hamel, 1991; Zuckerman & Bresnahan, 1991, for discussion). These and other difficulties associated with the conduct of well-controlled clinical studies are typically not an issue when conducting studies in laboratory animals. Thus, another approach that has been used to examine the consequences of early cocaine exposure for later offspring functioning has been to use animal models, with the results of these studies being used to confirm and extend clinical findings.

ANIMAL MODELS OF DEVELOPMENTAL
TOXICANTS: ARE THEY LIKELY
TO MODEL EFFECTS OBSERVED CLINICALLY?

The use of animal models to examine developmental neurotoxicants rests on the assumption that there will be good comparability of findings across species. But is this a reasonable assumption? This issue of across-species comparability of developmental toxicants was addressed in a 1989 workshop on the "Qualitative and Quantitative Comparability of Human and Animal Developmental Neurotoxicity," cosponsored by the Environmental Protection Agency and the National Institute on Drug Abuse (see Kimmel, Rees, & Francis, 1990). The goal of this workshop was to critically review and evaluate the consequences of a number of well-investigated developmental neurotoxicants (including ethanol, phenytoin, methylmercury, lead, polychlorinated biphenyls, and ionizing radiation), with a primary focus on comparing assessments of offspring function obtained in clinical studies with those obtained in animal (predominantly rodent) studies. Tests to assess functioning in each of five categories of functional effects (sensory, motivational/arousal, cognitive, motor, social) were identified in each species, although the specific tests used often varied markedly among the species. For instance, IQ tests or evaluation of language performance were often used to assess cognitive function in humans, whereas assessment of learning or retention of classical or operant conditioning tasks typically were examined in rodents.

Despite the notably different assessment methods that often were used to examine specific functions across species, review of the literature revealed remarkable qualitative comparability of findings across species for these known developmental toxicants. As summarized by the work group assigned the task of determining comparability of data across species:

> At the level of functional category, close agreement was found across species for all the neurotoxic agents reviewed at this Workshop. If a particular agent produced, for example, cognitive or motor deficits in humans, corresponding deficits were also evident in laboratory animals. This was true even when the specific endpoints used to assess these functions were often operationally quite different across species. (Stanton & Spear, 1990, p. 265)

In addition to comparing offspring outcome measures across species, doses necessary to produce adverse outcomes also have been compared (Rees, Francis, & Kimmel, 1990). In terms of delivered dose levels (amount of the substance entering the body in proportion to body weight), little correspondence was seen across species, with 100 to 10,000 times greater dose levels of the substances typically required in rodents to produce similar effects to those observed in humans (Rees et al., 1990). This perhaps should not be surprising given that the metabolic rate of rodents is substantially greater than that of humans. Indeed, if doses are expressed in terms of internal dose levels (tissue or blood concentrations of the substance), rodents and humans exhibit close comparability in terms of effective neurotoxic dose levels (Rees et al., 1990). Thus, when conducting work using animal models of developmental toxicants, it is critical to use a measure of internal dose levels rather than delivered dose per se to determine clinically relevant drug exposure levels.

To summarize, in these critical reviews of published data for known developmental toxicants, remarkable across-species comparability was obtained for both offspring outcome and the internal dose levels necessary to produce these adverse outcomes (e.g., see Driscoll, Streissguth, & Riley, 1990; Kimmel et al., 1990; Rees et al., 1990; Stanton & Spear, 1990). This does not mean, of course, that it necessarily can be concluded that the effects of other test substances such as cocaine will necessarily produce effects in animal studies that exactly mirror those obtained in humans. Rather, it would be highly atypical if good comparability of findings across species was not eventually obtained when assessing the developmental neurotoxicity of cocaine. Unfortunately, at this early stage in the examination of the developmental toxicity of cocaine, clinical and animal studies have largely focused on different dependent measures, with much of the clinical work to date focusing on reproductive and early infant outcomes, whereas animal studies have largely focused on offspring neurobehavioral function (see Spear, in press, for review). Ongoing efforts from both clinical and animal researchers in this area should result in a rapidly accumulating database of findings regarding outcomes associated with gestational cocaine exposure, data that can be used to determine the across-species comparability of cocaine's developmental toxicity and the ultimate outcome of individuals exposed prenatally to this drug of abuse.

ANIMAL MODELS OF DEVELOPMENTAL TOXICANTS: CHOICE OF ANIMAL MODEL

A variety of animal models of gestational cocaine exposure have been developed. These models differ in terms of the species used, the route of drug administration and the timing of the early cocaine exposure (see Spear, in press, for further discussion). In our work, like the majority of research in this area to date, we have chosen to use a rodent model. In our model, Sprague–Dawley rat dams are exposed chronically to cocaine beginning around the time of closure of the embryonic neural tube (embryonic Day 8—E8) until shortly before term (E20, with birth usually occurring on E22). It should be recognized that most rodents are born at a less mature stage than humans; for these altricial rodents, prenatal drug exposure typically models the first and second trimesters of human exposure, with drug exposure during the early postnatal period being necessary to model third trimester human exposure. Thus, the model system that we are using is roughly equivalent to human exposure beginning at the end of the first trimester and continuing through most of the second trimester. This exposure period encompasses early and critical stages of central nervous system development.

In our work, we have chosen to use the subcutaneous route for administering cocaine to our rat dams. Although this route induces some skin necrosis at injection sites (see Spear, in press, for further discussion), we chose this route because of the low toxicity of cocaine using this route relative to other routes, and because of data showing relatively sustained, dose-dependent, and clinically relevant plasma levels obtained using this procedure (e.g., Spear, Frambes, & Kirstein, 1989). For instance, dose-related increases in plasma and brain levels of cocaine were observed in chronically treated rat dams and their E20 fetuses following subcutaneous administration of 10, 20, or 40 mg/kg cocaine hydrochloride (Spear, Frambes, & Kirstein, 1989). Plasma levels of cocaine in the dams were in the range of those reported in human cocaine users, and significant levels of cocaine were observed in fetal brain (Spear, Frambes, & Kirstein, 1989). Given these findings, in much of our work we have focused on the 40 mg/kg dose, which is clearly above threshold for the production of neurobehavioral teratogenic effects.

Because cocaine is an anorexic agent, the dams typically exhibit a slight decrease in food intake at the start of treatment, although some degree of tolerance often develops to this effect. Hence, to determine whether alterations observed in cocaine-exposed offspring are related to the cocaine treatment per se or to the reduction in maternal weight gain during pregnancy, it is important to include nutritional controls. Typically we have included a pair-fed control group, with each dam in this group being fed only the amount of food consumed on the corresponding day of pregnancy by the cocaine-exposed dam to which it is paired. Offspring of cocaine-exposed and pair-fed dams can then be compared to offspring of a non-food-restricted control group to determine the impact, if any, of the reduction in maternal weight gain per se on the dependent measures of interest (see Spear & Heyser, 1993, for further discussion).

In our work, we typically foster each litter to a non-drug-treated surrogate mother at birth to control for possible residual effects of cocaine exposure on subsequent maternal behavior. Surrogate fostering appears to be important in that we have observed that rat dams exposed during pregnancy to cocaine exhibit subtle alterations in maternal behavior relative to control dams, and the behavior of offspring is likewise influenced by whether or not the dam that reared them was previously exposed to cocaine (Goodwin et al., 1992; Heyser, Molina, & Spear, 1992). As a final control issue, it should be noted that all of our testing procedures are conducted by experimenters who are blind to prenatal treatment condition.

OUR ANIMAL MODEL: BASIC FINDINGS

We obtained a relatively consistent set of findings regarding basic maternal–litter variables using the animal model already outlined. Typically, we see a slight (7%–10%) reduction in maternal weight gain during pregnancy at the 40 mg/kg dose of cocaine, which is presumably associated with a transient (3–5 day) reduction in food and water intake at the onset of drug treatment. In the dose range that we used, no alterations were seen in gestational length, number of fetal resorptions, number or gender of pups in the litter, offspring body weights from birth until adulthood, reflex development, or physical maturation. Whereas a number of laboratories have shown that higher doses of cocaine do induce maternal toxicity and reduce offspring body weights, it should be noted that the doses used in our model are below threshold for these effects, although well above threshold for inducing alterations in neurobehavioral function (see Spear, in press, for further discussion and references).

Whereas alterations in cognitive function are the focus of this review, these effects should be viewed within a context of other manifest neurobehavioral consequences of prenatal exposure to cocaine. In terms of neural alterations, we observed a variety of subtle alterations in the dopamine system in developing and adult offspring exposed prenatally to cocaine (Minabe, Ashby, Heyser, Spear, & Wang, 1992; Moody, Frambes, & Spear, 1992; Scalzo, Ali, Frambes, & Spear, 1990). Alterations in other neural systems are seen as well, including the opiate (Clow, Hammer, Kirstein, & Spear, 1991; Goodwin, Moody, & Spear, 1993) and serotonergic (Akbari, Kramer, Whitaker-Azmitia, Spear, & Azmitia, 1992) systems, along with age-dependent alterations in glycosphingolipids (Leskawa, Jackson, Moody, & Spear, 1994). Alterations are also seen outside the nervous system, such as age-related alterations in thymus weights (Spear, Kirstein, Frambes, & Moody, 1990).

In terms of behavioral alterations, we and others have observed that cocaine-exposed offspring exhibit characteristic alterations in their behavioral response to stress (Bilitzke & Church, 1992; Molina, Wagner, & Spear, 1994), which have been interpreted to suggest a reduced adaptability to stress in these offspring (Bilitzke & Church, 1992). We also observed subtle alterations in play behavior in these offspring (Wood, Molina, Wagner, & Spear, 1993), findings reminiscent of alterations in social and sexual behavior reported in such offspring by other laboratories (e.g., Johns et al., 1991; Raum, McGivern, Peterson, Shryne, & Gorski, 1990; Wood, Johanson, Bannoura, & Kendjelic, 1992). Cocaine-exposed offspring also are less sensitive to the discriminative stimulus effects of cocaine (Heyser, Rajachandran, Spear, & Spear, 1994) and are less predisposed than control animals to form cocaine-induced conditioned odor preferences in infancy (Heyser, Goodwin, Moody, & Spear, 1992) and cocaine-induced conditioned place preferences in adulthood (Heyser, Miller, Spear, & Spear, 1992), a pattern of psychopharmacological sensitivity suggestive of a potential alteration in later drug abuse liability. Thus, although the focus of this chapter is on cognitive alterations seen in cocaine-exposed offspring, these offspring vary behaviorally from control agemates in a number of other respects as well.

COGNITIVE ALTERATIONS SEEN
IN COCAINE-EXPOSED OFFSPRING

We have observed alterations in cognitive functioning in cocaine-exposed offspring in a number of conditioning situations. Our major findings in this area to date are outlined in the following.

Deficits in learning a simple classical conditioning task are evident during the early postnatal period in offspring exposed gestationally to cocaine. Early in life, if normal rat pups are given periodic intraoral infusions of milk in the presence of a particular odor and then are tested for their preference for that odor or another odor, they typically will spend more time over the odor previously paired with milk than rat pups that had been given equivalent but temporally separated (unpaired) exposures to both the odor and milk. Young cocaine-exposed rat pups appear to have difficulty learning this simple appetitive classical conditioning task. For instance, in some of our work (Spear, Kirstein, Bell, et al., 1989; see also Spear, Kirstein, & Frambes, 1989), 7-day-old offspring of cocaine-treated, pair-fed, and nontreated control dams were given three massed training trials, each consisting of a 3-min exposure to a novel odor not paired with reinforcement (the CS−) followed by a 3-min exposure to an odor (the CS+) paired with a 5-sec milk infusion every 30 sec. As can be seen in Fig. 11.1, pair-fed and nontreated lab chow control offspring receiving paired exposures of the milk and odor spent significantly more time over the CS+ odor than the CS− odor both immediately and 24 hrs after conditioning; in contrast, paired cocaine-exposed offspring did not exhibit a preference for the CS+ odor at either time interval. Similar conditioning deficits are also seen in 7- to 8-day-old cocaine-exposed offspring in an aversive classical conditioning task where the animals are trained to avoid an odor previously paired with foot shock (Goodwin et al., 1992; Heyser, Chen, Miller, Spear, & Spear, 1990).

Young cocaine-exposed offspring do not appear to be incapable of learning, but they may require more training to exhibit significant conditioning relative to control agemates. The classical conditioning deficits seen in young cocaine-exposed offspring may not reflect an absolute inability of these animals to learn a classical conditioning task early in life. Data to support this conclusion were obtained in a study by Goodwin et al. (1992) where we also examined the influence of fostering on behavioral functioning of the offspring. In this study, 7- to 8-day-old offspring were given either two, three, or four training trials of aversive (odor–foot shock) classical conditioning, or were given unpaired exposures to the odor and foot shock. Offspring examined in this study included cocaine-exposed offspring reared by their own dams (C40/C40) or foster dams (FOS/C40), lab chow control offspring reared by their own dams (LC/LC) or foster dams (FOS/LC), and untreated foster pups reared by lab chow control dams (LC/FOS) or by the previously cocaine-treated dams (C40/FOS).

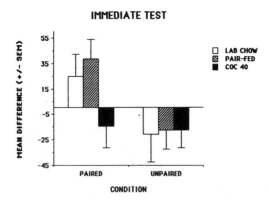

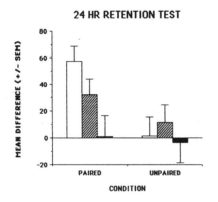

FIG. 11.1.   Mean time spent over the odor paired with milk minus the time spent over the nonreinforced odor [i.e., (CS+) – (CS–) difference scores] by 7-day-old cocaine-exposed (COC 40), pair-fed, and lab chow untreated control animals when tested immediately following conditioning (upper panel) and 24 hrs later (bottom panel). Animals received either paired exposure to the CS+ odor and milk (Paired) or explicitly unpaired exposure to these stimuli (Unpaired). The more positive the difference scores in Paired animals relative to Unpaired animals, the better the conditioning. Figure reprinted from Spear, Kirstein, and Frambes (1989), courtesy of the New York Academy of Sciences.

As can be seen in Fig. 11.2, all groups of control offspring (FOS/LC, LC/FOS, LC/LC) exhibited conditioning with as few as two training trials, with conditioning defined as a significant decrease in the time spent over the lemon odor previously paired with foot shock relative to the time spent over this odor by animals who previously received unpaired exposure to the odor and foot shock. Similarly, foster pups reared by previously cocaine-exposed mothers (C40/FOS) also learned the task in only two trials. In contrast, cocaine-exposed offspring

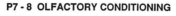

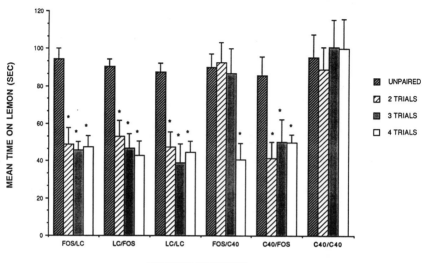

FIG. 11.2.   Mean time in seconds spent on the lemon side of the test apparatus by 7- to 8-day-old offspring from the various treatment groups who received either unpaired exposures to lemon and foot shock or two, three, or four training trials where lemon was paired with foot shock. Conditioning is inferred when animals that received paired exposure to the odor and foot shock spent significantly ($p <$ .05) less time over the lemon odor than their unpaired counterparts; such conditioning is indicated by a *. FOS = Foster; LC = Saline-injected controls; C40 = Cocaine group. Groups are designated by maternal treatment and pup origin (e.g., FOS/C40 reflects C40 pups reared by FOS dams). Figure reprinted from Goodwin et al. (1992), courtesy of Pergamon Press.

reared by foster dams (FOS/C40) required four trials to exhibit learning of the task, and cocaine-exposed offspring reared by their own dams (C40/C40) did not show significant conditioning on this task with even four training trials. These data illustrate that, although cocaine-exposed offspring do not exhibit conditioning on this task that is seen in control offspring following two or three training trials, if the number of training trials is increased, these offspring can exhibit significant conditioning. These data also suggest that cocaine-exposed offspring are even more impaired if they are reared by previously cocaine-exposed dams than non-drug-treated foster mothers.

Task difficulty and complexity may be an important factor in revealing conditioning deficits in cocaine-treated offspring, and this may in turn vary with age. Young cocaine-exposed offspring do not always exhibit cognitive deficits. One factor that may influence whether or not cognitive deficits are seen at a particular age is the difficulty and complexity of the task. Perceived task difficulty itself often appears to vary with age, with more complex tasks typically required to cognitively challenge older offspring than their infant counterparts. For instance, cocaine-exposed pups given two odor–foot shock training trials at postnatal Days 7 and 8 did not exhibit significant conditioning, although these offspring did develop an aversion to an odor paired with foot shock following only one training trial at postnatal Day 18 (Goodwin et al., 1992). Ontogenetic variations in odor–foot shock conditioning were examined systematically in Heyser et al. (1990). As can be seen in Fig. 11.3, 8-day-old cocaine-exposed offspring did not exhibit odor–foot shock conditioning that was evident in their

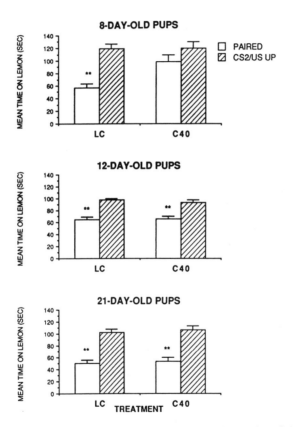

FIG. 11.3. Amount of time in seconds spent over the lemon side of the test apparatus by cocaine-exposed (C40) and saline-injected lab chow controls (LC) of the different test ages who received either unpaired exposures to lemon and foot shock (CS2/US UP) or two training trials where lemon was paired with foot shock (Paired). First-order conditioning was defined to occur if the paired animals spent significantly less time in the presence of the lemon odor than their unpaired counterparts (** = $p < .01$ for these comparisons). Figure reprinted from Heyser et al. (1990), courtesy of the American Psychological Association, Inc.

control counterparts, whereas cocaine-exposed pups given similar training at postnatal Day 12 or 21 did exhibit a significant aversion for the odor paired with foot shock (Heyser et al., 1990). These findings are reminiscent of those reported in offspring prenatally exposed to ethanol, where appetitive and aversive classical conditioning deficits were seen in 3- and 10-day-old exposed offspring, but not in exposed offspring tested later in life (Barron et al., 1988).

It is not simply the case that cocaine-exposed offspring "grow out of" their cognitive deficits later in life. When task complexity is increased, cognitive deficits are often evident in older cocaine-exposed offspring. For instance, as discussed later, deficits in higher order conditioning have been observed in cocaine-exposed offspring at postnatal Day 12 using a sensory preconditioning task (Heyser et al., 1990) and alterations in cognitive function have also been seen in these offspring in adulthood (Heyser, Spear, & Spear, 1992, 1994).

These conditioning deficits early in life do not appear to be related merely to a delay in cognitive development. In most conditioning tasks, performance improves with age, thus it is difficult to assess whether impaired performance reflects a delay in cognitive development or a fundamental alteration in cognitive functioning or information processing. There are a number of conditioning situations, however, in which young animals have been observed to learn more readily than older animals. One such task is sensory preconditioning, a task that is learned rapidly by normal rat pups in the age range from around 7 to 18 days postnatally, but not by weanling (postnatal Day 21) and older animals (Chen, Lariviere, Heyser, Spear, & Spear, 1991). If cocaine-exposed animals exhibit a delay in cognitive development, then it would be anticipated that at postnatal Day 21 they should perform like young animals on this task and hence exhibit better performance on this task than same-aged controls. If, however, there is a fundamental alteration in cognitive function, they should have difficulty performing this task regardless of age.

To examine these possibilities, Heyser et al. (1990) examined sensory preconditioning in cocaine-exposed and nontreated control offspring at 8, 12, and 21 days of age. There are two phases of conditioning in the sensory preconditioning paradigm. In the first phase, animals receive exposure to two odors simultaneously (e.g., banana and lemon) in the absence of any particular reinforcer. In the second phase, one of these odors (e.g., lemon) is paired with foot shock. To the extent that these animals learned an association between the two odors in Phase 1, when lemon is paired with foot shock in Phase 2, they should exhibit an aversion for banana on the preference test. Control groups include animals receiving unpaired exposures to the two odors in Phase 1 (CS1/CS2 UP) and unpaired exposures to the odor and foot shock in Phase 2 (CS2/US UP).

The results of this study are shown in Fig. 11.4. Focusing first on the data from the nontreated (LC) control animals, it can be seen that paired LC animals spent significantly less time over the test odor than both groups of unpaired animals when trained at postnatal Day 8 or 12, thereby exhibiting significant

SENSORY PRECONDITIONING

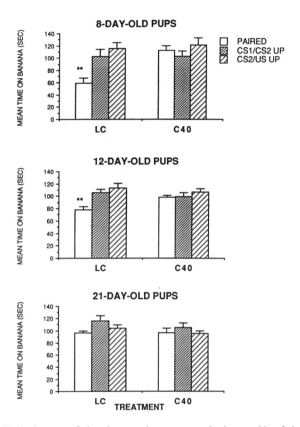

FIG. 11.4. Amount of time in seconds spent over the lemon side of the test apparatus by cocaine-exposed (C40) and saline-injected lab chow controls (LC) of the different test ages who received either unpaired exposure to lemon and banana in Phase 1 of conditioning (CS1/CS2 UP), unpaired exposure to lemon and foot shock in Phase 2 (CS2/US UP) or paired exposures in both phases (Paired). Sensory preconditioning was defined to occur if the paired animals spent significantly less time in the presence of the lemon odor than both unpaired groups (** = $p < .01$ for these comparisons). Figure reprinted from Heyser et al. (1990), courtesy of the American Psychological Association, Inc.

sensory preconditioning at these ages. No indication of conditioning was evident in LC animals at postnatal Day 21, confirming previous findings that there is an ontogenetic decline in performance of this task during ontogeny. In contrast, cocaine-exposed (C40) offspring did not show evidence of significant sensory preconditioning at any age. At postnatal Day 8, this absence of conditioning may be related to the cocaine-exposed animals' inability to exhibit odor–foot shock conditioning with the parameters used in Phase 2 (see Fig. 11.3). However, at

postnatal Day 12, cocaine-exposed animals still did not exhibit sensory preconditioning although they did demonstrate significant odor–foot shock conditioning
at this age (compare Figs. 11.3 and 11.4). These data from the 12-day-old
cocaine-exposed animals provide further support for the importance of task
difficulty in determining whether or not deficits in conditioning are seen in
cocaine-exposed offspring at a particular age. In addition, the finding that cocaine-exposed offspring do not demonstrate sensory preconditioning at any age
supports the hypothesis that these animals exhibit a fundamental alteration in
cognitive performance rather than merely a delay in cognitive development.

Alterations in cognitive performance are also evident in adult offspring
prenatally exposed to cocaine, particularly in terms of reversal performance. If
the conditioning deficits that cocaine-exposed offspring exhibit early in life are
related to a fundamental alteration in cognitive performance rather than a delay
in cognitive development, then it would be expected that cognitive deficits should
also be evident in these animals in adulthood. Indeed, we have seen alterations
in performance in two different tasks in cocaine-exposed male offspring in
adulthood, with these alterations being revealed in both studies particularly in
terms of reversal performance (Heyser, Spear, & Spear, 1992, 1994).

In a study by Heyser, Spear, and Spear (1992), we examined acquisition and
reversal of an operant conditional discrimination task in adult male cocaine-exposed and control offspring. Each animal was trained on an operant lever press
response for food reward, with every 10 presses on the correct lever resulting in
delivery of a food pellet. On each test day, an odor cue was placed in the chamber
to indicate which of the two levers would be reinforced on that day, with one
odor (banana or almond) indicating the right lever, and the other odor indicating
the left lever. Animals were trained on this rather difficult conditional discrimination until they reached the criteria of 80% correct in the first 10 responses,
and 90% correct over the entire session. Once that criterion was reached, each
animal was then placed into the reversal phase of the experiment where the odors
now predicted the opposite as previously; animals were trained on the reversal
task until the same criteria were reached. There were no differences among the
offspring in terms of their ability to learn the lever press response or with respect
to lever press response rates at any stage of the experiment; thus, the cocaine-
exposed offspring did not appear to differ from controls in basic performance
and motivational factors. Moreover, as can be seen in Fig. 11.5, there were no
differences in the number of sessions to reach criteria on the original discrimination task among the prenatal treatment groups. However, in the reversal phase,
offspring exposed gestationally to cocaine were substantially slower to learn the
reversal response than all the other groups of offspring.

A similar deficit in reversal performance was observed in a recent study
examining acquisition and reversal of a Morris water maze task in adult male
and female cocaine-exposed and control offspring (Heyser et al., 1994). During
acquisition, animals were trained to swim to a hidden platform in a fixed location

NUMBER OF SESSIONS TO CRITERION

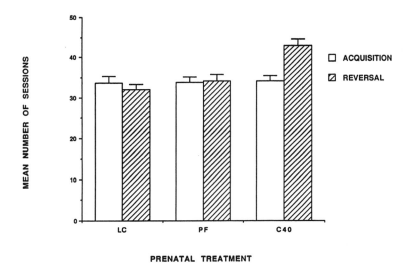

FIG. 11.5.   Mean number of sessions to reach criteria for acquisition and reversal
of the appetitive conditional discrimination task based on olfactory cues in adult
male offspring from the various treatment groups. LC = untreated lab chow control
group; PF = pair-fed control group; C40 = cocaine treatment group. * = C40 group
significantly different from all other groups. Data derived from Heyser, Spear, and
Spear (1992).

from one of two start positions at the edge of the swim tank; eight massed trials
were given daily for 3 days on this version of the task. Animals were then placed
on the training phase of the reversal task. Each animal received eight massed
trials per day for 3 days, with the fixed platform location repositioned in the
water maze to a location diametrically opposed to that used during training.
Numerous measures were assessed on each test trial and on several probe trials;
distance traveled to reach the platform on each trial is used to illustrate the
findings. Analyses of the acquisition data (Fig. 11.6) revealed that both male and
female cocaine-exposed offspring traveled slightly but significantly more distance
to find the platform on the first day of training when compared to both groups
of control offspring; distance traveled decreased across days indicating learning
in all groups, with no differences among the prenatal treatment groups revealed
on the second and third days of acquisition. These data, although not particularly
dramatic, are reminiscent of data discussed earlier (see Fig. 11.2) showing that
young cocaine-exposed offspring may exhibit slower acquisition than control
offspring (Goodwin et al., 1992). In terms of the reversal data (Fig. 11.7), although
all animals rapidly learned the new platform location, male cocaine-exposed
offspring traveled a significantly greater distance to find the new platform location
on the first reversal training trial when compared to both male LC and PF
offspring, with no differences observed among the female offspring. Gender-

MALE

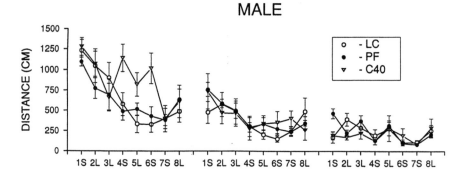

FEMALE

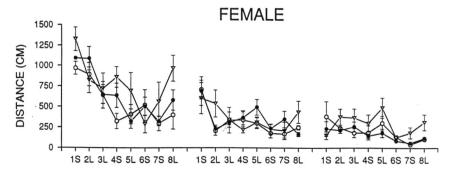

FIG. 11.6. Mean distance traveled to reach the hidden platform in the Morris water maze on the first 3 days of acquisition by adult male (top panel) and female (bottom panel) offspring from the various prenatal treatment groups. (Note that the letter designation following each trial number represents the relative distance from the start position to the platform: S = shorter distance; L = longer distance). LC = untreated lab chow control group; PF = pair-fed control group; C40 = cocaine treatment group.

specific findings also have been reported in various other studies investigating the effects of early cocaine exposure on later offspring neurobehavioral function (see Spear, in press, for review).

Although the tasks used in these two studies (Heyser, Spear, & Spear, 1992, 1994) were quite different, the findings from both studies provide evidence that deficits in reversal acquisition are seen in adult male offspring exposed gestationally to cocaine. It is as if these animals are perseverating/persisting in their behavior, and are having trouble modifying their behavior in response to a rule change. It is interesting that animals with certain kinds of brain damage, such as damage to the dopaminergic systems of the brain (e.g., see Simon & Le Moal, 1984; Le Moal & Simon, 1991, for references and discussion), also have trouble modifying their behavior in response to rule changes. As mentioned previously, we have data showing a variety of subtle alterations in the dopamine systems in these animals (e.g., Minabe et al., 1992; Moody et al., 1992; Scalzo et al., 1990).

MALE

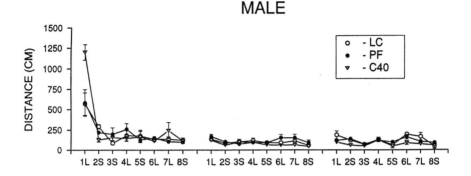

FEMALE

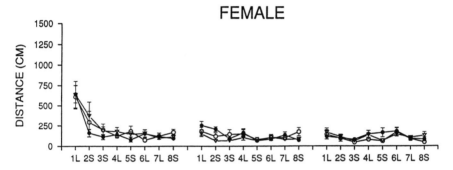

FIG. 11.7.   Mean distance traveled to reach the hidden platform in the Morris water maze following its repositioning (i.e., reversal acquisition) by adult male (top panel) and female (bottom panel) offspring from the various prenatal treatment groups. (Note that the letter designation following each trial number represents the relative distance from the start position to the platform: S = shorter distance; L = longer distance). LC = untreated lab chow control group; PF = pair-fed control group; C40 = cocaine treatment group.

Prenatal exposure to cocaine may not always result in impairments, but rather may sometimes be associated with an apparent facilitation of cognitive function. It is not always the case that cocaine-exposed offspring exhibit conditioning deficits when tested during the preweaning period. For instance, Heyser, McKinzie, Athalie, Spear, and Spear (1994) examined nonassociative learning and retention in terms of habituation of a heart rate (HR) orienting response (bradycardia) in 16-day-old cocaine-exposed and control offspring. Heart rate habituation was assessed by giving each pup 10 exposure trials to a 10-sec pulsed 80dB tone, with each tone presentation separated by a 60-sec interval. For each trial, heart rate was measured during a 5-sec pretone period and during the 10-sec tone presentation. The pups were then tested for retention of the habituated response by giving pups 10 additional trials at retention intervals of 1, 2, 4, or 6 hrs. The prenatal treatment groups did not differ in terms of HR habituation, with all groups showing initial HR deceleration to the tone and a reduction in the magnitude of this orienting response over trials. All groups showed good retention of the habituated HR response at 1 hr and 2 hrs and substantial forgetting by 6 hrs. However, as can be seen in Fig. 11.8, at the 4 hr retention interval, cocaine-exposed offspring exhibited better retention of the habituated response than pair-fed and untreated control offspring.

Thus, in this instance, cocaine-exposed offspring exhibited a *facilitated* retention of the habituated autonomic HR response when compared to control offspring. This facilitated retention may represent an alteration in the way information is processed in these animals, or may reflect perseverative behavior reminiscent of the reversal deficits seen in these animals in adulthood (as discussed earlier). Regardless of how these findings are interpreted, the data provide clear evidence that cocaine-exposed offspring are not always impaired in terms of cognitive performance, and may sometimes even exhibit facilitated perform-

HEART RATE CHANGE

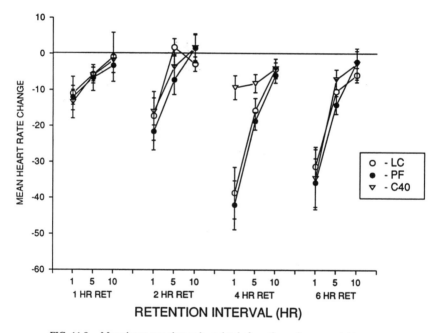

FIG. 11.8.   Mean heart rate change by animals from the various prenatal treatment groups during the tone presentation at 1, 2, 4, and 6 hrs after initial habituation of the heart rate orienting response. A greater negative change in heart rate reflects a greater orienting response, thus retention of the habituated heart rate orienting response to the tone is characterized by a smaller magnitude of heart rate deceleration. LC = untreated lab chow control group; PF = pair-fed control group; C40 = cocaine treatment group. Figure reprinted from Heyser, McKinzie, et al. (1994), courtesy of Wiley-Liss, Inc., a division of John Wiley & Sons, Inc.

ance relative to control animals. Similar findings have been reported in the literature with prenatal ethanol exposure: Although ethanol-exposed offspring exhibit cognitive deficits in a variety of tasks, on certain kinds of tasks ethanol-exposed offspring show facilitated acquisition or performance (see Riley, 1990, for references and discussion).

CONCLUSIONS AND FUTURE DIRECTIONS

In our work to date we have observed that offspring exposed gestationally to cocaine exhibit alterations in cognitive function in a variety of conditioning situations. These cognitive deficits do not appear to be related to a delay in cognitive development, and can be seen in adulthood as well as early in life. Whether or not such deficits will be evident in a particular task seems to depend on factors such as the amount of training, test age, and task complexity and difficulty.

With regard to possible implications of these findings for clinical populations of exposed offspring, one perspective would cautiously suggest potential optimism. On the positive side, it should be noted that these offspring often exhibit normal cognitive performance, and in instances where deficits are seen, they typically can be countered with additional training. In adulthood, few acquisition deficits were observed even on rather difficult conditional discrimination and spatial discrimination tasks, with deficits predominantly being seen in male cocaine-exposed offspring in terms of acquisition of reversal responses. Thus, one perspective of these data is that, although prenatal cocaine exposure may lead to some cognitive dysfunction, the deficits may be relatively subtle and may be counteracted by additional training.

On the other hand, these data can also be interpreted more pessimistically in terms of potential clinical implications. This interpretation rests on data showing that even mild disruptions obtained in simple tests of cognitive function in animal studies may be predictive of more severe cognitive dysfunctions in humans exposed to the same biological insult. For instance, untreated phenylketonuria (PKU) produces clear mental retardation in humans, whereas studies using animal models of PKU have found relatively mild disruptions in cognitive performance, with these impairments typically being evident predominantly only in tasks involving transfer of learning (e.g., see Strupp, Bunsey, Levitsky, & Hamberger, 1994).

Another approach that can be taken is to compare the effects of prenatal cocaine on cognitive performance observed to date with the more extensive literature available on cognitive effects of prenatal ethanol. In certain respects the consequences of early exposure to these two drugs bear similarities in animal studies. For instance, prenatal exposure to either drug results in classical conditioning deficits early in life that are not evident later in life (i.e., compare Barron et al., 1988; Heyser et al., 1990). Reversal deficits are also seen following prenatal exposure to either substance (Heyser, Spear, & Spear, 1992; Riley, Lochry, Shapiro, & Baldwin, 1979). These similarities in findings may have significant clinical implications for the prognosis of cocaine-exposed offspring given that individuals exposed to high levels of alcohol during gestation—that is, fetal alcohol syndrome (FAS) offspring—exhibit significant intellectual impairments that are evident not only during the early school-age years but also in adolescence and adulthood (e.g., see Streissguth, Sampson, & Barr, 1989). Yet, from the limited amount of data in cocaine-exposed animals to date, it appears that the effects of prenatal cocaine on conditioning may be somewhat less pronounced than those of prenatal ethanol exposure. Particularly in tasks (such as active and passive avoidance) where alterations in locomotor activity may influence performance, deficits have been reported in ethanol-exposed offspring (e.g., Lochry & Riley, 1980) that apparently are not seen in cocaine-exposed offspring (Riley & Foss, 1991). Whether these deficits seen in ethanol-exposed offspring are associative in nature or related to alterations in motor activity, however, is not clear; increases in locomotor activity are commonly seen following prenatal alcohol exposure (see Riley, 1990, for review), whereas alterations in baseline activity are not consistently seen in offspring prenatally exposed to cocaine (see Spear, in press, for review). Thus, it is possible that cocaine-exposed human offspring may exhibit cognitive deficits that are similar to but somewhat less pervasive than those seen in individuals prenatally exposed to high levels of ethanol.

Of course, these types of conclusions are quite speculative at this early stage in our investigation of the developmental toxicology of cocaine. It is hoped that the results from animal studies such as those reviewed here will encourage systematic assessment of cognitive function using a variety of conditioning tests in clinical populations of cocaine-exposed infants and children during their critical preschool and school-age years.

ACKNOWLEDGMENT

This work was supported by National Institute on Drug Abuse Grants R01 DA14478 and K02 DA00140.

REFERENCES

Akbari, H. M., Kramer, H. K., Whitaker-Azmitia, P. M., Spear, L. P., & Azmitia, E. C. (1992). Prenatal cocaine exposure disrupts the development of the serotonergic system. *Brain Research, 572,* 57–63.

Barron, S., Gagnon, W. A., Mattson, S. N., Kotch, L. E., Meyer, L. S., & Riley E. P. (1988). The effects of prenatal alcohol exposure on odor-associative learning in rats. *Neurotoxicology and Teratology, 10,* 333–339.

Bilitzke, P. J., & Church, M. W. (1992). Prenatal cocaine and alcohol exposures affect rat behavior in a stress test (The Porsolt Swim Test). *Neurotoxicology and Teratology, 14*, 359–364.

Chen, W. J., Lariviere, N. A., Heyser, C. J., Spear, L. P., & Spear, N. E. (1991). Age-related differences in sensory conditioning in rats. *Developmental Psychobiology, 24*, 307–325.

Clow, D. W., Hammer R. P., Jr., Kirstein, C. L., & Spear, L. P. (1991). Gestational cocaine exposure increases opiate receptor binding in weanling offspring. *Developmental Brain Research, 59*, 179–185.

Driscoll, C. D., Streissguth, A. P., & Riley, E. P. (1990). Prenatal alcohol exposure: Comparability of effects in humans and animal models. *Neurotoxicology and Teratology, 12*, 231–237.

Goodwin, G. A., Heyser, C. J., Moody, C. A., Rajachandran, L., Molina, V. A., Arnold, H. M., McKinzie, D. L., Spear, N. E., & Spear, L. P. (1992). A fostering study of the effects of prenatal cocaine exposure: II. Offspring behavioral measures. *Neurotoxicology and Teratology, 14*, 423–432.

Goodwin, G. A., Moody, C. A., & Spear, L. P. (1993). Prenatal cocaine exposure increases the behavioral sensitivity of neonatal rat pups to ligands active at opiate receptors. *Neurotoxicology and Teratology, 15*, 425–431.

Heyser, C. J., Chen, W. J., Miller, J., Spear, N. E., & Spear, L. P. (1990). Prenatal cocaine exposure induces deficits in Pavlovian conditioning and sensory preconditioning among infant rat pups. *Behavioral Neuroscience, 104*, 955–963.

Heyser, C. J., Goodwin, G. A., Moody, C. A., & Spear, L. P. (1992). Prenatal cocaine exposure attenuates cocaine-induced odor preference in infant rats. *Pharmacology, Biochemistry and Behavior, 42*, 169–173.

Heyser, C. J., McKinzie, D. L., Athalie, F., Spear, N. E., & Spear, L. P. (1994). Effects of prenatal exposure to cocaine on heart rate and nonassociative learning and retention in infant rats. *Teratology, 49*, 470–478.

Heyser, C. J., Miller, J. S., Spear, N. E., & Spear, L. P. (1992). Prenatal exposure to cocaine disrupts cocaine-induced conditioned place preference in rats. *Neurotoxicology and Teratology, 14*, 57–64.

Heyser, C. J., Molina, V. A., & Spear, L. P. (1992). A fostering study of the effects of prenatal cocaine exposure: I. Maternal behaviors. *Neurotoxicology and Teratology, 14*, 415–421.

Heyser, C. J., Rajachandran, L., Spear, N. E., & Spear, L. P. (1994). Responsiveness to cocaine challenge in adult rats following prenatal exposure to cocaine. *Psychopharmacology, 116*, 45–55.

Heyser, C. J., Spear, N. E., & Spear, L. P. (1992). Effects of prenatal exposure to cocaine on conditional discrimination learning in adult rats. *Behavioral Neuroscience, 106*, 837–845.

Heyser, C. J., Spear, N. E., & Spear, L. P. (1994). *The effects of prenatal exposure to cocaine on Morris water maze performance in adult rats.* Manuscript submitted for publication.

Hutchings, D. E. (1993). The puzzle of cocaine's effects following maternal use during pregnancy: Are there reconcilable differences? *Neurotoxicology and Teratology, 15*, 281–286.

Jacobson, J. L., & Jacobson, S. W. (1990). Methodological issues in human behavioral teratology. In C. Rovee-Collier & L. P. Lipsitt (Eds.), *Advances in infancy research* (Vol. 6, pp. 111–148). Norwood, NJ: Ablex.

Johns, J. M., Means, L. W., Bass, E. W., Means, M. J., Zimmerman, L. T., & McMillen, B. A. (1991, November). *Prenatal cocaine exposure alters aggressive behavior in adult Sprague-Dawley rat offspring.* Paper presented at the annual meeting of the Society for Neuroscience, New Orleans, LA.

Kimmel, C. A., Rees, D. C., & Francis, E. Z. (Eds.). (1990). Qualitative and quantitative comparability of human and animal developmental neurotoxicity [Special issue]. *Neurotoxicology and Teratology, 12*.

Koren, G., Shear, H., Graham, K., & Einarson, T. (1989). Bias against the null hypothesis: The reproductive hazard of cocaine. *Lancet, 2*, 1440–1442.

Le Moal, M., & Simon, H. (1991). Mesocorticolimbic dopaminergic network: Functional and regulatory roles. *Physiological Reviews, 71*, 155–234.

Leskawa, K. C., Jackson, G. H., Moody, C. A., & Spear, L. P. (1994). Cocaine exposure during pregnancy affects rat neonate and maternal brain glycosphingolipids. *Brain Research Bulletin, 33*, 195–198.

Lochry, E. A., & Riley, E. P. (1980). Retention of passive avoidance and T-maze escape in rats exposed to alcohol prenatally. *Neurobehavioral Toxicology, 2*, 107–115.

Minabe, Y., Ashby, C. R., Jr., Heyser, C. J., Spear, L. P., & Wang, R. Y. (1992). The effects of prenatal cocaine exposure on spontaneously active midbrain dopamine neurons in adult male offspring: An electrophysiological study. *Brain Research, 586*, 152–156.

Molina, V. A., Wagner, J. M., & Spear, L. P. (1994). The behavioral response to stress is altered in adult rats exposed prenatally to cocaine. *Physiology and Behavior, 55*, 941–945.

Moody, C. A., Frambes, N. A., & Spear, L. P. (1992). Psychopharmacological responsiveness to the dopamine agonist quinpirole in normal weanlings and in weanling offspring exposed gestationally to cocaine. *Psychopharmacology, 108*, 256–262.

Neerhof, M. G., MacGregor, S. N., Retzky, S. S., & Sullivan, T. P. (1989). Cocaine abuse during pregnancy: Peripartum prevalence and perinatal outcome. *American Journal of Obstetrics and Gynecology, 161*, 633–638.

Neuspiel, D. R., & Hamel, S. C. (1991). Cocaine and infant behavior. *Journal of Developmental and Behavioral Pediatrics, 12*, 55–64.

Raum, W. J., McGivern, R. F., Peterson, M. A., Shryne, J. H., & Gorski, R. A. (1990). Prenatal inhibition of hypothalamic sex steroid uptake by cocaine: Effects on neurobehavioral sexual differentiation in male rats. *Developmental Brain Research, 53*, 230–236.

Rees, D. C., Francis, E. Z., & Kimmel, C. A. (1990). Qualitative and quantitative comparability of human and animal developmental neurotoxicants: A workshop summary. *Neurotoxicology, 11*, 257–270.

Riley, E. P. (1990). The long-term behavioral effects of prenatal alcohol exposure in rats. *Alcoholism: Clinical and Experimental Research, 14*, 670–673.

Riley, E. P., & Foss, J. A. (1991). The acquisition of passive avoidance, active avoidance, and spatial navigation tasks by animals prenatally exposed to cocaine. *Neurotoxicology and Teratology, 13*, 559–564.

Riley, E. P., Lochry, E. A., Shapiro, N. R., & Baldwin, J. (1979). Response perseveration in rats exposed to alcohol prenatally. *Pharmacology, Biochemistry and Behavior, 10*, 255–259.

Scalzo, F. M., Ali, S. F., Frambes, N. A., & Spear, L. P. (1990). Weanling rats exposed prenatally to cocaine exhibit an increase in striatal D2 dopamine binding associated with an increase in ligand affinity. *Pharmacology, Biochemistry and Behavior, 37*, 371–373.

Simon, H., & Le Moal, M. (1984). Mesencephalic dopaminergic neurons: Functional role. In E. Usdin, A. Carlsson, A. Dahlstrom, & J. Engel (Eds.), *Catecholamines: Neuropharmacology and central nervous system—Theoretical aspects* (pp. 293–307). New York: Liss.

Spear, L. P. (in press). Neurobehavioral consequences of gestational cocaine exposure: A comparative analysis. In C. Rovee-Collier & L. P. Lipsitt (Eds.), *Advances in infancy research*.

Spear, L. P., Frambes, N. A., & Kirstein, C. L. (1989). Fetal and maternal brain and plasma levels of cocaine and benzoylecgonine following chronic subcutaneous administration of cocaine during gestation in rats. *Psychopharmacology, 97*, 427–431.

Spear, L. P., & Heyser, C. J. (1993). Is use of a cellulose-diluted diet a viable alternative to pair-feeding? *Neurotoxicology and Teratology, 15*, 85–89.

Spear, L. P., Kirstein, C. L., Bell, J., Yoottanasumpun, V., Greenbaum, R., O'Shea, J., Hoffmann, H., & Spear, N. E. (1989). Effects of prenatal cocaine exposure on behavior during the early postnatal period. *Neurotoxicology and Teratology, 11*, 57–63.

Spear, L. P., Kirstein, C. L., & Frambes, N. A. (1989). Cocaine effects on the developing central nervous system: Behavioral, psychopharmacological, and neurochemical studies. In D. E. Hutchings (Ed.), *Annals of the New York Academy of Sciences: Vol. 562. Prenatal abuse of licit and illicit drugs* (pp. 290–307). New York: New York Academy of Sciences.

Spear, L. P., Kirstein, C. L., Frambes, N. A., & Moody, C. A. (1990). Neurobehavioral teratogenicity of gestational cocaine exposure. *NIDA Research Monograph (Problems of Drug Dependence, 1989), 95*, 232–238.

Stanton, M. E., & Spear, L. P. (1990). Workshop on the qualitative and quantitative comparability of human and animal developmental neurotoxicity, Work Group I Report: Comparability of measures of developmental neurotoxicity in humans and laboratory animals. *Neurotoxicology and Teratology, 12*, 261–267.

Streissguth, A. P., Grant, T. M., Barr, H. M., Brown, Z. A., Martin, J. C., Maycock, D. E., Ramey, S. L., & Moore, L. (1991). Cocaine and the use of alcohol and other drugs during pregnancy. *American Journal of Obstetrics and Gynecology, 164*, 1239–1243.

Streissguth, A. P., Sampson, P. D., & Barr, H. M. (1989). Neurobehavioral dose-response effects of prenatal alcohol exposure in humans from infancy to adulthood. In D. E. Hutchings (Ed.), *Annals of the New York Academy of Sciences: Vol. 562. Prenatal abuse of licit and illicit drugs* (pp. 145–158). New York: New York Academy of Sciences.

Strupp, B. J., Bunsey, M., Levitsky, D. A., & Hamberger, K. (1994). Deficient cumulative learning: An animal model of retarded cognitive development. *Neurotoxicology and Teratology, 16*, 71–79.

Wood, R. D., Johanson, I. B., Bannoura, M. D., & Kendjelic, E. M. (1992, June). *Prenatal cocaine effects on sexually dimorphic behaviors in the young rat*. Poster presented at the annual meeting of the Neurobehavioral Teratology Society, Boca Raton, FL.

Wood, R. D., Molina, V. A., Wagner, J. M., & Spear, L. P. (1993, November). *Play behavior in the juvenile rat following prenatal exposure to cocaine and postnatal stress*. Poster presented at the annual meeting of the International Society for Developmental Psychobiology, Alexandria, VA.

Zuckerman, B., & Bresnahan, K. (1991). Developmental and behavioral consequences of prenatal drug and alcohol exposure. *Pediatric Clinics of North America, 38*, 1387–1406.

12

▼▼▼▼▼▼▼

Neurophysiological Effects of Prenatal Cocaine Exposure: Comparison of Human and Animal Investigations

Robert Needlman
Case Western Reserve University School of Medicine

Deborah A. Frank
Marilyn Augustyn
Barry S. Zuckerman
Boston University School of Medicine

Among the proposed teratogenic effects of prenatal exposure to cocaine, effects on neurological structure and function are of particular interest. Cocaine is known to block the reuptake by the presynaptic neuron of the monoamines norepinephrine, dopamine, and serotonin. As a consequence, exposure to cocaine during a period of rapid neuronal growth and elaboration may result in longstanding or irreversible changes in the brain. From the social perspective, the widely embraced stereotype of "crack kids" implies that these children suffer from an immutable neurologic derangement that renders them inattentive, disruptive, and potentially dangerous. This chapter reviews selected clinical and animal research studies that speak to the question of neurophysiological effects of prenatal cocaine exposure, both in the immediate neonatal period and beyond. The term *effect* is used loosely. In the clinical studies cited, the findings actually represent correlates, inasmuch as causality is exceptionally difficult to establish. Experimental studies, however, do make claims of cause and effect.

A large number of phenomena can be gathered under the umbrella of *neurophysiological effects*, including such diverse topics as brain growth and injury, neurochemistry, electroencephalographic activity, and autonomic nervous system control. On a more clinical level, phenomena such as habituation, learning, and behavioral regulation can also be accommodated under the same heading. From the cellular to the social, proposed effects or correlates of prenatal cocaine exposure can be arranged along a continuum. This organizational schema, which

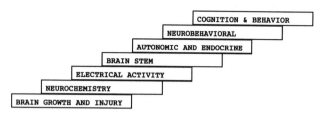

FIG. 12.1.   Levels of proposed neurophysiological effects.

provides the conceptual backbone of this chapter, is presented in Fig. 12.1. At each step, research from both human and animal studies is discussed and an attempt is made to point out areas of concordance and discordance, as well as areas where there is information from one but not the other realm of investigation. Areas of overlap between animal and human studies are presented in Table 12.1. Due to the large body of data in the animal area, and the representation in this volume of a number of researchers who have contributed significantly to that corpus, special attention is paid to studies in humans.

Before beginning this survey, it is important to point out that on the question of greatest social concern—that is, the potential existence of permanent cognitive or behavioral sequelae in humans—there are still no reliable data. No prospective study has followed exposed children from birth into elementary school. The controlled study with the longest follow-up to date includes children aged 3½, and the existence of large and differential attrition from the exposed and control groups renders its findings suspect (Chasnoff, Griffith, & Freier, 1992). The complex methodological and logistical issues that preclude any easy answer to this question have been extensively reviewed, as have the temptations and dangers of reaching a premature conclusion (Mayes, Granger, Bornstein, & Zuckerman, 1992; Zuckerman & Bresnahan, 1991). Animal studies that speak to the issue of long-lasting behavioral and cognitive changes are described later, and in other chapters of this book. Provocative as they are, these studies must be considered hypothesis generating with respect to humans. The intent of this chapter is to outline a context for such hypotheses.

BRAIN GROWTH AND INJURY

Prenatal cocaine exposure is consistently linked with decreased neonatal head circumference. Brain growth is the main stimulus to cranial growth. Therefore, decreased head circumference is thought to reflect a deficit in brain growth. Perhaps the best estimate of the magnitude of this effect comes from our study of 1,226 mothers attending a general prenatal clinic. Gestational cocaine exposure was independently associated with a decrement in head circumference of .43 cm, after controlling statistically for 13 potential confounding factors, including gestational age, maternal characteristics, and other substances of abuse (Zuckerman

TABLE 12.1

Correlates of In Utero Cocaine Exposure: Human and Animal Research

Level	Human Outcome Measures	Animal Outcome Measures
Brain growth and injury	Head circumference Cranial ultrasound, MRI	Head circumference DNA and protein synthesis No studies
Neurochemistry	CSF monoamines, precursors, and metabolites (neonatal only)	Brain concentrations, turnover, receptor number and activity, spontaneous electrical activity, glucose metabolism
Electrical activity	EEG Auditory evoked potentials Visual evoked potentials	EEG Auditory brain stem responses
Brain stem Startle Respiratory control Cry	Glabellar tap ± sound Hypoxic, hypercapneic challenge airstream stimulation Acoustic cry analysis	Acoustic startle Hypoxic, hypercapneic challenge No studies
Autonomic and endocrine	Circulating catecholamines and receptors Blood pressure and pulse Cortisol response to stress	No studies In utero studies, only Cortisol response (acute administration, only)
Neurobehavioral organization	NBAS clusters: habituation, orientation, motor, state, autonomic, and reflex	Reflex development, motor activity, response to stress
Cognition and behavior	IQ (DQ) tests (e.g., the Bayley)	Operant conditioning Maze learning Aggression, exploration

et al., 1989). Among the methodological strengths of this study were the large sample size and ascertainment of drug exposure both during pregnancy and after birth, by both standardized interviews and biological screening.

Cocaine has also been linked with prenatal brain injury. Chasnoff and colleagues reported a single case of cerebral infarction in a 1-day-old infant whose mother admitted to intranasal cocaine use during the first 5 weeks of pregnancy, as well as heavy use during the 3 days prior to delivery (Chasnoff, Bussey, Savich, & Stack, 1986). However, in an uncontrolled series of nine cocaine-exposed infants studied by cranial MRI, no abnormalities of white or gray matter were detected (Link, Weese-Mayer, & Byrd, 1991). The authors acknowledge that small sample size and subject self-selection may have limited the validity of this result.

In contrast, multiple cranial ultrasound abnormalities were reported in a series of 74 full-term infants who had been exposed to cocaine, methamphetamine, or some combination of drugs of abuse (Dixon, 1989). Sonographic abnormalities were found in 35.1% (26 of 74) of drug-exposed infants, significantly more than in a group of drug-free, healthy newborns (5.3%), and similar to the rate in a group of critically ill drug-free infants (27.6%). A variety of lesions were found. In 8.1% of the drug-exposed infants, characteristic 3- to 10-mm echolucencies were found in the periventricular areas, frontal lobes, and basal ganglia, suggesting small prior hemorrhage or ischemia. The location and nature of these lesions were consistent with a postulated mechanism of either increased blood pressure (hemorrhage) or decreased blood flow (ischemia). As in other studies, drug-exposed infants had significantly decreased head size, but no association was found between head circumference and sonographic abnormalities, suggesting that these effects may occur by different mechanisms.

The inclusion of infants exposed to multiple drugs, and lack of details about subject and control group selection, dosage, and potential confounding factors make interpretation of this study problematic: It is possible that the effects reported occur only in children exposed to unusually high doses of cocaine, or when cocaine was combined with, say, a high level of cigarette or alcohol use. Evidence of a synergistic constricting effect of cocaine and cigarette smoking on coronary arteries highlights the potential importance of multiple drug interactions (Moliterno et al., 1994).

A longitudinal, controlled study by our group at Boston City Hospital has attempted to address these methodological concerns. Cocaine-exposed infants were identified by maternal history and use of biologic markers, including meconium testing. Meconium testing identifies cocaine exposure that occurred during at least the third, and possibly the second trimester, compared to urine testing which only identifies use in the last 3 or 4 days (Ostrea, Parks, & Brady, 1988). Infants exposed to amphetamines or opiates were excluded. Control subjects were recruited from the same maternity ward, matched for ethnicity. In addition to biological screening, detailed interviews were used to assess the dosage of cocaine and other substance use, maternal mental health, and social stressors.

In an initial analysis no significant difference in the number of intracranial abnormalities was found between cocaine-exposed and nonexposed infants (Frank, McCarten, Cabral, & Zuckerman, 1992). However, an analysis of the full data set ($N = 240$) found evidence of a dose effect: Echodensities in the caudate nucleus were found in 48% of infants of heavy cocaine users (defined as > 75th percentile in either self-reported days of use or meconium benzoylecgonine concentration), compared to 22% of infants exposed to lesser amounts of cocaine, and 23% of cocaine-nonexposed infants. The difference was significant after statistically controlling for birth weight and maternal parity, age, ethnicity, cigarettes, alcohol, and marijuana use (Frank, McCarten, Cabral, Levenson, & Zuckerman, 1994).

The animal literature offers few direct parallels to the findings in humans of altered head growth and brain injury. The findings for brain growth are equivocal: In one rabbit study, continuous subcutaneous cocaine from Day 10 of pregnancy failed to produce differences in snout-occiput head circumference (Weese-Mayer, Klemka-Walden, Chan, & Gingras, 1991). Few studies in rats have reported data on head circumference or overall brain weights. Administration of 30 mg/kg/day of cocaine to pregnant rats resulted in "little or no" effect on brain weights or DNA content of forebrain or cerebellum (Seidler & Slotkin, 1993). This effect was not accounted for by ischemia, a local anesthetic effect, or general inhibition of macromolecule synthesis, suggesting a specific action on cell replication. We are not aware of an animal model that parallels the ultrasonographic changes observed in humans.

NEUROCHEMISTRY

In human infants, the inaccessibility of brain tissue for study has limited research on brain metabolic correlates of prenatal cocaine exposure. The only available data are from a single pilot study of monoamine precursors and metabolites in cocaine-exposed neonates (Needlman, Zuckerman, Anderson, Mirochnik, & Cohen, 1993). Cerebrospinal fluid (CSF) was obtained from 31 infants at the time of lumbar punctures undertaken to rule out central nervous system (CNS) infection. The 11 exposed infants had documented cocaine exposure, either by maternal history or drug testing; the 20 unexposed infants had both negative histories and at least one biological assay (meconium or urine) negative for cocaine. Cocaine-exposed children had significantly lower weights and smaller heads, and were of lower gestational age than controls, but were similar in other respects. There was no difference in the rate of perinatal complications or Apgar scores, and none of the infants had CNS infection.

The major finding was lower homovanillic acid (HVA) among cocaine-exposed infants; the difference, 148 ng/ml versus 219 ng/ml, was significant at the $p = .01$ level, even in this small sample. Other substances—tyrosine, trypto-phan, 3-methoxy-4-hydroxyphenylglycol (MHPG), and 5-hydroxyindoleacetic acid (5HIAA)—did not differ between groups. The association between cocaine and lower HVA remained significant at the $p = .03$ level, after removing from the analysis mothers who used other illegal substances. Cigarette smoking, almost universal among the cocaine-using mothers, was controlled by removing from the analysis subjects who were *not* exposed to cigarettes. In this analysis, the association between cocaine and lower HVA remained significant at $p = .002$. As a further control for potential confounding factors, bivariate analyses were carried out, each time controlling for a single factor, including birth weight, length, head circumference, and gestational age. With these factors controlled, the association between cocaine and lower HVA no longer reached the usual level of statistical significance, although the adjusted mean HVA among exposed children remained, in all cases, about 50 points lower than that among unexposed.

HVA is the principal metabolite of dopamine (DA) in the CNS, and the finding of decreased CSF HVA among cocaine-exposed infants is consistent with de-creased brain production or turnover of DA. Interpretation of these findings is problematic, however, because of the small sample size. A more fundamental problem is the uncertain the relationship between concentrations of substances in the CSF and actual alterations in structure or function in the brain (Commis-siong, 1985; Westerink, & Kikert, 1986). For example, decreased levels of HVA could be due to decreased production globally, or only in specific brain regions, or to increased clearance. Finally, these findings relate to the immediate newborn period only: Whether or not differences in CSF monoaminergic metabolites persist later in life remains an open question. Depressed brain dopamine levels were reported in autopsies of two adult chronic cocaine users, compared to age-matched controls, although the specific sites of dopamine depletion differed in the two cocaine-using subjects (Wilson et al., 1992). No similar data are available from children exposed prenatally.

In the animal literature, neurochemical changes have been documented by direct analysis of brain tissue, rather than CSF assays. As a result, there are no published animal data that are directly comparable with the human CSF findings already described. Studies of neurochemical changes in mature animals after withdrawal from chronic cocaine may be analogous, in some respects, to the situation of the prenatally exposed infant. Chronic administration of cocaine to adult rats resulted in decreased extracellular DA 5 days after withdrawal (Rossetti, Melis, Carboni, & Gessa, 1992), but *increased* extracellular DA following a challenge dose (Akimoto, Hamamura, & Otsuki, 1989). Sixty days after chronic cocaine administration (20 mg/kg/day of cocaine for 10 days), tyrosine hydroxy-lase activity and dopamine synthesis were decreased (Trulson, Joe, Babb, & Raese, 1987; Trulson, & Ulissey, 1987), although a different laboratory found unchanged concentrations of dopamine and its metabolites (Kleven, Woolverton, & Seiden, 1988).

There is a rapidly expanding literature on the neurochemical effects of in utero cocaine exposure in laboratory animals. In some instances, this exposure has been shown to affect the developing nervous system differently than the mature brain. For example, repeated administration of DA antagonists during the third trimester results in decreased DA receptors (down-regulation), whereas postnatal administration increases receptors (up-regulation; Miller & Friedhoff, 1988). A wide range of outcomes has been investigated in rat pups at various ages following administration to the mother of 10 to 50 mg/kg/day of cocaine. These outcomes include number and function of dopaminergic and other receptors (Fung, Reed, & Lau, 1989; Henderson, McConnaughey, & McMillen, 1991; Scalzo, Ali, Frambes, & Spear, 1990), dopamine concentration and turnover (Seidler & Slotkin, 1993; Weese-Mayer et al., 1993; Yablonsky-Alter et al., 1991), dopaminergic and serotonergic fiber density (Akbari, Kramer, & Azmitia, 1991; Kramer, Azmitia, & Akbari, 1991), spontaneous electrical activity of dopaminergic neurons (Minabe, Ashby, Heyser, Spear, & Wang, 1992), and brain glucose metabolism (Dow-Edwards, Freed, & Fico, 1990; Dow-Edwards, Freed, & Milhorat, 1988). A full review of this literature is beyond the scope of this chapter (see the chapters in this volume by Dow-Edwards and Spear).

BRAIN ELECTRICAL ACTIVITY

A limited number of studies have looked at brain electrical activity in cocaine-exposed infants. The earliest report, a nonblinded, uncontrolled series of 39 full-term infants exposed to cocaine but no other illicit substances, found a high incidence of abnormal EEGs—17 of 38 in the first week of life—most characterized by "irritability." The degree of abnormality did not correlate with the dose or timing of cocaine use reported by the mothers. By the second week, however, only nine tracings were abnormal, and all but one had normalized between 3 and 12 months of age. These findings were considered consistent with transient neurotransmitter changes (Doberczak, Shanzer, Senie, & Kandall, 1988). A subsequent, controlled study found no significant association between prenatal exposure to cocaine and abnormal EEG findings (Legido, Clancy, Spitzer, & Finnegan, 1992). However, at younger conceptual ages more drug-exposed infants showed a continuous slow-wave sleep pattern than did controls, suggesting accelerated maturation. Because this study was cross-sectional, no information is available about the time course of sleep EEG abnormalities; also, no attempt was made to distinguish between cocaine exposure and polydrug exposure.

Auditory brain-stem evoked responses have been looked at as an index of brain myelination and neurological maturity. In an initial study, delayed absolute and interpeak latencies were found in a group of 18 cocaine-exposed infants of 32 to 40 weeks gestational age (Shih, Cone-Wesson, & Reddix, 1988). However, in a cross-sectional study of 64 infants at multiple postconceptual ages, prolonged latencies were evident in premature and term cocaine-exposed infants but not in infants assessed at 52 to 65 weeks postconceptual age (equivalent to 1 month old in a full-term infant; Salamy, Eldredge, Anderson, & Bull, 1990). This study included only 24 cocaine-exposed term infants, and only 6 in the oldest group. In a cross-sectional study of 50 cocaine-exposed term neonates, with matched controls, no abnormality of auditory brain-stem evoked potentials was found, and no cocaine-exposed infant had evidence of sensorineural hearing impairment (Carzoli, Murphy, Hammer-Knisely, & Houy, 1991). Visual evoked potentials (VEP) were looked at in a convenience sample of 16 4- to 5-month-old full-term infants, half of whom were cocaine exposed. No differences in VEP latencies were found, although the cocaine-exposed infants scored significantly lower on a test of visual recognition memory (Hansen, Struthers, & Gospe, 1993).

The animal literature offers few direct analogues to human EEG studies and studies of cortical or brain-stem evoked responses. In chronically catheterized fetal sheep, .5 mg/kg of cocaine resulted in transient decreases in low-voltage electrocortical activity; a larger dose (1.0 mg/kg) resulted in decreased low-voltage activity that did not remit (Chan et al., 1992). Fetal sheep in another laboratory also showed EEG changes during cocaine infusion, but not afterwards. These changes, which were associated with changes in behavior, did not appear to be associated with cerebral hypoxia (Abrams, Burchfield, Gerhardt, & Peters, 1992). One study of rats chronically exposed to cocaine during gestation and lactation has shown prolonged auditory brain-stem evoked response latencies, suggesting delayed myelinization (Salamy, Dark, Salfi, Shah, & Peeke, 1992). Visual evoked response changes in cocaine-exposed animals have not been reported.

BRAIN STEM

Startle Response

The intensity of eyeblink and startle reflexes may be an indicator of activity in the brain stem centers controlling sensorimotor reactivity and arousal. Eyeblink following a controlled tap between the eyes was significantly greater in 19 cocaine-exposed infants compared to 19 age-matched controls, and the difference was increased when paired with a loud (90 dB) tone (Anday, Cohen, Kelley, & Leitner, 1989).

In laboratory animals, there is evidence that the effect of cocaine on the acoustic startle response is mediated by dopaminergic neurons. Acute administration of cocaine to previously unexposed adult rats increased the acoustic startle response, and this effect was blocked by dopamine receptor inhibitors but not by local anesthetics (Davis, 1985).

However, prenatal cocaine exposure does not appear to have long-term effects on the startle response in the laboratory. A series of carefully designed experiments failed to demonstrate differences between gestationally exposed versus unexposed rats in acoustic startle response, modulation of startle by a prestartle sound pulse, habituation to startle, or augmentation of the startle response following an acute dose of cocaine (Foss, 1991; Foss & Riley, 1991).

Respiratory Control

Alterations in respiratory control have also been correlated with prenatal cocaine exposure. During the first week of life, sleeping cocaine-exposed infants had a greater frequency of respiratory pauses and depression of minute ventilation elicited by a stream of air blown at the face, but there were no differences in heart rate either at rest or following stimulation, or in the hyperventilatory response to elevated carbon dioxide (hypercapnia; Chen et al., 1991). Subjects for this study were 21 full-term infants with histories and urine testing consistent with exposure to cocaine but not alcohol, tobacco, and other illicit drugs, and the control group was closely matched for gestational age, birth weight, and age.

Blunted responses to hypoxia and hypercapnia during sleep were documented in a group of 23 cocaine-exposed infants between 1 and 4 months of age (Davidson-Ward et al., 1992). However, a number of polydrug-exposed infants were included in the drug-exposed group, and it is therefore impossible to assess the contribution of exposure to phencyclidine, opiates, alcohol, and cigarettes. Birth weight was not controlled, although drug-exposed infants were significantly smaller, and other potential confounding factors such as ethnicity were not reported. Another group found no correlation between prenatal cocaine exposure and response to hypoxia in full-term infants (McCann & Lewis, 1991).

Two animal studies of respiratory control following cocaine exposure have been reported, both using rabbit pups as the model. In the first, 2-day-old cocaine-exposed pups showed increased minute ventilation at baseline and in response to hypoxia and hypercapnia (Wasiewski & Hasen, 1989). In the second, 4- to 5-day-old cocaine-exposed pups showed no increase in minute ventilation either at baseline or in response to hypoxia, whereas controls showed significant hyperventilation (Weese-Mayer, Klemka-Walden, Barkov, & Gingras, 1992). These opposite results may be explained by differences between these studies in the dosage and timing of the cocaine, or perhaps the age at testing, but it is not clear which most closely approximates the typical human situation.

Cry

Acoustic analysis of infant cry may reveal components, such as fundamental frequency or pitch, that reflect underlying neural control at the level of the midbrain and brain stem (Lester et al., 1991). Physiologically, these neural mechanisms determine cry characteristics by controlling laryngeal muscle tension, airway constriction, and force of expiration. Cries were recorded on the second day of life from 80 cocaine-exposed infants and 80 controls. Cocaine exposure was determined on the basis of information in the medical record; a minority of mothers admitted to other substance use, and controls were matched for maternal age, ethnicity, and substance use (other than cocaine).

Based on a statistical equation modeling procedure, cocaine-exposed infants were felt to fall into two groups: an "excitable" group characterized by longer duration, higher fundamental frequency, and more variable first formant, and a "depressed" group characterized by longer latency to cry, fewer cry utterances, lower amplitude cries, and more dysphonation. "Excitability" was interpreted as a direct neurological effect of cocaine, whereas "depressed" status was interpreted as a secondary effect of cocaine exposure, mediated by placental insufficiency and intrauterine growth retardation (Lester et al., 1991). The authors speculated that these different behavioral syndromes might be related to different exposure to timing of the exposure. Other possible explanations include differential exposure to other drugs of abuse, the use of which may well have gone undetected, because of the lack of systematic maternal interviews and biological testing, or differences in infant state at the time of the cry sampling. To date, no published research has investigated cry characteristics of cocaine-exposed infants beyond the immediate neonatal period, so the temporal stability of the "excitable" and "depressed" syndromes is unknown.

Acoustic analysis of laboratory animal vocalizations has not been reported.

AUTONOMIC AND ENDOCRINE

A variety of measures reflecting autonomic nervous system activity and reactivity have been used in clinical studies of prenatal cocaine exposure, including measurement of circulating catecholamines and receptors, blood pressure and pulse, and endocrine responses. There are few directly analogous studies in the animal literature.

Circulating Catecholamines

Circulating catecholamines were measured in the immediate neonatal period (24–48 hrs after birth) in a group of 12 cocaine-exposed infants and 8 controls (Mirochnick, Meyer, Cole, Herren, & Zuckerman, 1991). Cocaine exposure was documented by history and urine screens, together with negative histories and toxicology screens for opiates or other illicit drugs; control infants had both negative histories and meconium assays for drugs of abuse. Dopamine (DA) and norepinephrine (NE) were not different between groups, however the mean concentration of dihydroxyphenalanine (DOPA) was increased nearly twofold (10.3 versus 5.9, $p = .055$). DOPA is the precursor of both DA and NE, and DOPA levels may reflect neuronal catecholamine production (Mirochnick et al., 1991).

The potential confounding effects of gestational age and intrauterine growth were not controlled in this small pilot study.

Similar results were obtained in a study of neonates between 1 and 3 months of age. Plasma catecholamine levels were measured in 22 infants who had been exposed prenatally to a variety of substances including cocaine, opiates, phencyclidine, alcohol, and tobacco, and in 15 infants with negative drug histories (Davidson-Ward et al., 1991). NE was elevated by a factor of 1.8 in exposed infants. No differences were found in either epinephrine or dopamine, or in measures of alpha and beta adrenergic receptor binding on blood platelets. These findings were interpreted as evidence of increased sympathetic tone, possibly compounded by a failure of the expected receptor down-regulation. However, no attempt was made to separate out the effects of cocaine from those of other drugs of abuse, and both ethnicity and birth weight differed significantly between the exposed and control groups. Plasma norepinephrine was actually associated more strongly with socioeconomic status (SES), as indicated by whether the family received federal assistance, than with the history of substance exposure. The possibility of confounding by factors associated with low SES, such as the level of environmental stressors, cannot be excluded.

Animal studies have not reported circulating catecholamines or receptors in older animals following gestational cocaine exposure.

Blood Pressure and Pulse

Administered acutely, cocaine is known to cause increased pulse rate and blood pressure. The effects of repeated prenatal exposure are less clear. Elevated blood pressure with depressed cardiac output and stroke volume were documented in 15 cocaine-exposed infants on Day 1 of life compared to controls. By Day 2, however, the differences were no longer significant (van-de-Bor, Walther, & Ebrahimi, 1990).

One study has reported elevated blood pressure among cocaine-exposed children between 1 month and 4 years of age (Horn, 1992). Manual blood pressure measurements were obtained in a group of 12 prenatally exposed children. Four had hypertension, based on published population norms. Only 1 of 24 children not identified as cocaine exposed was found to have hypertension during the same period. These results were interpreted as evidence of a persistent autonomic nervous system abnormality (Horn, 1992). However, the study suffered from a number of methodological weaknesses, including manual (and therefore subjective) measurement of blood pressures by a nonblinded observer, and the absence of statistical analysis.

An attempt to replicate the finding using automated blood pressure measurement and blinded observers showed no group differences in blood pressure or pulse. The subjects were being followed as part of our follow-up study of cocaine-exposed infants at Boston City Hospital. Measurements were obtained from 32 cocaine-exposed and 23 nonexposed children between 9 and 24 months of age using an oscillometric blood pressure gauge and observers blinded to the children's cocaine status. We found no difference in systolic pressure ($M \pm SD$ 102.6 ± 9.4 in exposed vs. 101.8 ± 8.1 in nonexposed), diastolic pressure (945.0 ± 14.5 in exposed vs. 51.2 ± 10.6 in nonexposed), or pulse rate (113.6 ± 19.1 in exposed vs. 119.1 ± 19.4 in nonexposed). The study had adequate power to detect a difference of 6.3 blood pressure points or greater, with alpha = .05 and beta = .8 (Needlman, Kwon, Mirochnick, Zuckerman, & Frank, 1994).

Numerous studies have documented transient elevations in blood pressure and pulse after acute cocaine administration both in adult and fetal animals (Chan et al., 1992; Moore, Sorg, Miller, Key, & Resnik, 1986; Pitts & Marwah, 1989), but long-term changes following chronic in utero exposure in animals have not been reported.

Endocrine Changes

Endocrinologic effects of post- and prenatal exposure to opiates, alcohol, and marijuana have been demonstrated in laboratory animals, and to a much lesser extent in humans (Di Paolo, Rouillard, Morissette, & Levesque, 1989; Kuhn, Ignar, & Windh, 1992). Changes in the endocrine system may reflect direct actions on developing neural circuits, or effects secondary to changes in maternal hormones, stress, nutrition, or other factors (Kuhn, Ignar, & Windh, 1991). Correlates of prenatal cocaine exposure have been less extensively studied. In humans, one report has shown decreased cortisol response to stress in cocaine-exposed infants (Magnano, Gardner, & Karmel, 1992). Salivary cortisol levels in preterm infants exposed to cocaine but not to other drugs of abuse were compared with levels in nonexposed infants at baseline, following a mild stressor (a physical examination), and following a moderate stressor (a routine heel-stick). Basal cortisol levels did not differ between groups. Nonexposed infants showed a monotonic rise in cortisol following the mild and moderate stressors, but the cocaine-exposed infants showed no increase following the mild stressor, and a significantly attenuated rise following the moderate stressor. These results were interpreted to indicate either a direct effect of cocaine on the hypothalamic pituitary axis (HPA), or down-regulation of the HPA secondary repeated to in utero hypoxic stress. The authors speculated that the decreased cortisol response in cocaine-exposed infants might be related to decreased ability to regulate arousal (Magnano et al., 1992).

Immediate effects of maternal cocaine on fetal cortisol have been documented in sheep (Owiny, Sadowsky, Massmann et al., 1991). Fetal plasma cortisol rose significantly following maternal administration of higher dose (2 mg/kg) cocaine, but not lower. There was a concomitant reduction in fetal oxygen concentration after the higher dose, and it is unclear whether the rise in cortisol was due to hypoxia or to a central action of the cocaine (Owiny, Jones, Sadowsky, Myers et al., 1991). Endocrinologic effects of chronic in utero exposure have not been documented in animals.

NEUROBEHAVIORAL ORGANIZATION—NEONATAL

A number of studies have rated neurobehavioral correlates of prenatal cocaine in newborns using the Brazelton Neonatal Behavioral Assessment Scale (NBAS; Brazelton, 1984). The NBAS consists of a standardized sequence of observations under conditions of controlled stress. For example, the infant is first observed sleeping, then is aroused by a series of stimuli of increasing intensity, from a light shown in the eyes, to a bell, to being unwrapped. Items on the exam can be clustered to reflect six discreet neurobehavioral domains, including habituation, orientation, motor control, state control, autonomic control, and reflexes (Lester, Als, & Brazelton, 1982).

A summary of findings from six studies using the NBAS (Table 12.2) shows no clear-cut pattern of neurobehavioral correlates. Most studies found significant differences in no more than two domains. These disparate results may reflect underlying differences in the populations studied, in terms of dose and timing of cocaine exposure and other substances used, or differences in the administration or scoring of the NBAS. Although there has not been convincing evidence for a cocaine withdrawal syndrome in infants similar to opiate withdrawal, it is possible that some of the behaviors noted in the immediate newborn period are

TABLE 12.2
Results of Studies Using the NBAS

Study	Habituation	Orientation	Motor	State	Autonomic	Reflex
Chasnoff, Hunt, Kletter, & Kaplan (1989) $n = 79$	0	+	+	+	0	+
Eisen et al. (1991) $n = 52$	+	0	0	0	0	0
Neuspiel, Hamel, Hochberg, Greene, & Campbell (1991) $n = 111$	0	0	+	0	0	0
Richardson & Day (1991) $n = 24$	0	0	0	0	0	0
Coles, Platzman, Smith, James, & Falek (1992) $n = 107$	0	0	0	0	+	+
Mayes, Granger, Bornstein, & Zuckerman (1992) $n = 86$	+	0	0	0	0	0

due to recent cocaine exposure. The NBAS is not sensitive beyond 1 month of age, so these studies cannot provide information about the persistence of behavioral changes in later development.

Animal studies of neurobehavioral organization following in utero cocaine have focused on somewhat different outcomes, generally at later ages. Direct parallels to the NBAS studies described previously are not found. Outcomes have included, for example, development of reflexes (Sobrian et al., 1990; Spear, Kirstein, & Frambes, 1989), activity and righting behavior in immature rats (Henderson, & McMillen, 1990; Johns, Means, Means, & McMillen, 1992; Zmitrovich, Hutchings, Dow-Edwards, Malowany, & Church, 1992), and response to a stressful situation (Bilitzke & Church, 1992; Johns, Means, Anderson, Means, & McMillen, 1992). As with the human studies, no clear-cut picture has emerged. Effects have generally been subtle, and have not been noted consistently at multiple ages.

COGNITION AND BEHAVIOR

Data on the developmental progress of cocaine-exposed children beyond the newborn period are just beginning to appear in print. As noted earlier, studies attempting to correlate prenatal cocaine with postnatal development must contend with myriad methodological difficulties, including: (a) the impossibility of accurately determining the dose and timing of exposure; (b) the potentially confounding effects of variables such as other substances of abuse, maternal health and nutrition, and the postnatal childrearing environment; and (c) the necessity to follow large numbers of children for long periods of time (Mayes et al., 1992; Zuckerman & Bresnahan, 1991). As a result, no statements can be made with confidence about developmental outcomes correlated specifically with prenatal cocaine exposure in humans.

Limited data, however, are available from a handful of studies: Chasnoff's group reported on 3-year follow-up of a cohort of polydrug-exposed infants, including 92 exposed to cocaine and other drugs, 25 exposed to cigarettes, alcohol, and marijuana, but no cocaine, and 45 controls judged "drug free" (Azuma & Chasnoff, 1993). A statistical path analysis indicated main effects on Stanford–Binet IQ scores for exposure to all of the substances (drugs, alcohol, and cigarettes) together, although not for cocaine singly, as well as effects mediated through head circumference, home environment, and task perseverance as rated during the testing. These findings, however, do not speak to the question of cocaine per se. Also, high subject attrition and unclear criteria for selection for testing hamper interpretation of the results (Frank et al., 1994). An analysis of the same subject cohort at 2 years of age found no overall difference in scores on the Bayley Scales of Infant Development (BSID), although a higher percentage of cocaine and polydrug-exposed infants scored below the mean than did non-drug-exposed controls (Chasnoff et al., 1992). Again, selective sample retention and selection for testing could have biased the results in either direction, accounting for this modest correlation.

Another follow-up study, this one in a predominantly White, middle- and working-class cohort, has not found long-term effects of relatively light cocaine exposure. Children of women admitting to "social" cocaine use in the first trimester only and who stopped when they learned they were pregnant ($n = 30$), were compared with matched nonexposed controls ($n = 30$), and controls exposed only to marijuana ($n = 20$). BSID scores and scores on the Vineland Adaptive Behavior Scale at 19 to 20 months did not differ between cocaine-exposed children and either of the control groups, despite higher reported use of alcohol and cigarettes and lower SES and education among the cocaine-using mothers (Graham et al., 1992). There were no differences in the acquisition of social, motor, and language developmental milestones. The study had the power to detect an effect size as large as 0.8 *SD*.

Traditional developmental and IQ tests, such as the Stanford–Binet and Bayley, measure performance but do not illuminate the processes of cognition itself (Stanton & Spear, 1990). Few studies have appeared in print relating cocaine exposure and cognitive processes such as attention, short- and long-term memory, the acquisition of conditioned responses, and the ability to change learned behaviors in response to changing contingencies. One exception is the report of significantly lower scores on a visual recognition memory test, the Fagan Test of Infant Intelligence, noted earlier (Hansen et al., 1993). In that test, the child's preference for novelty is gauged by measuring the relative amounts of time spent looking at novel versus familiar pictures; relatively strong correlations with later IQ have been reported. The study included a convenience sample of eight term infants exposed to cocaine and/or amphetamines, drawn from a special high-risk nursery, and eight controls matched for ethnicity. The children were tested between 6 and 12 months of age, however the actual ages of the exposed and control group are not reported. Birth weight, maternal age, and exposure to marijuana and cigarettes also differed between the groups, making interpretation problematic.

Reliable data about other aspects of behavior, such as aggression, play, and emotional development, are not yet available for clinical populations.

In the animal literature, studies of rats who were prenatally exposed to cocaine indicate the persistence of abnormal cognition and behavior, although the results are varied. Spear et al. (1989) reported a series of experiments using classical conditioning in gestationally cocaine-exposed rat pups. At 7 to 8 days of age, exposed pups did not learn to associate an odor with milk when they were presented together, although control animals did so readily. At 17 to 18 days of age, exposed pups also showed impaired ability to associate an odor with a foot shock when these stimuli were presented together. However, under similar conditions at 7 days of age, there was no difference between cocaine-exposed and control pups' acquisition of the aversive stimulus conditioning (Spear et al., 1989).

Gestationally exposed rats took no longer to learn a conditioned discrimination task (bar press), but were less accurate, and were less able to change their response to the conditional stimulus when the contingency was changed (Heyser, Molina, & Spear, 1992). However, performance on a water maze test that required learning and memory of the position of a submerged platform was not changed by prenatal cocaine exposure (Johns, Means, Anderson, Means, & McMillen, 1992). In another study, operant learning was impaired by prenatal cocaine exposure coupled with rearing by the cocaine-exposed dam, but not by cocaine exposure alone (Goodwin et al., 1992).

Other behaviors investigated include exploratory behavior and aggression. Faced with a novel environment, prenatally cocaine-exposed rats were significantly less likely to explore it than were controls (Johns, Means, Means, & McMillen, 1992). Forced to negotiate a water maze, cocaine-exposed animals in the same laboratory were described (by blinded observers) as "swimming frantically." The importance of postnatal environmental factors in animal behavior studies was highlighted by a cross-fostering study, in which cocaine-exposed and nonexposed rat pups were reared either by cocaine-treated or untreated dams. The pups reared by cocaine-exposed dams showed aggressive behavior in response to a foot shock stimulus, regardless of whether or not the pups had been exposed in utero (Goodwin et al., 1992). The complex and growing body of studies in this area has been added to by other contributors to this volume, and is beyond the scope of this review.

SUMMARY AND CONCLUSIONS

A small but growing body of clinical and experimental data addresses the question of lasting neurophysiological effects or correlates of prenatal cocaine exposure. Much more is known about acute and chronic effects of cocaine in mature humans and laboratory animals. This chapter has surveyed available information at various levels along the continuum from the cellular and neurochemical to the behavioral and cognitive. At each level, clinical findings have been compared with information from the animal literature. With a few exceptions, these two domains of research have used qualitatively different outcomes, even when studying conceptually similar phenomena.

Two recent reviews have directly addressed the issue of animal models of prenatal cocaine exposure. Dow-Edwards (1991) compared clinical and animal studies of prenatal cocaine exposure along a number of dimensions, including maternal factors such as undernutrition and premature delivery, physical growth and anomalies, and neurologic sequelae, although differences in measurement were not explored. Stanton and Spear, writing for a larger working group, proposed that endpoints in developmental neurotoxicology be compared along five functional categories: sensory, motivational/arousal, cognitive, motor, and

TABLE 12.3
Comparison of Endpoints in Published Clinical and Animal Studies
by Functional Category

Functional Category	Clinical	Animal
Sensory	Auditory evoked potential Visual evoked potential Orientation (NBAS)	Auditory evoked potentials
Motivational/Arousal	Eyeblink, with and without sound Cry	Acoustic startle response, with prepulse inhibition
Cognitive	IQ and developmental quotient (DQ) tests (e.g., the Bayley) Visual recognition memory	Retention of learned conditioning
Motor	BNBAS[a] motor and reflex clusters	Activity Reflex maturation
Social		Aggression

[a]BNBAS = Brazelton Neonatal Behavior Assessment Scale.

social (Stanton & Spear, 1990). Their review demonstrates that available measures for animal and clinical studies of several developmental toxins are closely comparable at the level of functional categories, even though specific endpoints frequently differ. However, cocaine is not discussed in the paper. When outcome measures from the studies reviewed here are arranged according to the functional categories proposed in Stanton and Spear's review (Table 12.3), it is apparent that there are many functional categories in which the correspondence between clinical and animal cocaine research warrants further investigation.

The organizational schema proposed in this chapter leads to a similar conclusion: At several levels, animal models might be made more directly analogous to clinical studies by employing more closely matched outcomes (e.g., CSF measures). By the same token, clinical outcome studies could be made more relevant to the experimental literature (and, arguably, more sensitive to the actual effects of prenatal cocaine exposure) by examining neurodevelopmental phenomena such as learning and memory, rather than the traditional global measures of IQ (Mayes et al., 1992). This chapter has presented, for the most part, only published studies. Newer clinical and animal research, some of which appears elsewhere in this volume, will fill in many of the gaps. As the body of data on the effects and correlates of prenatal cocaine grows, it will be even more useful, periodically, to impose order.

REFERENCES

Abrams, R. M., Burchfield, D. J., Gerhardt, K. J., & Peters, A. J. (1992). Effect of cocaine on electrocortical activity in fetal sheep. *Brain Research, 70,* 97–102.

Akbari, H. M., Kramer, H. K., & Azmitia, E. C. (1991). Prenatal cocaine and fenfluramine administration inhibit serotonin and dopamine fiber growth. *Society for Neuroscience Abstracts, 17,* 1182.

Akimoto, K., Hamamura, T., & Otsuki, S. (1989). Subchronic cocaine treatment enhances cocaine-induced dopamine efflux, studied by in vivo intracerebral dialysis. *Brain Research, 490*, 339–344.

Anday, E. K., Cohen, M. E., Kelley, N. E., & Leitner, D. S. (1989). Effect of in utero cocaine exposure on startle and its modification. *Developmental Pharmacologic Therapy, 12*(3), 137–145.

Azuma, S. D., & Chasnoff, I. J. (1993). Outcome of children prenatally exposed to cocaine and other drugs: A path analysis of three-year data. *Pediatrics, 92*, 396–402.

Bilitzke, P. J., & Church, M. W. (1992). Prenatal cocaine and alcohol exposures affect rat behavior in a stress test (the Porsolt swim test). *Neurotoxicology and Teratology, 14*, 359–364.

Brazelton, T. B. (1984). *Neonatal Behavioral Assessment Scale* (2nd ed.). Philadelphia: Lippincott.

Carzoli, R. P., Murphy, S. P., Hammer-Knisely, J., & Houy, J. (1991). Evaluation of auditory brain-stem response in full-term infants of cocaine-abusing mothers. *American Journal of Diseases of Children, 145*(9), 1013–1016.

Chan, K., Dodd, P. A., Day, L., Kullama, L., Ervin, M. G., Padbury, J., & Ross, M. G. (1992). Fetal catecholamine, cardiovascular, and neurobehavioral responses to cocaine. *American Journal of Obstetrics and Gynecology, 167*(6), 1616–1623.

Chasnoff, I. J., Griffith, D. R., & Freier, C. (1992). Cocaine/polydrug use in pregnancy. *Pediatrics, 89*, 284–289.

Chasnoff, I. J., Hunt, C., Kletter, R., & Kaplan, D. (1989). Prenatal cocaine exposure is associated with respiratory pattern abnormalities. *American Journal of Diseases of Children, 143*, 583–587.

Chasnoff, M. D., Bussey, M. E., Savich, R. W., & Stack, C. M. (1986). Clinical and laboratory observations: Perinatal cerebral infarction and maternal cocaine use. *Journal of Pediatrics, 108*(3), 456–459.

Chen, C., Duara, S., Neto, G. S., Tan, S., Bandstra, E. S., Gerhardt, T., & Bancalari, E. (1991). Clinical and laboratory observations: Respiratory instability in neonates with in utero exposure to cocaine. *Journal of Pediatrics, 119*(1), 111–113.

Coles, C. D., Platzman, K. A., Smith, I., James, M. E., & Falek, A. (1992). Effects of cocaine and alcohol use in pregnancy on neonatal growth and neurobehavioral status. *Neurotoxicology and Teratology, 14*, 23–33.

Commissiong, J. W. (1985). Monoamine metabolites: Their relationship and lack of relationship to monoaminergic neuronal activity. *Biochemistry and Pharmacology, 34*(8), 1127–1131.

Davidson-Ward, S. L., Bautista, D. B., Woo, M. S., Chang, M., Schuetz, S., Wachsman, L., Sehgal, S., & Bean, X. (1992). Responses to hypoxia and hypercapnia in infants of substance-abusing mothers. *Journal of Pediatrics, 121*(5), 704–709.

Davidson-Ward, S. L., Schuetz, S., Wachsman, L., Bean, X., Bautista, D., Buckley, S., Sehgal, S., & Warburton, D. (1991). Elevated plasma norepinephrine levels in infants of substance-abusing mothers. *American Journal of Diseases of Children, 145*, 44–48.

Davis, M. (1985). Cocaine: Excitatory effects on sensorimotor reactivity measured with acoustic startle. *Psychopharmacology, 86*(1–2), 31–36.

Di Paolo, T., Rouillard, C., Morissette, M., & Levesque, D. (1989). Endocrine and neurochemical actions of cocaine. *Canadian Journal of Physiology and Pharmacology, 67*, 1177–1181.

Dixon, S. D. (1989). Echoencephalographic findings in neonates associated with maternal cocaine and methamphetamine use: Incidence and clinical correlates. *Journal of Pediatrics, 115*(5), 770–778.

Doberczak, T. M., Shanzer, S., Senie, R. T., & Kandall, S. (1988). Neonatal neurologic and electroencephalographic effects of intrauterine cocaine exposure. *Journal of Pediatrics, 113*(2), 354–358.

Dow-Edwards, D. L. (1991). Cocaine effects on fetal development: A comparison of clinical and animal research findings. *Neurotoxicology and Teratology, 13*, 347–352.

Dow-Edwards, D. L., Freed, L. A., & Fico, T. A. (1990). Structural and functional effects of prenatal cocaine exposure in adult rat brain. *Brain Research and Developmental Brain Research, 57*, 263–268.

Dow-Edwards, D. L., Freed, L. A., & Milhorat, T. H. (1988). Stimulation of brain metabolism by perinatal cocaine exposure. *Developmental Brain Research, 42,* 137–141.

Eisen, L. N., Field, T. M., Bandstra, E. S., Roberts, J. P., Morrow, C., Larson, S. K., & Steele, B. M. (1991). Perinatal cocaine effects on neonatal stress behavior and performance on the Brazelton Scale. *Pediatrics, 88*(3), 477–480.

Foss, J. A. (1991). Elicitation and modification of the acoustic startle reflex in animals prenatally exposed to cocaine. *Neurotoxicology and Teratology, 13,* 541–546.

Foss, J. A., & Riley, E. P. (1991). Failure of acute cocaine administration to differentially affect acoustic startle and activity in rats prenatally exposed to cocaine. *Neurotoxicology and Teratology, 13,* 547–551.

Frank, D. A., McCarten, K., Cabral, H., Levenson, S., & Zuckerman, B. S. (1994). Association of heavy in-utero cocaine exposure with caudate hemmorhage in term newborns: Abstract. *Pediatric Research, 35*(4), 269A.

Frank, D. A., McCarten, K., Cabral, H., & Zuckerman, B. S. (1992). Cranial ultrasound in term newborns: Failure to replicate excess abnormalities in cocaine-exposed newborns. *Pediatric Research, 31,* 247A.

Fung, Y. K., Reed, J. A., & Lau, Y.-S. (1989). Prenatal cocaine exposure fails to modify neurobehavioral responses and the striatal dopaminergic system in newborn rats. *General Pharmacology, 20*(5), 689–693.

Goodwin, G. A., Heyser, C. J., Moody, C. A., Rajachandran, L., Molina, V. A., Arnold, H. M., McKinzie, D. L., Spear, N. E., & Spear, L. P. (1992). A fostering study of the effects of prenatal cocaine exposure: Offspring behavioral measures. *Neurotoxicology and Teratology, 14,* 423–432.

Graham, K., Feigenbaum, A., Pastuszak, A., Nulman, I., Weksberg, R., Einarson, T., Goldberg, S., Ashby, S., & Koren, G. (1992). Pregnancy outcome and infant development following gestational cocaine use by social cocaine users in Toronto, Canada. *Clinical Investigations in Medicine, 15,* 384–394.

Hansen, R. L., Struthers, J. M., & Gospe, S. M. (1993). Visual evoked potentials and visual processing in stimulant drug-exposed infants. *Developmental Medicine in Child Neurology, 35,* 798–805.

Henderson, M. G., McConnaughey, M. M., & McMillen, B. A. (1991). Long-term consequences of prenatal exposure to cocaine or related drugs: Effects on rat brain monoaminergic receptors. *Brain Research Bulletin, 26,* 941–945.

Henderson, M. G., & McMillen, B. A. (1990). Effects of prenatal exposure to cocaine or related drugs on rat developmental and neurological indices. *Brain Research Bulletin, 24,* 207–212.

Heyser, C. J., Molina, V. A., & Spear, L. P. (1992). A fostering study of the effects of prenatal cocaine exposure: I. Maternal behaviors. *Neurotoxicology and Teratolgy, 14,* 415–421.

Horn, P. T. (1992). Persistent hypertension after prenatal cocaine exposure. *The Journal of Pediatrics, 121,* 288–291.

Johns, J. M., Means, L. W., Means, M. J., & McMillen, B. A. (1992). Prenatal exposure to cocaine I: Effects of gestation, development, and activity in Sprague–Dawley rats. *Neurotoxicology and Teratology, 14,* 337–342.

Johns, J. M., Means, M. J., Anderson, D. R., Means, L. W., & McMillen, B. A. (1992). Prenatal exposure to cocaine II: Effects on open-field activity and cognitive behavior in Sprague–Dawley rats. *Neurotoxicology and Teratology, 14,* 343–349.

Kleven, M. S., Woolverton, W. L., & Seiden, L. S. (1988). Lack of long-term monoamine depletions following repeated or continuous exposure to cocaine. *Brain Research Bulletin, 21,* 233–237.

Kramer, H. K., Azmitia, E. C., & Akbari, H. M. (1991). Early postnatal cocaine exposure fails to modify cortical serotonin and dopamine innervation. *Society for Neuroscience Abstracts, 17,* 1182.

Kuhn, C., Ignar, D., & Windh, R. (1991). Endocrine function as a target of perinatal drug effects: Methodologic issues. *NIDA Research Monograph, 114,* 206–232.

Legido, A., Clancy, R. R., Spitzer, A. R., & Finnegan, L. P. (1992). ELectroencephalographic and behavioral-state studies in infants of cocaine-addicted mothers. *American Journal of Diseases of Children, 146,* 748–752.

Lester, B. M., Als, H., & Brazelton, T. B. (1982). Regional obstetric anesthesia and newborn behavior: A reanalysis towards synergistic effects. *Child Development, 53*, 687–692.

Lester, B. M., Corwin, M. J., Sepkoski, C., Seifer, R., Peucker, M., McLaughlin, S., & Golub, H. L. (1991). Neurobehavioral syndromes in cocaine-exposed newborn infants. *Child Development, 62*(4), 694–705.

Link, E. A., Weese-Mayer, D. W., & Byrd, S. E. (1991). Magnetic resonance imaging in infants exposed to cocaine prenatally: A preliminary report. *Clinical Pediatrics Philadelphia, 30*, 506–508.

Magnano, C. L., Gardner, J. M., & Karmel, B. Z. (1992). Differences in salivary cortisol levels in cocaine-exposed and noncocaine-exposed NICU infants. *Developmental Psychobiology, 25*(2), 93–103.

Mayes, L. C., Granger, R. H., Bornstein, M. H., & Zuckerman, B. S. (1992). The problem of prenatal cocaine exposure: A rush to judgment. *Journal of the American Medical Association, 267*(3), 406–408.

McCann, E. M., & Lewis, K. (1991). Control of breathing in babies of narcotic- and cocaine-abusing mothers. *Early Human Development, 27*, 175–186.

Miller, J. C., & Friedhoff, A. J. (1988). Prenatal neurotransmitter programming of postnatal receptor function. In G. J. Boer, M. G. P. Feenstra, M. Mirmiran, D. F. Swaab, & F. Van Haaren (Ed.), *Progress in brain research* (Vol. 73, pp. 509–522). New York: Elsevier Science.

Minabe, Y., Ashby, C. R., Jr., Heyser, C., Spear, L. P., & Wang, R. Y. (1992). The effects of prenatal cocaine exposure on spontaneously active midbrain dopamine neurons in adult male offspring: An electrophysiological study. *Brain Research, 586*, 152–156.

Mirochnick, M., Meyer, J., Cole, J., Herren, T., & Zuckerman, B. (1991). Circulating catecholamines in cocaine-exposed neonates: A pilot study. *Pediatrics, 88*, 481–485.

Moliterno, D. J., Willard, J. E., Lange, R. A., Negus, B. H., Boehrer, J. D., Glamann, D. B., Landau, C., Rossen, J. D., Winniford, M. W., & Hillis, L. D. (1994). Coronary-artery vasoconstriction induced by cocaine, cigarette smoking, or both. *New England Journal of Medicine, 330*, 454–459.

Moore, T. R., Sorg, J., Miller, L., Key, T., & Resnik, R. (1986). Hemodynamic effects of intravenous cocaine on the pregnant ewe and fetus. *American Journal of Obstetrics and Gynecology, 155*, 883–888.

Needlman, R., Kwon, C., Mirochnick, M., Zuckerman, B., & Frank, D. (1994). *Blood pressure in infants exposed prenatally to cocaine.* Manuscript submitted for publication.

Needlman, R., Zuckerman, B., Anderson, G. M., Mirochnick, M., & Cohen, D. J. (1993). Cerebrospinal fluid monoamine precursors and metabolites in human neonates following in-utero cocaine exposure: A preliminary study. *Pediatrics, 92*(1), 55–60.

Neuspiel, D. R., Hamel, C., Hochberg, E., Greene, J., & Campbell, D. (1991). Maternal cocaine use and infant behavior. *Neurotoxicology and Teratology, 13*, 229–233.

Ostrea, E. M., Parks, P., & Brady, M. (1988). Rapid isolation and detection of drugs in meconium of drug-dependent infants. *Clinical Chemistry, 34*, 2372–2373.

Owiny, J. R., Jones, M. T., Sadowsky, D., Massmann, A., Ding, X. Y., & Nathanielsz, P. W. (1991). Lack of effect of fetal administration of cocaine on maternal and fetal plasma adrenocorticotropin, cortisol and lactate concentrations at 127–138 days gestational age. *Gynecology and Obstetric Investigation, 32*, 196–199.

Owiny, J. R., Jones, M. T., Sadowsky, D., Myers, T., Massman, A., & Nathanielsz, P. W. (1991). Cocaine in pregnancy: The effect of maternal administration of cocaine on the maternal and fetal pituitary-adrenal axes. *American Journal of Obstetrics and Gynecology, 164*, 658–663.

Pitts, D. K., & Marwah, J. (1989). Autonomic action of cocaine. *Canadian Journal of Physiology and Pharmacology, 67*, 1168–1176.

Richardson, G. A., & Day, N. L. (1991). Maternal and neonatal effects of moderate cocaine use during pregnancy. *Neurotoxicology and Teratology, 13*, 455–460.

Rossetti, Z. L., Melis, F., Carboni, S., & Gessa, G. L. (1992). Dramatic depletion of mesolimbic extracellular dopamine after withdrawal from morphine, alcohol or cocaine: A common neurochemical substrate for drug dependence. *Annals of the New York Academy of Science, 654*, 513–516.

Salamy, A., Dark, K., Salfi, M., Shah, S., & Peeke, H. V. (1992). Perinatal cocaine exposure and functional brainstem development in the rat. *Brain-Research, 598,* 307–310.

Salamy, A., Eldredge, L., Anderson, J., & Bull, D. (1990). Clinical and laboratory observations: Brain-stem transmission time in infants exposed to cocaine in utero. *Journal of Pediatrics, 117*(4), 627–629.

Scalzo, F. M., Ali, S. F., Frambes, N. A., & Spear, L. P. (1990). Weanling rats exposed prenatally to cocaine exhibit an increase in striatal D2 dopamine binding associated with an increase in ligand affinity. *Psychopharmacology Biochemistry and Behavior, 37,* 371–373.

Seidler, F. J., & Slotkin, T. A. (1993). Prenatal cocaine and cell development in rat brain regions: Effects on ornithine decarboxylase and macromolecules. *Brain Research Bulletin, 30*(1–2), 91–99.

Shih, L., Cone-Wesson, B., & Reddix, B. (1988). Effects of maternal cocaine abuse on the neonatal auditory system. *International Journal of Pediatric Otorhinolaryngology, 15,* 245–251.

Sobrian, S. K., Burton, L. E., Robinson, N. L., Ashe, W. K., James, H., Stokes, D. L., & Turner, L. M. (1990). Neurobehavioral and immunological effects of prenatal cocaine exposure in rat. *Pharmacology, Biochemistry and Behavior, 35,* 617–629.

Spear, L. P., Kirstein, C. L., & Frambes, N. A. (1989). Cocaine effects on the developing central nervous system: Behavioral, psychopharmacological, and neurochemical studies. *Annals of the New York Academy of Sciences, 562,* 290–307.

Stanton, M. E., & Spear, L. P. (1990). Workshop on the qualitative and quantitative comparability of human and animal developmental neurotoxicity, Work Group I report: Comparability of measures of developmental neurotoxicity in humans and laboratory animals. *Neurotoxicology and Teratology, 12,* 261–267.

Trulson, M. E., Joe, J. C., Babb, S., & Raese, J. (1987). Chronic cocaine administration depletes tyrosine hydroxylase immunoreactivity in the meso-limbic dopamine system in rat brain: Quantitative light microscopic studies. *Brain Research Bulletin, 19,* 39–45.

Trulson, M. E., & Ulissey, M. J. (1987). Chronic cocaine administration decreases dopamine synthesis rate and increases [3H] spiroperidol binding in rat brain. *Brain Research Bulletin, 19,* 35–38.

van-de-Bor, M., Walther, F. J., & Ebrahimi, M. (1990). Decreased cardiac output in infants of mothers who abused cocaine. *Pediatrics, 85,* 30–32.

Wasiewski, W. W., & Hasen, T. N. (1989). Intrauterine cocaine exposure alters respiratory control in newborn rabbit pups. *Pediatric Research, 25,* 74A.

Weese-Mayer, D. E., Klemka-Walden, L. M., Barkov, B. A., & Gingras, J. L. (1992). Effects of prenatal cocaine on the ventilatory response to hypoxia in newborn rabbits. *Developmental Pharmacology Therapy, 18*(1–2), 116–124.

Weese-Mayer, D. E., Klemka-Walden, L. M., Chan, M. K., & Gingras, J. L. (1991). Effects of prenatal cocaine exposure on perinatal morbidity and postnatal growth in the rabbit. *Developmental Pharmacology Therapy, 16,* 221–230.

Weese-Mayer, D. E., Silvestri, J. M., Lin, D., Buhfiend, C. M., Lo, E. S., & Carvey, P. M. (1993). Effect of cocaine in early gestation on striatal dopamine and neurotrophic activity. *Pediatric Research, 34,* 389–392.

Westerink, B., & Kikert, R. (1986). Effect of various centrally acting drugs on the efflux of dopamine metabolites from the rat brain. *Journal of Neurochemistry, 46,* 1145–1152.

Wilson, J. M., Nobrega, J. N., Corrigall, W., Shannak, K., Deck, J. H. N., & Kish, S. J. (1992). Influence of chronic cocaine on monoamine neurotransmitters in human brain and animal model: Preliminary observations. *Annals of the New York Academy of Sciences, 654*(28), 461–463.

Yablonsky-Alter, E., Belenky, Y., Nathan, M. A., Glezer, I., Lidsky, T. J., & Banerjee, S. P. (1991). Effects of pre- and post-natal cocaine exposure on the striatal dopaminergic system in newborn mice. *Society for Neuroscience Abstracts, 17,* 823.

Zmitrovich, A. C., Hutchings, D. E., Dow-Edwards, D. L., Malowany, D., & Church, S. (1992). Effects of prenatal exposure to cocaine on the rest–activity cycle of the preweanling rat. *Pharmacology, Biochemistry and Behavior, 43,* 1059–1064.

Zuckerman, B. S., & Bresnahan, K. (1991). Developmental and behavioral consequences of prenatal drug and alcohol exposure. *Pediatric Clinics of North America, 38,* 1387–1406.

Zuckerman, B. S., Frank, D. A., Hingson, R., Amaro, H., Levenson, S. M., Kayne, H., Parker, S., Vinci, R., Aboagye, K., Fried, L., Cabral, H., Timperi, R., & Bauchner, H. (1989). Effects of maternal marijuana and cocaine use on fetal growth. *New England Journal of Medicine, 320,* 762–768.

Developmental Dilemmas for Cocaine-Abusing Parents and Their Children

Linda C. Mayes
Yale Child Study Center

Marc H. Bornstein
National Institute of Child Health and Human Development

Cocaine abuse is an old problem with a special contemporary theme. Familiar, often cited examples of the persistent popularity of cocaine in the last century include Freud's letters about his own use for "heartburn" and his prescription to others, before unfortunate consequences with a colleague persuaded him to abandon the drug (Byck, 1974). In the United States of the late 1800s, cocaine was widely available to both women and men of all social classes. It was used as a tonic for hay fever and recommended as a cure for addiction to alcohol or opiates (Musto, 1973). Concern about the effects of widespread cocaine abuse on individual functioning and social morality as expressed in public health records of the period presages contemporary worries about the "new" epidemic that threatens 20th-century families and communities. The consensus of a survey of physicians along the East Coast conducted by the Committee on the Acquirement of the Drug Habit in the late 1800s was that "The use of cocaine by unfortunate women generally ... in certain parts of the country is simply appalling. ... The police officers of these questionable districts tell us that the [addicts] are made wild by cocaine, which they have no difficulty at all in buying, sometimes peddled around from door to door" (Musto, 1973, p. 17). The number of children cared for by these women was not recorded, nor has there been a systematic historical study of how families were affected by these earlier patterns of cocaine abuse. That women addicts, regardless of social class, had children and that these children were affected in various ways by their mothers' addictions is certain, though not documented except in case studies and anecdotal accounts. These individual accounts do, however, reveal that cocaine abuse often left its participants, and thus their children, impoverished and involved in crime, prostitution, and other addictions including alcohol and opiates. Cocaine addiction was tenacious and debilitating, and there was considerable social stigma and isolation associated with prolonged cocaine abuse (Courtwright, 1982).

The more extensive study and concern about the effects of cocaine abuse on children and on maternal and family functioning are special themes of contemporary focus on the so-called "crack/cocaine epidemic." These concerns extend to both pre-and postnatal exposure to cocaine and crack abuse among women who are also parents. Estimates of the number of infants and young children affected by parental cocaine abuse in today's society vary widely. A study of consecutively recruited women in routine prenatal care reported that 17% had used cocaine during pregnancy (Frank et al., 1988), and national estimates across all socioeconomic groups estimate that 10% to 20% of infants are exposed to cocaine prenatally (Chasnoff, Landress, & Barrett, 1990). In some geographic areas, childbearing populations are at much greater risk for abusing drugs (Amaro, Zuckerman, & Cabral, 1989; Zuckerman, Frank, Hingson, & Amaro, 1989). For example, in many inner-city populations, nearly 50% of women giving birth report or test positive for cocaine use at the time of delivery (Amaro, Fried, Cabral, & Zuckerman, 1990; Osterloh & Lee, 1989). Estimates suggest that a minimum of 40,000 to 80,000 infants (Scherling, 1994), or maximally 375,000 infants, are born yearly in the United States who have been exposed prenatally to crack or cocaine, often in conjunction with alcohol, tobacco, and other drugs (Besharov, 1990; Gomby & Shiono, 1991).

This chapter reviews the effects of cocaine[1] on infant development at three different levels. First is a brief survey of the effects of cocaine on central nervous system (CNS) functioning and on developing fetal brain. Second is a summary of available data on developmental outcomes in infants and children exposed prenatally to cocaine with a particular focus on the effects of prenatal cocaine exposure on infant attention and arousal regulation. The ways in which cocaine abuse affects parental functioning is the third area reviewed. We conclude with an overview of some prominent pathways through which the effects of prenatal cocaine exposure on basic neurodevelopmental functions may be mediated. This overview of pathways of effect also serves to underscore why the problem of prenatal cocaine exposure poses developmental dilemmas. Investigators seeking to understand the effects of prenatal cocaine exposure on children's psychological development face the dilemma that cocaine affects development through multiple pathways and that rarely, if ever, is it possible to speak of a "pure" cocaine effect or a singular and identifiable effect on one aspect of brain development. Further, no one pathway of the effect of cocaine exposure on development is primary, each contributes variance to the relation between prenatal exposure and the child's

---

[1]Throughout this review, cocaine refers to both cocaine and crack insofar as the two agents are psychoactively equivalent.

developmental status, and an adequate study of the prenatally cocaine-exposed child must involve studies of parenting and the general environment as well. In other words, because cocaine is a teratologic agent with profound effects on the child's immediate parental and more global social environment, as well as the child's prenatal development, studies of the outcome of prenatally cocaine-exposed infants necessarily involve biologic–environment interaction models (Bergeman & Plomin, 1989). Finally, for the child and parent, the multiple pathways of effect of prenatal cocaine exposure pose dilemmas because each represents risks for multiple other problems, such as involvement in violence and crime, homelessness, poor school performance and early school drop-out, and multigenerational drug abuse, problems that trap both parent and child in poverty and discord.

COCAINE AND BRAIN DEVELOPMENT

Cocaine influences brain development directly through effects on developing neurotransmitter systems critical to neuronal differentiation and brain structure formation and indirectly through effects on blood flow to the developing fetal brain (see review by Mayes, in press-b; Mayes & Bornstein, in press). Cocaine is a central nervous system stimulant that acts through the monoaminergic neuro-transmitter systems including dopamine, norepinephrine, and serotonin (5-HT) (Gawin & Ellinwood, 1988; Wise, 1984). The primary CNS action of cocaine occurs at the level of neurotransmitter release, reuptake, and recognition at the synaptic junction. Cocaine blocks the reuptake of dopamine, norepinephrine, and 5-HT by the presynaptic neuron (Swann, 1990), a process that is primarily re-sponsible for inactivation of neurotransmitters. Blocking reuptake leaves more dopamine, norepinephrine, and 5-HT available within the synaptic space (and thus, in the peripheral blood as well) and results in enhanced activity of these agents in the CNS (Goeders & Smith, 1983) with associated physiologic reactions (e.g., tachycardia and vasoconstriction with hypertension—see Richie & Greene, 1985) and behaviors (e.g., euphoria and increased motor activity).

Within the various dopamine-rich areas of the brain, certain areas of the prefrontal cortex (mesocortical system) are somewhat insensitive to the effects of cocaine on dopamine reuptake, whereas the corpus striatum (nigrostriatal system) is 100% sensitive to the effect (Hadfield & Nugent, 1983). The dopamine-rich nigrostriatal system projects from cell bodies in the substantia nigra to the corpus striatum and innervates the prefrontal cortex, nucleus accumbens, amygdala, and septum (Goeders & Smith, 1983; Shepherd, 1988). Each of these areas is involved in a number of basic neuropsychological functions including arousal and attentional modulation, the regulation of anxiety and other emotional states, and the reinforcing properties basic to stimulant addiction in adults.

The norepinephrine system arising in the locus coeruleus also plays a crucial role in the regulation of reactivity, or the level of arousal induced by novel stimulation, and in turn the maintenance of alert states (Posner & Petersen, 1990) in the face of arousal-activating, novel stimulation (Rothbart & Posner, 1985). Norepinephrine pathways are strongly present in the posterior parietal lobe, pulvinar, and superior colliculus (Morrison & Foote, 1986). In animal models, prenatal cocaine exposure appears to result in increased catecholaminergic fiber densities in selected brain areas including the posterior parietal cortex (Akbari & Azmitia, 1992). These brain areas are related to the posterior attention system, which is involved in the orienting response to novel information (Posner & Petersen, 1990). The posterior attentional system gates the processing of novel stimuli and the ability to move on to another situation (Posner & Peterson, 1988). A curvilinear relation obtains between optimal levels of arousal and attention (Field, 1981), and excessively increased levels of arousal may impede the gating function of the posterior attention system. Pharmacologically blocking norepinephrine activity at the neural junction in effect produces increased distractibility on attention tasks in human subjects (Clark, Geffen, & Geffen, 1989). Thus, on account of the effect of cocaine on central noradrenergic as well as dopaminergic systems, we might expect prenatally exposed infants to show altered arousal regulation and overall to be more easily overaroused when orienting in a novel situation.

In fetal brain development, monoaminergic neurotransmitters are critical for the definition of brain structure and neuronal formation through their effects on cell proliferation, neural outgrowth, and synaptogenesis (Lauder, 1988; Mattson, 1988). Cocaine readily crosses the placenta and the blood–brain barrier. Brain concentrations of cocaine have been reported as high as four times that of peak plasma levels (Farrar & Kearns, 1989). Thus, cocaine may alter the formation and remodeling of brain structures through this effect on the release and metabolism of monoamines. Additionally, cocaine may alter the actual ontogeny of the monoaminergic neurotransmitter systems and thus again modify a number of critical processes in brain development. Prenatal treatment of the pregnant rat with cocaine results in an increase in monoaminergic fiber densities in selected brain areas including the parietal cortex, the hippocampus, and the cingulate cortex (Akbari & Azmitia, 1992; Akbari, Kramer, Whitaker-Azmitia, Spear, & Azmitia, 1992). Similarly, cocaine administration to the rat during the early postnatal period of synaptogenesis in the forebrain, a period roughly equivalent to the third trimester for the human fetus, shows greatest change in glucose metabolism in those dopaminergic-rich areas of the brain (Dow-Edwards, 1989; Dow-Edwards, Freed, & Milhorat, 1988).

Effects on developing monoaminergic neurotransmitter systems have far-reaching implications, for they may lead to mistimed neurogenesis between the affected and unaffected areas of the brain with resultant alterations in synaptic connections (Lauder, 1991), and those dopaminergic areas involved in arousal and attention seem 100% sensitive to the cocaine-related inhibition of dopamine reuptake in the synaptic junction. By altering monoaminergic neurotransmitter control of morphogenesis, chronic exposure to cocaine in utero may adversely affect autonomic function, state regulation, and regulation of attention by the developing nervous system. Also, exposure during particular phases of fetal development may be more critical for teratogenic effects than others—the so-called critical phase or sensitive period concept (Bornstein, 1989). For example, because monoaminergic neurotransmitters appear in the first trimester, exposure at this time may continue to have effects later in pregnancy even without further exposure because of the first trimester effects on monoaminergic neurogenesis. (Similarly, because processes of postnatal brain development including synaptic formation and remodeling are timed in part by monoaminergic neurotransmitters, exposure in the first months after birth may represent a sensitive period for postnatal brain development (see below).

Through cocaine-related effects on norepinephrine, prenatal cocaine exposure also alters blood flow to the developing fetal brain. Norepinephrine-related vascular effects of cocaine are seen in decreased uteroplacental blood flow, severe uteroplacental insufficiency (acute and chronic), maternal hypertension, and fetal vasoconstriction (Moore, Sorg, Miller, Key, & Resnik, 1986; J. R. Woods, Plessinger, & Clark, 1987). These, in turn, result in a relative state of fetal hypoxia. Various congenital malformations seen among infants who were prenatally exposed to cocaine have been linked to the effects of cocaine on fetal vascular tone at critical times in morphogenesis (Bingol, Fuchs, Diaz, Stone, & Gromisch, 1987; Hoyme et al., 1990; Zuckerman & Frank, 1992). Similarly, the effect of cocaine use on placental blood flow probably contributes to the relation between cocaine and fetal growth—low birth weight and microcephaly—reported now by several investigators (Fulroth, Phillips, & Durand, 1989; Hadeed & Siegel, 1989; MacGregor et al., 1987; Mayes, Granger, Frank, Bornstein, & Schottenfeld, 1993; Oro & Dixon, 1987; Ryan, Ehrlich, & Finnegan, 1987).

Chronic cocaine users frequently report marked appetite reduction (Scherling, 1994) as well as regular use of other drugs including alcohol, tobacco, and opiates (Amaro, Zuckerman, & Cabral, 1989; Frank et al., 1988). Both alcohol and tobacco adversely affect fetal growth, and there are potentially direct effects of alcohol exposure on the developing fetal brain (Day, 1992; Streissguth, 1992). Children exposed to alcohol prenatally show more difficulties with impulse regulation and are more distractible with poorer concentration by school age (Day, 1992). Combinations of poor nutrition, uteroplacental insufficiency, and polydrug use during pregnancy further contribute to an overall poorer state of maternal health and increased risk for fetal growth retardation and impaired fetal outcome.

In summary, on account of inhibition of monoaminergic neurotransmitter systems, neurodevelopmental functioning in prenatally cocaine-exposed infants might be expected to be compromised specifically in areas such as reactivity, capacity to modulate levels of arousal in response to stimulation, and attentional regulation. Further, on account of reduction in placental and fetal blood flow, prenatally cocaine-exposed infants might be expected to be compromised generally in functions reflecting information processing or in terms of problem solving. Effects on arousal or reactivity are different from effects on information processing or cognition. The regulation of arousal influences the capacity to sustain attention which, in turn, supports the processing of novel information, but the effect on cognition is not primary. Given that cocaine potentially affects fetal brain development at two different levels, it may be that there are (at least two) different groups of prenatally exposed infants—children with impairments of regulatory systems such as arousal and attention and children with more general impairments in information processing. Issues of timing and amount of exposure are particularly critical and pose a primary methodologic dilemma for sorting through predictors of these different outcomes, but few data are yet available to permit closer evaluation of possible subgroup effects among prenatally exposed infants. Nevertheless, some findings from outcome studies lend tentative support.

PRENATAL COCAINE EXPOSURE AND INFANT OUTCOME

Behavioral and cognitive outcome measures beyond the neonatal period in studies of children exposed to cocaine prenatally have for the most part utilized general measures of developmental competency (Mayes, in press-a), such as the *Bayley Scales of Infant Development* (BSID; Bayley, 1969, 1993). In early reports of infants exposed to cocaine as well as combinations of heroin, methadone, and marijuana, cocaine exposure was predictively linked to moderate to severe developmental delays across diverse developmental domains (see Mayes, 1992). However, subsequent studies have reported mild to no impairments in overall developmental functioning in cocaine-exposed children compared to non-exposed groups (Mayes, in press-a; Scherling, 1994; Zuckerman & Frank, 1992). Chasnoff, Griffith, McGregor, Dirkes, and Burns (1989) reported on the developmental profiles of a group of cocaine/alcohol-exposed 24-month-olds followed from birth compared with the performance of a non-cocaine-, but marijuana- and/or alcohol-, exposed group (Chasnoff, Griffith, Freier, & Murray, 1992). Mothers of infants in the non-cocaine-using comparison groups were similar to the cocaine-using mothers in socioeconomic status (SES), age, marital status, and tobacco use during pregnancy. On repeated developmental assessments using the BSID at 3, 6, 12, 18, and 24 months, albeit with a high rate of attrition from the original cohort, there were no mean differences across groups in either the mental or motor domains. The investigators cautioned, however, that a higher percentage of cocaine-exposed infants scored two standard deviations below the mean (Chasnoff et al., 1992).

Three other investigative groups have reported similar failures to find differences on general measures of developmental competency in cocaine-exposed children in the first, second, and third years of life (e.g., Anisfeld et al., 1991; Arendt, Singer, & Minnes, 1993; Billman, Nemeth, Heimler, & Sasidharan, 1991). Findings such as these have resulted in a reevaluation of early concerns about global developmental delay in prenatally cocaine-exposed children. However, studies of more specific developmental functions suggest that cocaine-exposed infants and young children may have impairments in attention and state or arousal regulation (Mayes & Bornstein, in press). For example, it has been reported that, despite no apparent differences on either motor or mental indices on the BSID, cocaine-exposed 24-month-olds appear to have more difficulty attending to several objects at the same time, and they fail more often in structuring an approach to a nonfamiliar task in the context of developmental assessment (Hawley & Disney, 1992).

In the few studies examining functional components, such as attention or state and arousal regulation, differences between cocaine-exposed and non-cocaine-exposed infants have been reported in startle responsivity, neonatal orientation, motor and state regulatory capacities, habituation, recognition memory, and reactivity to novelty. Anday, Cohen, Kelley, and Leitner (1989) observed that cocaine-exposed newborns were more reactive to reflex-eliciting stimuli as well as to specific auditory stimuli. In the neonatal period, findings of neurobehavioral impairments as measured by the *Brazelton Neonatal Behavioral Assessment Scales* (NBAS; Brazelton, 1984) have been reported but are inconsistent. Chasnoff and colleagues (1989) found impairments of orientation, motor, and state regulatory behaviors on the NBAS. In contrast, C. D. Coles, Platzman, Smith, James, and Falek (1992) reported that NBAS scores (for some, but not all clusters) for all infants fell within a clinically normal range regardless of cocaine or alcohol exposure. Eisen and colleagues (1990), studying neonates who were urine-screen positive only for cocaine at birth and whose mothers denied opiate use, and Mayes et al. (1993) found significant deficits in cocaine-exposed infants in habituation performance as assessed by the NBAS.

Habituation and the complementary processes of novelty responsiveness and recognition memory provide information about the organization of looking behavior and attention in the first years of life, and the habituation process represents an early form of some type of information processing and encoding by the infant and child (Bornstein, 1985a; Bornstein & Mayes, 1992; Colombo & Mitchell, 1990; Lewis & Brooks-Gun, 1981; Lewis, Goldberg, & Campbell, 1969). Habituation measures discriminate among samples of infants differing in risk status (reviewed in Bornstein, 1985a; Mayes & Bornstein, in press). Attention indexed by habituation also involves arousal and arousal regulation (Mayes & Bornstein, in press), and the development of attention is directly linked to the development of control of states of sleep and wakefulness (see Thoman & Ingersoll, 1989). Sustained attention to a novel stimulus entails not only the active intake of information but also requires more tonic alteration in state or arousal. A deficit in the modulation of arousal or in the activation of states of arousal will influence attentional processes and habituation performance (Pribram & McGuiness, 1975; Ruff, 1988). Links between the dopaminergic system and arousal regulation as well as attentional mechanisms that are indexed by the habituation process (B. J. Coles & Robbins, 1989) make it plausible to hypothesize that prenatal cocaine exposure could affect the infant's early habituation performance, the processes related to habituation such as recognition memory or novelty responsiveness, and the infant's reactivity or regulation of arousal to novel stimulation.

Studies examining habituation and its related processes in cocaine-exposed infants have suggested specific impairments in recognition memory, novelty responsiveness, and arousal and reactivity to novel stimuli in infants 3 to 12 months of age. Struthers and Hansen (1992) reported impaired recognition memory among cocaine- or amphetamine-exposed infants compared with a non-drug-exposed group between 7 and 8 months of age. Similarly, Alessandri, Sullivan, Imaizumi, and Lewis (1993) reported impaired contingent learning well into the second half of the first year of life in cocaine-exposed infants. Recognition memory tasks rely in part on habituation processes and, while measuring infant responsiveness to novel versus familiar stimuli rather than decrement of attention over time, nevertheless require an integrated capacity to attend selectively to novel information. Mayes, Bornstein, Chawarska, and Granger (in press) found that, compared to a non-drug-exposed group, infants exposed prenatally to cocaine are significantly more likely to fail to begin a habituation procedure and significantly more likely to react with irritability early in the procedure. However, the majority of even cocaine-exposed infants reach a habituation criterion, and among those who do, there are no significant differences between cocaine- and non-cocaine-exposed infants in habituation or in recovery to a novel stimulus. Thus, for at least a subgroup of cocaine-exposed infants, initial reactivity and selectivity toward novel stimuli appear to be impaired.

In summary, available findings suggest that the neurodevelopmental effects of prenatal cocaine exposure may be expressed primarily in the general area of arousal regulation in novel or stimulating situations. Impaired arousal regulation, in turn, influences attention and reactivity and the child's response to both nonsocial and social situations. However, the biologically or genetically based developmental trajectory of capacities for the regulation of states of arousal and of attention is also sensitive to environmental influences. Infants exposed prenatally to cocaine are exposed to a number of environmental risk factors that may impair the development of attention and arousal regulatory mechanisms (Mayes, 1992, in press-a; Mayes, Granger, Bornstein, & Zuckerman, 1992). These include prenatal exposure to other substances of abuse including alcohol and tobacco as well as opiates, marijuana, and amphetamines. Mothers who abuse cocaine often have associated health problems including a higher incidence of HIV-positive titers with or without AIDS related illnesses, and they have pregnancies more often complicated by preterm delivery and intrauterine growth retardation. Postnatally, infants exposed to cocaine continue to be exposed to ongoing parental substance abuse, they are more often neglected and abused, and they have parents with more frequent depression and higher overall stress and anxiety (Mayes, in press-c; Zuckerman, Amaro, Bauchner, & Cabral, 1989). Any one of these factors may compound cocaine effects on the development of early attentional and arousal regulatory functions in infants. Thus, the dilemma for understanding the relation of prenatal cocaine exposure to impairments in such basic functions as arousal or state regulation is that the cocaine-related effect may be mediated through effects on brain development and through effects on the child's parenting environment.

THE PARENTING ENVIRONMENT
OF COCAINE-EXPOSED INFANTS

Perhaps the most methodologically problematic area in the study of prenatal cocaine exposure in infants and young children has been comprehensive evaluation of the parenting environment (Mayes, in press-c). A central methodologic dilemma for the question of how the effects of cocaine exposure on children's development are mediated by the effects of substance abuse on parenting is: Do cocaine-abusing parents have impaired relationships with their children that are different from impairments found in other dysfunctional or disadvantaged families not affected by substance abuse, and if so, are the patterns of parenting impairment uniquely related to the effects of cocaine on adult psychological functioning? Stated another way, cocaine abuse in an adult may or may not indicate that he or she is a dysfunctional parent but rather may mark other conditions that negatively affect parenting, such as depression, or that indicate increased risk for severe disruptions in parenting, such as child abuse and neglect.

Observations of parenting behaviors based on cocaine exposure of animal models suggest that cocaine use during pregnancy alters mothers' behavior when caring for their own infants and that such alterations also influence the behavior of the offspring. For example, in the rat, cocaine-treated mothers were significantly more aggressive to intruders when protecting their young than either non-cocaine-treated mothers or cocaine- or non-cocaine-treated foster mothers (Heyser, Molina, & Spear, 1992). Infant behavior was also altered in that, regardless of the prenatal exposure conditions, infants reared by cocaine treated mothers were more quickly aggressive to challenge (Goodwin, Heyser, Moody, & Rajachandran, 1992). Animal models for parenting behavior in substance-abusing conditions are only recently being developed. They may find value in suggesting hypotheses for interactive effects between pre- and postnatal exposure conditions on both infant outcomes and parenting behaviors (Mayes, in press-c).

Parenting functions among substance-abusing human adults have been examined primarily with indirect measures, such as surveys of the incidence of child abuse and of the home environment, to assess the adequacy of the child's physical care. That parents who are actively abusing cocaine and other substances have problems caring for their children is indicated in part by the increased incidence of physical abuse and neglect in such families, and by the proportionately higher than national average numbers of children from substance-abusing families who are in foster care or other types of placements (Lawson & Wilson, 1980; Rogosch, Cicchetti, Shields, & Toth, in press). In a case-control study of all consecutive emergency room or hospital evaluations of injuries thought to be secondary to abuse, children who were physically abused were significantly more likely to come from households with cocaine-abusing adults as parents (Wasserman & Leventhal, in press). Black and Mayer (1980) reported on a sample of 200 addicted parents, 92 of whom were alcoholics and 108 opiate addicts. In 22.5% of the families, a child was physically or sexually abused, and in 41%, children had been physically neglected.

Other commonly used measures of parenting function among substance-abusing adults include questionnaires that assess the level of stress or competency parents experience in caring for their children, the adult's own experience of being parented (e.g., Bernardi, Jones, & Tennant, 1989), or the parent's perception of his or her role. For example, the *Parental Attitudes Research Instrument* provides factors describing the degree of parental control, use of supports, and reliance on authoritarian techniques for discipline (Wellisch & Steinberg, 1980). On measures such as this, substance-abusing mothers report a broad range of parenting difficulties including reliance on a more disciplinarian, threatening style of parenting and negative reinforcement (Bauman & Dougherty, 1983). However, such measures do not usually examine how mothers perceive the effects of their substance abuse on their parenting. For example, maternal attitudes toward the child are influenced in part by worries and guilt over potentially damaging her child through cocaine use. Such worries may be sufficient to discourage maternal participation in treatment programs for herself or for her child for fear that others will remind her of what she believes she has done through her addiction. Moreover, self-report instruments are often distorted or inaccurate when completed by substance-abusing adults and do not address the question of whether or not active cocaine abuse limits or distorts a mother's immediate interactions with her children.

Studies of interactions between substance-abusing parents and their children have utilized direct observations of children's and mothers' responses to brief separations and of play interactions between mothers and infants. Studies of separation paradigms and attachment patterns among the children of substance-abusing adults suggest an increased incidence of disrupted or disturbed relationships between parents and children and higher rates of disorganized attachment behaviors (Group D; Main & Solomon, 1986; Rodning, Beckwith, & Howard, 1989, 1991). Higher rates of insecure attachment may be related more to postnatal environmental conditions than to the effects of prenatal drug exposure on infant behavior. Drug-exposed children reared in foster care may be less likely to be insecurely attached than those living with their biological mothers (Rodning et al., 1989), although these differences in attachment patterns by rearing conditions have not been found consistently (Rodning et al., 1991). However, failure to find a difference between prenatally exposed infants in foster care and those in the care of their biological mothers does not provide sufficient evidence for a relation between prenatal cocaine exposure and overall attachment inasmuch as children in foster care have often been in their biological parents' care for months to years and have experienced more than one foster placement. The child's caregiving situation at the time of the attachment assessment does not necessarily reflect the situation even a month earlier. (Indeed, defining who is the primary caregiver is a difficult problem in studies of substance-abusing parents and reflects a difficult dilemma in all studies of parenting of cocaine-exposed children because in many substance-abusing families, a child may be in the care of many different adults in the course of a day or week.) Moreover, disordered attachment patterns may not be specific to substance abuse but more reflective of the overall increased disorganization, stress, abuse, and exposure to violence among drug-using families (Carlson, Cicchetti, Barnett, & Braunwald, 1989; O'Connor, Sigman, & Brill, 1987).

Direct observational measures of child and parent together have been employed less often with substance-abusing families and have mainly included measures of parental involvement and intrusiveness (e.g., for heroin/methadone using families, Bernstein, Jeremy, Hans, & Marcus, 1984, and Bernstein, Jeremy, & Marcus, 1986; for cocaine using adults, Burns, Chethik, Burns, & Clark, 1991). Bernstein and colleagues (1984) reported that mothers participating in a methadone-maintenance program in comparison to a non-opiate-addicted group reacted less often and less contingently to their 4-month-old infants' communicative bids and less often tried to elicit or encourage communicative play with their infants. Similar impairments in maternal responsiveness and reciprocity were reported by Burns and colleagues (1991) in a group of five polydrug-using mothers, two of whom used cocaine primarily, with no comparison group. Polydrug- (including cocaine-) abusing mothers showed a reduction in reciprocal behaviors with their infants and infrequently structured and mediated the environment, findings suggestive of problems with attention directing, structuring activities. Far more work is needed using direct observational measures of interactions between cocaine-using parents and their children.

Importantly, although substance-abusing mothers generally engage in more impaired interactions than comparison groups, not all substance-abusing parents interact poorly with their children. A number of associated factors in addition to, or instead of, substance abuse seem to predict dysfunctional parenting behaviors. For example, Bernstein and colleagues (1984) reported that 47% of a group of methadone-maintained women received adequate scores for their interaction and communication with their infants. Women with poor interaction scores showed lower IQs, lower SES (based on a combination of maternal education and family income), and had fewer contacts with their child's father (methods described in Marcus, Hans, Patterson, & Morris, 1984). Similarly, Johnson and Rosen (1990), examining the maternal behaviors of a sample of 75 multirisk infants, half of whom were methadone exposed, found no relation between the severity of maternal drug abuse and the degree of maternal responsiveness toward the infant. Co-existing maternal psychopathology contributes to greater impairments in parenting interactions among substance-abusing adults compared to both non-substance abusers and substance-abusing adults with no co-existing psychiatric disturbance. Hans and colleagues (Hans, Bernstein, & Henson, 1990, reported in Griffith & Freier, 1992) reported that mothers using methadone who were also diagnosed as having antisocial personality disorders were significantly more dysfunctional in their interactions with their 24-month-olds than were methadone-maintained mothers either having no significant psychopathology or affective disorders alone.

Infant behavior may also affect parenting behaviors (Lewis & Rosenblum, 1974). Diverse infant characteristics, and thus infant behaviors, related to the effects of prenatal drug exposure as with fetal alcohol effects or narcotic withdrawal or the more general contributions of prenatal drug exposure to prematurity and intrauterine growth retardation (Zuckerman, Frank et al., 1989) may make an infant more difficult to care for. Only recently have investigators of parenting among substance-abusing mothers begun to employ interactive models that examine how variations in infant characteristics also influence maternal behaviors (Griffith & Freier, 1992). For example, in a study of maternal alcohol use, maternal–infant interaction, and infant cognitive development, O'Connor, Sigman, and Kasari (1992, 1993) reported that the direction of strongest association was between maternal prenatal alcohol use and the effects on infant affective regulation, which in turn influenced mother–infant interaction and subsequent infant cognitive outcome. Postnatal maternal alcohol consumption did not relate to maternal interactive characteristics.

More detailed studies of the specific alterations in parenting associated with substance abuse are needed not only to guide the design of more effective interventions for substance-abusing parents but also because developmental trajectories for domains such as attention and arousal regulation in infants are influenced by parental interactions (Bornstein, 1985b; Bornstein & Lamb, 1992; Bornstein & Tamis-LeMonda, 1990; Tamis-LeMonda & Bornstein, 1989). Infant attention, exploration, and use of language are influenced by maternal activity including such behaviors as directing the infant's attention to a new toy, naming and pointing, or elaborating on the child's play. Although attention and reactivity reflect neuropsychological functions that are biologically based, these functions are sensitive to the level of environmental organization, responsivity, and adaptability. The degree of sensitivity is individually variable among infants but those with problems in reactivity to novelty or in the regulation of states of arousal may be overall more sensitive to parental disorganization and inconsistency.

Problems in the regulation of arousal in infants may also contribute to an infant's being more difficult to care for, which further influences the potentially compromised cocaine-abusing adult's ability to respond to and support that particular infant's needs. Finally, because of the debilitating effects of chronic cocaine abuse on overall adult psychological and physical health, parental responsiveness and adaptation may deteriorate over time or vary depending on the severity of the cocaine abuse and intoxication.

PATHWAYS OF COCAINE EFFECTS
ON CHILDREN'S DEVELOPMENT

In the preceding sections, several pathways have been suggested that partially explain the effects of cocaine on children both in terms of general developmental outcome and specific functions such as attention and reactivity or arousal regulation. In this section, we make explicit four possible pathways of cocaine-related developmental effects; they are additional to direct effects of cocaine on developing monoaminergic neurotransmitter systems in fetal brain and on overall fetal brain and physical growth through placental vasoconstriction. Any one of these pathways may both express its effect in functions such as attention and arousal regulation and have its effect shaped by the infant's difficulties with attention and arousal. Thus, these pathways are deemed to be both bidirectional and interactive. Each of these pathways also carries considerable risk or is a marker for the parent's continued involvement with drugs and deteriorating parenting function. They also increase the child's likelihood of later involvement in substance abuse, poor school performance and early drop-out, and chronic entrapment in poverty, unemployment, and social isolation.

The first pathway for the effect of cocaine on development is through continued postnatal cocaine exposure for the infant via passive absorption of crack smoke (Kjarasch, Glotzer, Vinci, Wietzman, & Sargent, 1991). Brain development continues through at least the first 12 months postnatally with extensive synaptic remodeling, pruning, and actual structural refinement, and monoaminergic neurotransmitter systems are involved in aspects of the postnatal brain growth (Goldman-Rakic, 1987). Because of the effect of cocaine on monoaminergic neurotransmitter levels and receptor sensitivity, passive exposure postnatally to cocaine may affect these processes of synaptic remodeling, loss, and formation.

The second pathway relates to issues that bring adults to cocaine abuse in the first place. For many substance-abusing adults, psychiatric disorders, such as depression or even attention deficit disorder, appear to predate substance abuse per se and, at least for some, they may represent a significant factor in the adult's initial experimentation with cocaine or other substances (Khantzian, 1985; Khantzian & Khantzian, 1984; N. S. Woods, Eyler, Behnke, & Conlon, 1991). This circumstance will have two consequences: (a) Drug-abusing parents will suffer other psychiatric symptoms and associated psychological and social disorders; and (b) drug-abusing parents may pass to their offspring an increased genetic risk for these psychiatric conditions.

The association between active substance abuse and major psychopathology has been noted by several investigators. Among substance-abusing adults, the incidence of major depression, recurrent and early psychiatric hospitalizations, and, for men, conduct problems often resulting in criminal prosecution is higher than that of the general population (Mirin, Weiss, Griffin, & Michael, 1991; Rounsaville et al., 1991). Among substance abusers' parents and siblings, there is also a high rate of psychiatric disorders such as depression and antisocial personality disorder which are comorbid with substance abuse (Mirin et al., 1991; Rounsaville et al., 1991). The comorbidity appears not to be an aggregation of specific disorders, that is, a concordance for depression or antisocial personality, but rather a general conveyance of risk and an elevation in the incidence of several disorders (Luthar, Anton, Merikangas, & Rounsaville, 1992; Merikangas, Rounsaville, & Prusoff, 1992). Parental death or desertion, marital discord, divorce, substance abuse, and high rates of physical and sexual abuse have also been identified as characteristics of the families of origin of substance abusers (Chambers, Hinesby, & Moldestad, 1970; Raynes, Clement, Patch, & Ervin, 1974). Rounsaville, Weissman, Wilber, and Kleber (1982) reported that disruptive events such as family violence, hospitalizations, or unexpected separations were common historical incidents in the early experiences of substance abusers.

This comorbidity of substance abuse with other psychiatric conditions will have implications as well for the genetic transmission of disorders in the second-generation offspring of these families (Pauls, 1991). In particular, both affective disorders and impairments in attention regulation may be at least partially genetically transmitted from the substance-abusing adult to his or her offspring. Thus, though not directly related to the cocaine exposure itself, maternal cocaine addiction may serve as a marker for genetic loading for such disorders in the newborn.

The third level of effect of cocaine on developmental outcome relates to the effects of these comorbid psychiatric disorders on the substance-abusing adult's parenting behaviors. Impairments in parenting by a cocaine-abusing adult may reflect preexisting psychological and psychiatric conditions that contributed to the individual's addiction. An extensive literature is available describing the early effects of maternal postpartum depression on maternal responsivity and sensitivity to the infant and, in turn, on the infant's active engagement and affective range (Field, in press). The substance-abusing adult's depression may be worsened by poor social supports, the repeated stress of violence and poverty, and the often poor physical health associated with addiction. Severe depression may also make it more difficult for an adult to decrease or stop cocaine use. Thus, the adult becomes more dysfunctional because of both depression and worsening drug abuse, resulting in disordered parenting.

Similar impairments in the substance-abusing adult's capacity to respond to the child may also reflect the effects of chronic cocaine use on specific neuropsychological domains that are crucial for certain aspects of parenting (Bauman & Dougherty, 1983; Mayes, in press-c). All substances of abuse alter the individual's state of consciousness, memory, affect regulation, and impulse control in varying degrees and may become so addictive that the adult's primary goal is to supply his or her addiction to the exclusion of other activities and other people in his or her life. These types of alterations will markedly influence the adult's capacity, for example, to sustain important responsive interactions with an infant and young child at any given moment (Bornstein, in press). No studies have specifically examined how the duration of an adult's cocaine abuse impacts on the degree of parenting dysfunction. However, neuropsychological impairments in memory, verbal fluency, attention, persistence, and task orientation associated with chronic cocaine abuse might be expected to influence certain parenting behaviors such as the capacity to sustain interaction (Ardila, Rosselli, & Strumwasser, 1991; Berry et al., 1993; Manschreck et al., 1990; O'Malley, Adamse, Heaton, & Gawin, 1992). Parenting infants and older children relies extensively on remembering previous experiences—familiar routines that support the infant's emerging regulation of states and later anticipation of mother's responsiveness. Both are rooted in part in parental consistency. Similarly, the neuropsychological effects of prolonged addiction on memory, persistence, and concentration may also impede an adult's response to drug-treatment interventions and contribute to an intractable addiction involving multiple drugs in addition to cocaine including alcohol, marijuana, and tobacco (which also precludes attributing any developmental effects on child or parent to cocaine alone).

The fourth potential pathway of cocaine effect on infant and child relates to the global amount of family discord, virtual homelessness, poverty, and on a more basic level, chronic uncertainty, despair, and fear in both adults and children that characterize the cocaine-using world. Abuse of cocaine often involves the user directly or indirectly in criminal activities such as prostitution, theft, or drug dealing (Boyd & Mieczkowski, 1990) and exposes the user as well as her or his children to personal and property violence. Because of these activities, cocaine-abusing adults are more likely to be arrested and incarcerated repeatedly, exposing their children to multiple episodes of parental separation and placements usually with different foster families or with other (often substance-abusing) neighbors or relatives (Lawson & Wilson, 1980). The levels and types of violence which the children of cocaine-abusing mothers are exposed to range from verbal abuse between adults to physical fights with deadly weapons. Children 5 to 6 years of age have also seen and participated in scenes well beyond their psychological capacities either to understand or cope.

Acute and chronic trauma affect children's brain development and psychological function. We might readily surmise that children developing amidst drug-associated violence, poverty, discord, neglect, and uncertainty experience a level of acute and ongoing stress and trauma of potentially sufficient intensity and chronicity to alter the development of centrally regulated, basic psychophysiological functions. Moreover, many of these children may have impairments in the capacity to regulate states of arousal in response to novel or highly stimulating situations and are thus exposed to conditions which further stress dysfunctional regulatory systems. In instances of severely overwhelming, and perhaps chronically stressful trauma, stress-related neurotransmitters potentially contribute to increased CNS sensitivity to stimulating and novel events and altered arousal regulatory mechanisms (Pittman, 1988). Compromise secondary to traumatic events may further impede the child's already compromised ability to respond to ongoing discord and chaos in the world around him or her.

CONCLUSION

Study of the developmental effects of prenatal exposure to cocaine requires investigators to examine interactions among conditions of risk due to prenatal exposure to a potential teratogen and various environmental disruptions ascribable also to the effects of cocaine abuse. The developmental dilemmas posed for substance-abusing families and their prenatally exposed children involve the multiple bidirectional and interactive pathways through which cocaine exposure pre- and postnatally may affect the child and family. Cocaine exposure may directly affect fetal and postnatal brain development and adult neuropsychological functions requisite to adequate parenting. Moreover, the cocaine-associated environment is characterized by increased parental psychopathology, abuse and violence, and poverty and homelessness, each of which threatens the child's cognitive and social development and traps both parent and child in a deteriorating cycle of chronic substance abuse, poor health, and social isolation.

Despite these dilemmas, the problem of prenatal cocaine exposure submits to modeling of biologic–environment interaction. The following areas are either potentially fruitful or much needed lines of investigation with ongoing studies of prenatally cocaine-exposed infants and preschool-aged children: (a) studies of reactivity, arousal, and attention regulation and the stability of such capacities from infancy into the second and third year of life; (b) studies of language and communication with attention to early communicative precursors; (c) direct observations of parent–child interaction with emphasis on parental attention directing and structuring activities, and (d) studies of the effects of chronic exposure to violence on such functions as a capacity for empathy or for mediating aggression. Closer studies of basic functions such as attention and the regulation of arousal that underlie broader developmental competencies and the interaction of such functions with the parental environment will provide a more adequate profile of the potentially specific and nonspecific problem areas for prenatally cocaine-exposed children as they reach school age.

ACKNOWLEDGMENTS

This chapter summarizes selected aspects of our collaborative research; portions of the text have appeared in our previous scientific publications cited in the references. We thank K. Chawarska, O. M. Haynes, D. Cohen, and R. Schottenfeld for their support of our studies of prenatal cocaine exposure.

REFERENCES

Akbari, H. M., & Azmitia, E. C. (1992). Increased tyrosine hydroxylase immunoreactivity in the rat cortex following prenatal cocaine exposure. *Developmental Brain Research, 66*, 277–281.

Akbari, H. M., Kramer, H. K., Whitaker-Azmitia, P. M., Spear, L. P., Azmitia, E. C. (1992). Prenatal cocaine exposure disrupts the development of the serotonergic system. *Brain Research, 572*, 57–63.

Alessandri, S. M., Sullivan, M. W., Imaizumi, S., & Lewis, M. (1993). Learning and emotional responsivity in cocaine-exposed infants. *Developmental Psychology, 29*, 989–997.

Amaro, H., Fried, L. E., Cabral, H., & Zuckerman, B. (1990). Violence during pregnancy and substance use. *American Journal of Public Health, 80*, 575–579.

Amaro, H., Zuckerman, B., & Cabral, H. (1989). Drug use among adolescent mothers: Profile of risk. *Pediatrics, 84*, 144–151.

Anday, E. K., Cohen, M. E., Kelley, N. E., & Leitner, D. S. (1989). Effect of in utero cocaine exposure on startle and its modification. *Developmental Pharmacology and Therapeutics, 12*, 137–145.

Anisfeld, E., Cunningham, N., Ferrari, L., Melendez, M., Ruesch, N., Soto, L., & Wagner, D. (1991). Infant development after prenatal cocaine exposure (Abstract). *Society for Research in Child Development.*

Ardila, A., Rosselli, M., & Strumwasser, S. (1991). Neuropsychological deficits in chronic cocaine abusers. *International Journal of Neuroscience, 57*, 73–79.

Arendt, R., Singer, L., & Minnes, S. (1993). Development of cocaine exposed infants (Abstract). *Society for Research in Child Development.*

Bauman, P. S., & Dougherty, F. E. (1983). Drug-addicted mothers' parenting and their children's development. *International Journal of the Addictions, 18*, 291–302.

Bayley, N. (1969). *Manual for the Bayley Scales of Infant Development.* New York: Psychological Corporation.

Bayley, N. (1993). *Bayley Scales of Infant Development* (rev. ed.). New York: Psychological Corporation.

Bergeman, C. S., & Plomin, R. (1989). Genotype-environment interaction. In M. H. Bornstein & J. S. Bruner (Eds.), *Interaction in human development* (pp. 157–171). Hillsdale, NJ: Lawrence Erlbaum Associates.

Bernardi, E., Jones, M., & Tennant, C. (1989). Quality of parenting in alcoholics and narcotic addicts. *British Journal of Psychiatry, 154*, 677–682.

Bernstein, V., Jeremy, R. J., Hans, S., & Marcus, J. (1984). A longitudinal study of offspring born to methadone-maintained women: II. Dyadic interaction and infant behavior at four months. *American Journal of Drug and Alcohol Abuse, 10*, 161–193.

Bernstein, V., Jeremy, R. J., & Marcus, J. (1986). Mother–infant interaction in multiproblem families: Finding those at risk. *Journal of the American Academy of Child Psychiatry, 25*, 631–640.

Berry, J., Van, G. W. G., Herzberg, D. S., & Hinkin, C. E. (1993). Neuropsychological deficits in abstinent cocaine abusers: Preliminary findings after two weeks of abstinence. *Drug and Alcohol Dependence, 32*, 231–237.

Besharov, D. J. (1990). Crack children in foster care. *Children Today, 19*(4), 21–25, 35.

Billman, D., Nemeth, P., Heimler, R., & Sasidharan, P. (1991). Prenatal cocaine exposure: Advanced Bayley Psychomotor Scores. *Clinical Research, 39,* 697A.

Bingol, N., Fuchs, M., Diaz, V., Stone, R. K., & Gromisch, D.S. (1987). Teratogenicity of cocaine in humans. *Journal of Pediatrics, 110,* 93–96.

Black, R., & Mayer, J. (1980). Parents with special problems: Alcoholism and opiate addiction. *Child Abuse and Neglect, 4,* 45–54.

Bornstein, M. (1985a). Habituation as a measure of visual information processing in human infants: Summary, systemization, and synthesis. In G. Gottlieb & N. Krasnegor (Eds.), *Development of audition and vision during the first year of postnatal life: A methodological overview* (pp. 253–295). Norwood, NJ: Ablex.

Bornstein, M. H. (1985b). How infant and mother jointly contribute to developing cognitive competence in the child. *Proceedings of the National Academy of Science* (U.S.A.), *85,* 7470–7473.

Bornstein, M. H. (1989). Sensitive periods in development: Structural characteristics and causal interpretations. *Psychological Bulletin, 105,* 179–197.

Bornstein, M. H. (in press). Parenting infants. In M. H. Bornstein (Ed.), *Handbook of parenting* (Vol. 1). Hillsdale, NJ: Lawrence Erlbaum Associates.

Bornstein, M. H., & Lamb, M. E. (1992). *Development in infancy: An introduction* (3rd ed.). New York: McGraw-Hill.

Bornstein, M. H., & Mayes, L. C. (1992). Taking a measure of the infant mind. In F. Kessell, M. H. Bornstein, & A. Sameroff (Eds.), *Contemporary constructions of the child: Essays in honor of William Kessen* (pp. 45–56). Hillsdale, NJ: Lawrence Erlbaum Associates.

Bornstein, M. H., & Tamis-LeMonda, C. S. (1990). Activities and interactions of mothers and their firstborn infants in the first six months of life: Covariation, stability, continuity, correspondence, and prediction. *Child Development, 61,* 1206–1217.

Boyd, C. J., & Mieczkowski, T. (1990). Drug use, health, family, and social support in "crack" cocaine users. *Addictive Behaviors, 15,* 481–485.

Brazelton, T. B. (1984). *Neonatal Behavioral Assessment Scale* (2nd ed.) (Clinics in Developmental Medicine, No. 88). Philadelphia: Lippincott.

Burns, K., Chethik, L., Burns, W. J., & Clark, R. (1991). Dyadic disturbances in cocaine-abusing mothers and their infants. *Journal of Clinical Psychology, 47,* 316–319.

Byck, R. (1974). *Cocaine papers: Sigmund Freud.* New York: Stonehill.

Carlson, V., Cicchetti, D., Barnett, D., & Braunwald, K. (1989). Disorganized/ disoriented attachment relationships in maltreated infants. *Developmental Psychology, 25,* 525–531.

Chambers, C. D., Hinesby, R. K., & Moldestad, M. (1970). Narcotic addiction in females: A race comparison. *International Journal of the Addictions, 5,* 257–278.

Chasnoff, I. J., Griffith, D. R., Freier, C., & Murray, J. (1992). Cocaine/ polydrug use in pregnancy: Two-year follow-up. *Pediatrics, 89,* 284–289.

Chasnoff, I, Griffith, D. R., MacGregor, S., Dirkes, K., & Burns, K. (1989). Temporal patterns of cocaine use in pregnancy. *Journal of the American Medical Association, 261,* 1741–1744.

Chasnoff, I. J., Landress, H. J., & Barrett, M. E. (1990). Prevalence of illicit drugs or alcohol abuse during pregnancy and discrepancies in mandatory reporting in Pinellas County, Florida. *New England Journal of Medicine, 322,* 102–106.

Clark, C. R., Geffen, G. M., & Geffen, L. B. (1989). Catecholamines and the covert orientation of attention in humans. *Neuropsychologia, 27,* 131–139.

Coles, B. J., & Robbins, T. W. (1989). Effects of 6-hydroxydopamine lesions of the nucleus accumbens septi on performance of a 5-choice serial reaction time task in rats: Implications for theories of selective attention and arousal. *Behavioral Brain Research, 33,* 165–179.

Coles, C. D., Platzman, K. A., Smith, I., James, M. E., & Falek, A. (1992). Effects of cocaine and alcohol use in pregnancy on neonatal growth and neurobehavioral status. *Neurotoxicology and Teratology, 14,* 23–33.

Colombo, J., & Mitchell, D. W. (1990). Individual differences in early visual attention. In J. Colombo & J. Fagen (Eds.), *Individual differences in infancy: Reliability, stability, and prediction* (pp. 193–227). Hillsdale, NJ: Lawrence Erlbaum Associates.

Courtwright, D. T. (1982). *Dark paradise*. Cambridge, MA: Harvard University Press.

Day, N. L. (1992). Effects of prenatal alcohol exposure. In I. S. Zagon & T. A. Slotkin (Eds.), *Maternal substance abuse and the developing nervous system* (pp. 27–44). Boston: Academic.

Dow-Edwards, D. (1989). Long-term neurochemical and neurobehavioral consequences of cocaine use during pregnancy. *Annals of the New York Academy of Science, 562*, 280–289.

Dow-Edwards, D., Freed, L. A., & Milhorat, T. H. (1988). Stimulation of brain metabolism by perinatal cocaine exposure. *Brain Research, 470*, 137–141.

Eisen, L. N., Field, T. M., Bandstra, E. S., Roberts, J. P., Morrow, C., Larson, S. K., & Steele, B. M. (1990). Perinatal cocaine effects on neonatal stress behavior and performance on the Brazelton Scale. *Pediatrics, 88*, 477–480.

Farrar, H. C., & Kearns, G. L. (1989). Cocaine: Clinical pharmacology and toxicology. *Journal of Pediatrics, 115*, 665–675.

Field, T. F. (1981). Infant arousal, attention, and affect during early interactions. In L. Lipsitt & C. Rovee-Collier (Eds.), *Advances in infancy research* (Vol. 1, pp. 57–100). Norwood, NJ: Ablex.

Field, T. M. (in press). Psychologically depressed parents. In M. H. Bornstein (Ed.), *Handbook of parenting, Vol. 3. Status and social conditions of parenting*. Hillsdale, NJ: Lawrence Erlbaum Associates.

Frank, D. A., Zuckerman, B. S., Amaro, H., Aboagye, K., Bauchner, H., Cabral, H., Fried, L., Hingson, R., Kayne, H., & Levenson, S. M. (1988). Cocaine use during pregnancy: Prevalence and correlates. *Pediatrics, 82*(6), 888–895.

Fulroth, R., Phillips, B., & Durand, D. J. (1989). Perinatal outcome of infants exposed to cocaine and/or heroin in utero. *American Journal of Diseases of Children, 143*, 905–910.

Gawin, F. H., & Ellinwood, F. H. (1988). Cocaine and other stimulants. *New England Journal of Medicine, 318*, 1173–1182.

Goeders, N. E., & Smith, J. E. (1983). Cortical dopaminergic involvement in cocaine reinforcement. *Science, 221*, 773–775.

Goldman-Rakic, P. S. (1987). Development of cortical circuitry and cognitive function. *Child Development, 58*, 601–622.

Gomby, D. S., & Shiono, P. H. (1991). Estimating the number of substance-exposed infants. *The Future of Children, 1*(1), 17–25. (Available from Center for the Future of Children, David & Lucille Packard Foundation, Los Alto, CA)

Goodwin, G. A., Heyser, C. J., Moody, C. A., & Rajachandran, L. (1992). A fostering study of the effects of prenatal cocaine exposure: II. Offspring behavioral measures. *Neurotoxicology and Teratology, 14*, 423–432.

Griffith, D., & Freier, C. (1992). Methodological issues in the assessment of the mother–child interactions of substance-abusing women and their children. *NIDA Research Monograph, 117*, 228–247.

Hadeed, A. J., & Siegel, S. R. (1989). Maternal cocaine use during pregnancy: Effect on the newborn infant. *Pediatrics, 84*, 205–210.

Hadfield, M. G., & Nugent, E. A. (1983). Cocaine: Comparative effect on dopamine uptake in extrapyramidal and limbic systems. *Biochemical Pharmacology, 32*, 744–746.

Hans, S. L., Bernstein, V. J., & Henson, L. G. (1990). *Interaction between drug-using mothers and their toddlers*. Paper presented at the seventh International Conference on Infant Studies, Montreal.

Hawley, T. L., & Disney, E. R. (1992). Crack's children: The consequences of maternal cocaine abuse. *Social Policy Report of the Society for Research in Child Development, 6*(4), 1–22.

Heyser, C. J., Molina, V. A., & Spear, L. P. (1992). A fostering study of the effects of prenatal cocaine exposure: I. Maternal behaviors. *Neurotoxicology and Teratology, 14*, 415–421.

Hoyme, H. E., Jones, K. L., Dixon, S. D., Jewett, T., Hanson, J. W., Robinson, L. K., Msall, M. E., & Allanson, J. E. (1990). Prenatal cocaine exposure and fetal vascular disruption. *Pediatrics, 85*, 743–747.

Johnson, H. L., & Rosen, T. S. (1990). Difficult mothers of difficult babies: Mother–infant interaction in a multi-risk population. *American Journal of Orthopsychiatry, 60*, 281–288.

Khantzian, E. J. (1985). The self-medication hypothesis of addictive disorders: Focus on heroin and cocaine dependence. *American Journal of Psychiatry, 142*, 1259–1264.

Khantzian, E. J., & Khantzian, N. J. (1984). Cocaine addiction: Is there a psychological predisposition? *Psychiatric Annals, 14*, 753–759.

Kjarasch, S. J., Glotzer, D., Vinci, R., Wietzman, M., & Sargent, T. (1991). Unsuspected cocaine exposure in children. *American Journal of Diseases of Children, 145*, 204–206.

Lauder, J. M. (1988). Neurotransmitters as morphogens. *Progressive Brain Research, 73*, 365–387.

Lauder, J. M. (1991). Neuroteratology of cocaine: Relationship to developing monamine systems. *National Institute of Drug Abuse Research Monographs, 114*, 233–247.

Lawson, M., & Wilson, G. (1980). Parenting among women addicted to narcotics. *Child Welfare, 59*, 67–79.

Lewis, M., & Brooks-Gunn, J. (1981). Visual attention at three months as a predictor of cognitive functioning at two years of age. *Intelligence, 5*, 131–140.

Lewis, M., Goldberg, S., & Campbell, H. (1969). A developmental study of information processing within the first three years of life: Response decrement to a redundant signal. *Monographs of the Society for Research in Child Development, 39* (9, Serial No. 133).

Lewis, M., & Rosenblum, L. A. (1974). *The effect of the infant on its caregiver.* New York: Wiley.

Luthar, S., Anton, S. F., Merikangas, K. R., & Rounsaville, B. J. (1992). Vulnerability to substance abuse and psychopathology among siblings of opioid abusers. *Journal of Nervous and Mental Disorders, 180*, 153–161.

MacGregor, S. N., Keith, L. G., Chasnoff, I. J., Rosner, M. A., Chisum, R. N., Shaw, P., & Minogue, J. (1987). Cocaine use during pregnancy: Adverse perinatal outcome. *American Journal of Obstetrics and Gynecology, 157*, 686–690.

Main, M., & Solomon, J. (1986). Discovery of an insecure-disorganized/ disoriented attachment pattern. In T. B. Brazelton & M. Yogman (Eds.), *Affective development in infancy.* New Jersey: Ablex.

Manschreck, T., Schneyer, M., Weisstein, C., Laughery, J., Rosenthal, J., Celada, T., & Berner, J. (1990). Freebase cocaine and memory. *Comprehensive Psychiatry, 31*, 369–375.

Marcus, J., Hans, S. L., Patterson, C. B., & Morris, A. J. (1984). A longitudinal study of offspring born to methadone-maintained women. I. Design, methodology, and description of women's resources for functioning. *American Journal of Drug and Alcohol Abuse, 10*, 135–160.

Mattson, M. P. (1988). Neurotransmitters in the regulation of neuronal cytoarchitecture. *Brain Research Reviews, 13*, 179–212.

Mayes, L. C. (1992). The effects of prenatal cocaine exposure on young children's development. *The Annals of the American Academy of Political and Social Science, 521*, 11–27.

Mayes, L. C. (in press-a). Exposure to cocaine: Behavioral outcomes in preschool aged children. In L. Finnegan (Ed.), *Behaviors of drug-exposed offspring* (NIDA Technical Symposium).

Mayes, L. C. (in press-b). Neurobiology of prenatal cocaine exposure: Effect on developing monoaminergic systems. *Infant Mental Health.*

Mayes, L. C. (in press-c). Substance abuse and parenting. In M. H. Bornstein (Ed.), *The handbook of parenting.* Hillsdale, NJ: Lawrence Erlbaum Associates.

Mayes, L. C., & Bornstein, M. (in press). Attention regulation in infants born at risk: Preterm and prenatally cocaine exposed infants. In J. Burak & J. Enns (Eds.), *Development, attention, and psychopathology.* New York: Guilford.

Mayes, L. C., Bornstein, M. H., Chawarska, K., & Granger, R. H. (in press). Information processing and developmental assessments in three month olds exposed prenatally to cocaine. *Pediatrics.*

Mayes, L. C., Granger, R. H., Bornstein, M. H., & Zuckerman, B. (1992). The Problem of Intrauterine Cocaine Exposure. *Journal of the American Medical Association, 267*, 406–408.

Mayes, L. C., Granger, R. H., Frank, M. A., Bornstein, M., & Schottenfeld, R. (1993). Neurobehavioral profiles of infants exposed to cocaine prenatally. *Pediatrics, 91*, 778–783.

Merikangas, K. R., Rounsaville, B. J., & Prusoff, B. A. (1992). Familial factors in vulnerability to substance abuse. In M. Glantz & R. Pickens (Eds.), *Vulnerability to drug abuse* (pp. 75–98). Washington, DC: American Psychiatric Association.

Mirin, S. M., Weiss, R. D., Griffin, M. L., & Michael, J. L. (1991). Psychopathology in drug abusers and their families. *Comprehensive Psychiatry, 32*, 36–51.

Moore, T. R., Sorg, J., Miller, L., Key, T., & Resnik, R. (1986). Hemodynamic effects of intravenous cocaine on the pregnant ewe and fetus. *American Journal of Obstetrics and Gynecology, 155*, 883–888.

Morrison, J. H., & Foote, S. I. (1986). Noradrenergic and serotonergic innervation of cortical, thalamic, and tectal visual structures in old and new world monkeys. *Journal of Comparative Neurology, 243*, 117–128.

Musto, D. (1973). *The American disease: Origins of narcotic control.* New Haven: Yale University Press.

O'Connor, M. J., Sigman, N., & Brill, N. (1987). Disorganization of attachment in relation to maternal alcohol consumption. *Journal of Consulting and Clinical Psychology, 55*, 831–836.

O'Connor, M. J., Sigman, M., & Kasari, C. (1992). Attachment behavior of infants exposed prenatally to alcohol: Mediating effects of infant affect and mother–infant interaction. *Development and Psychopathology, 4*, 243–256.

O'Connor, M. J., Sigman, M., & Kasari, C. (1993). Maternal alcohol use and infant cognition. *Infant Behavior and Development, 16*, 177–193.

O'Malley, S., Adamse, M., Heaton, R. K., & Gawin, F. H. (1992). Neuropsychological impairments in chronic cocaine abusers. *American Journal of Drug and Alcohol Abuse, 18*, 131–144.

Oro, A. S., & Dixon, S. D. (1987). Perinatal cocaine and methamphetamine exposure: Maternal and neonatal correlates. *Journal of Pediatrics, 111*, 571–578.

Osterloh, J. D., & Lee, B. L. (1989). Urine drug screening in mothers and newborns. *American Journal of Diseases of Children, 143*, 791–793.

Pauls, D. (1991). Genetic influences on child psychiatric conditions. In M. Lewis (Ed.), *Child and adolescent psychiatry: A comprehensive textbook* (pp. 351–363). Baltimore: Williams and Wilkins.

Pittman, R. K. (1988). Post-traumatic stress disorder, conditioning, and network theory. *Psychiatric Annals, 18*, 182–189.

Posner, M. I., & Petersen, S. E. (1988). Structures and functions of selected attention. In T. Boll & B. Bryant (Eds.), *Master lectures of clinical neuropsychology* (pp. 173–202). Washington, DC: American Psychological Association.

Posner, M. I., & Petersen, S. E. (1990). The attention system of the human brain. *Annual Review of Neuroscience, 13*, 25–42.

Pribram, K. H., & McGuiness, D. (1975). Arousal, activation, and effort in the control of attention. *Psychological Review, 82*, 116–149.

Raynes, A. E., Clement, C., Patch, V. D., & Ervin, F. (1974). Factors related to imprisonment in female heroin addicts. *International Journal of the Addictions, 9*, 145–150.

Richie, J. M., & Greene, N. M. (1985). Local anesthetics. In A. G. Gilman, L. S. Goodman, T. N. Rall, & F. Murad (Eds.). *The pharmacologic basis of therapeutics* (7th ed., pp. 309–310). New York: Macmillan.

Rodning, C., Beckwith, L., & Howard, J. (1989). Characteristics of attachment organization and play organization in prenatally drug-exposed toddlers. *Development and Psychopathology, 1*, 277–289.

Rodning, C., Beckwith, & Howard, J. (1991). Quality of attachment and home environments in children prenatally exposed to PCP and cocaine. *Development and Psychopathology, 3*, 351–366.

Rogosch, F. A., Cicchetti, D., Shields, A., & Toth, S. L. (in press). Parenting dysfunction in child maltreatment. In M. H. Bornstein (Ed.), *Handbook of parenting* (Vol. 4). Hillsdale, NJ: Lawrence Erlbaum Associates.

Rothbart, M. K., & Posner, M. I. (1985). Temperament and the development of self regulation. In H. Hartlage & C. E. Telzrow (Eds.), *Neuropsychology of individual differences: A developmental perspective* (93–123). New York: Plenum.

Rounsaville, B. J., Kosten, T. R., Weissman, M. M., Prusoff, B., Pauls, D., Foley, S., & Merikangas, K. (1991). Psychiatric disorders in the relatives of probands with opiate addicts. *Archives of General Psychiatry, 48*, 33–42.

Rounsaville, B. J., Weissman, M. M., Wilber, C. H., & Kleber, H. D. (1982). Pathways of opiate addiction: An evaluation of differing antecedents. *British Journal of Psychiatry, 141*, 437–466.

Ruff, H. A. (1988). The measurement of attention in high-risk infants. In P. M. Vietze & H. G. Vaughan (Eds.), *Early identification of infants with developmental disabilities* (pp. 282–296). New York: Grune and Stratton.

Ryan, L., Ehrlich, S., & Finnegan, L. (1987). Cocaine abuse in pregnancy: Effects on the fetus and newborn. *Neurotoxicology and Teratology, 9*, 295–299.

Scherling, D. (1994). Prenatal cocaine exposure and childhood psychopathology. *American Journal of Orthopsychiatry, 64*, 9–19.

Shepherd, G. M. (1988). *Neurobiology.* (2nd ed.). New York: Oxford University Press.

Streissguth, A. P. (1992). Fetal alcohol syndrome and fetal alcohol effects: A clinical perspective on later developmental consequences. In I. S. Zagon & T. A. Slotkin (Eds.), *Maternal substance abuse and the developing nervous system* (pp. 5–26). Boston: Academic.

Struthers, J. M., & Hansen, R. L. (1992). Visual recognition memory in drug-exposed infants. *Journal of Developmental and Behavioral Pediatrics, 13*, 108–111.

Swann, A. C. (1990). Cocaine: Synaptic effects and adaptations. In N. D. Volkow & A. C. Swann (Eds.), *Cocaine in the brain* (pp. 58–94). New Brunswick, NJ: Rutgers University Press.

Tamis-LeMonda, C. S., & Bornstein, M. H. (1989). Habituation and maternal encouragement of attention in infancy as predictors of toddler language, play, and representational competence. *Child Development, 60*, 738–751.

Thoman, E. B., & Ingersoll, E. W. (1989). The human nature of the youngest humans: Prematurely born babies. *Seminars in Perinatology, 13*, 482–494.

Wasserman, D. R., & Leventhal, J. M. (in press). Maltreatment of children born to cocaine-abusing mothers. *American Journal of Diseases of Children.*

Wellisch, D. K., & Steinberg, M. R. (1980). Parenting attitudes of addict mothers. *International Journal of the Addictions, 15*, 809–819.

Wise, R. A. (1984). Neural mechanisms of the reinforcing action of cocaine. *National Institute of Drug Abuse Research Monograph, 50*, 15–33.

Woods, J. R., Plessinger, M. A., & Clark, K. E. (1987). Effect of cocaine on uterine blood flow and fetal oxygenation. *Journal of the American Medical Association, 257*, 957–961.

Woods, N. S., Eyler, F. D., Behnke, M., & Conlon, M. (1991, April). Cocaine use during pregnancy: Maternal depressive symptoms and neonatal neurobehavior over the first month. Paper presented at the meeting of the Society for Research in Child Development, Seattle, WA.

Zuckerman, B., Amaro, H., Bauchner, H., & Cabral, H. (1989). Depressive symptoms during pregnancy: Relationships to poor health behaviors. *American Journal of Obstetrics and Gynecology, 160*, 1107–1111.

Zuckerman, B., & Frank, D. A. (1992). Prenatal cocaine and marijuana exposure: Research and clinical implications. In I. S. Zagon & T. A. Slotkin (Eds.), *Maternal substance abuse and the developing nervous system* (pp. 125–154). Boston: Academic.

Zuckerman, B., Frank, D. A., Hingson, R., & Amaro, H. (1989). Effects of maternal marijuana and cocaine use on fetal growth. *New England Journal of Medicine, 320*, 762–768.

14

▼▼▼▼▼▼▼

Temperament in Cocaine-Exposed Infants

Steven M. Alessandri
Medical College of Pennsylvania

Margaret Wolan Sullivan
Margaret Bendersky
Michael Lewis
Robert Wood Johnson Medical School

An infant cries in a high-pitched voice, sleeps irregularly and feeds poorly, rarely smiles, and does not seem very responsive to stimuli. A preschooler can never seem to sit still, often changes mood without any apparent reason, and has a very short attention span even during play. A child is easily distracted in school by outside noises, gives up easily when an answer to a question is not known, and shows very little interest in learning. Can the concept of temperament provide a framework to better understand these behavioral differences? We believe that it can. There is converging evidence that suggests that cocaine exposure may affect behavioral domains linked to underlying temperamental differences. In this chapter, we employ the framework of infant temperament to examine the behavior of cocaine-exposed infants. The particular focus is on the temperament of cocaine-exposed infants and on the role it plays in learning, emotional responsivity, and social functioning. Is there a cluster of temperamental characteristics that typifies the cocaine-exposed infant? If so, is the cocaine-exposed child's ability to learn, emotional expression, and regulation compromised as a function of these characteristics? We begin with a selective review of the temperament literature, emphasizing the role of temperament in learning and emotional behavior and prenatal and postnatal factors that influence temperament. We then explore the interplay between temperament, learning, and emotional responsivity in cocaine-exposed infants. Finally, the relation between temperament and caregiver–infant interactions is discussed.

TEMPERAMENT IN INFANCY

Much attention has been given to the definition and measurement of temperament in infancy, with numerous reviews of the construct and its assessment appearing in recent years (Bates, 1987; Bornstein, Gaughran, & Homel, 1985; Goldsmith & Campos, 1982, 1986). Although no single definition of temperament has gained universal acceptance, most researchers would agree that temperament includes individual behavioral differences in attention, affective expressiveness, motor activity, soothability, and self-regulation (Campos, Barrett, Lamb, Goldsmith, & Stenberg, 1983; Derryberry & Rothbart, 1984; Goldsmith et al., 1987; Thomas & Chess, 1989). Thus, temperament can be observed behaviorally at all ages as individual differences in patterns of emotionality, activity, and self-regulation. Such individual differences are presumed to have genetic and psychobiological bases, although the environment is seen as a factor that molds temperament styles (Buss & Plomin, 1984; Rothbart & Derryberry, 1981; Thomas & Chess, 1980).

A wide variety of instruments have been developed to measure temperament in infants and young children. Assessment of infant temperament is typically based on parental report (questionnaires more than interviews), observer ratings, and direct behavioral recording. The most prevalent type of temperament measure in infancy is parental report. Parental reports are used because they allow sampling of the infant's behavior over a range of occasions and situations that are difficult to achieve in laboratory and home visits. Direct observations of temperament in the laboratory or home have been proposed as a means of validating maternal assessment. These methods are vulnerable to distortion because the period of observation is short and the range of behavior may be constricted. Moreover, there are few standard contexts for measuring temperament in the laboratory though there are several currently being developed (Bates, 1989). Parental report of their experiences with their infants are, therefore, of value in the measurement of temperament. In a review of studies that have compared maternal ratings of infants with observational data, Bates (1989) concluded that there is a modest to moderate objective basis in parental perceptions.

On an intrapersonal basis, temperamental behavioral tendencies show some degree of stability and cross-sectional generality (Goldsmith & Campos, 1986). Continuity in temperament beginning in early infancy and over several years has been found for "behavioral inhibition" (Garcia-Coll, Kagan, & Reznick, 1984; Kagan, Reznick, Clarke, Snidman, & Garcia-Coll, 1984). Moreover, individual differences in anger and sadness expressions have been reported to persist over the first 18 months (Izard, Hembree, Dougherty, & Spizzirri, 1983). Several studies show continuity in maternal reports of activity level throughout the first year (McDevitt & Carey, 1981; Peters-Martin & Wachs, 1984; Rothbart, 1981). Other data based on parental report rather than behavioral coding are consistent with this view of continuity (Izard & Malatesta, 1987, for a review). Thus, there is evidence that the major temperament concepts are somewhat stable during infancy, whether measured by parent report or direct observation.

Temperament and Learning

There is converging evidence to support the assertion that learning performance is related to individual differences in behavioral style. For example, Piagetian levels of sensorimotor performance are significantly correlated with several dimensions of infant temperament such as attention and persistence (Carey & McDevitt, 1978). Similarly, Bayley Scale mental performance scores were positively correlated with temperament dimensions such as reactivity, persistence, and attention span (Matheney, Dolan, & Wilson, 1974). In addition, Keogh (1982) found that persistence not only predicted IQ and grades in school but also correlated with teachers' estimates of ability when IQ was held constant.

Undesirable temperamental characteristics, on the other hand, such as susceptibility to distress, fear of novel stimuli, and low frustration tolerance can result in behavioral disorganization, which can be disruptive in an immediate learning situation and possibly limit future opportunities for cognitive growth through faulty parent–child interactions. There is some data to support the notion that "difficult" infants show cognitive delays (Field, Hallock, Ting et al., 1978; Sostek & Anders, 1977; Thomas & Chess, 1977). Taken as a whole, it appears that at least some temperamental factors influence performance on cognitive tasks, especially those that require attention and persistence.

In this regard, there is some evidence to indicate that temperament may be related to the ease with which infants learn a simple operant response. The infant's rate of learning may reflect a psychobiological preparedness to learn. This does not refer to cognitive capacity but to the infant's ability to engage in arousing and challenging environmental events. Theorists who advocate a biological–evolutionary perspective of temperament (e.g., Buss & Plomin, 1984) argue that genetic factors influence individual differences in behavioral styles, which, in turn, would be expected to influence predispositions to learn. In instrumental conditioning studies, however, the relation between learning and temperament is inconsistent. Krafchuk, Sameroff, and Barkow (1976) reported that high activity level was significantly correlated with operant learning. Dunst and Lingerfelt (1985) also reported that the temperament dimensions of persistence and rhythmicity were significant correlates of learning rates during conditioning. On the other hand, Alessandri, Sullivan, and Lewis (1990) found that the ease with which infants learned an operant response did not depend on the behavioral styles they brought to the situation.

Rothbart and Derryberry (1981) hypothesized that attention span and duration of orienting along with latency to approach sudden or novel stimuli (fearfulness) are behavioral processes that promote self-regulation in learning situations. For example, Fagen and Ohr (1985) found that crying in response to changes in mobile complexity could reliably be predicted by the temperamental dimensions of activity level, duration of orienting, and distress to sudden or novel stimuli. However, a subsequent study revealed that the prediction of group membership (criers/noncriers) was more reliable only for females (Fagen, Ohr, Singer, & Fleckenstein, 1987). Further studies that examine the use of temperament measures as part of infant conditioning studies are needed to determine the mutual contributions of individual differences and environmental factors in learning.

Temperament and Emotional Behavior

Although the concepts of temperament and emotion have been linked by many theorists, Goldsmith and Campos (1982, 1986) offered a direct link between temperament and emotion. They viewed temperament as interacting with or as a moderator of other intraindividual variables such as emotion. In fact, they have provided a theoretical mapping of the major temperament dimensions and their correspondence to discrete emotions described by Ekman and Friesen (1975) and Izard (1983). It is possible, therefore, to match temperament dimensions, particularly those of Rothbart (1986) with the facial expressions of Izard (1983). For example, the temperament dimension of smiling or laughter is likely to correspond to joy, distress to limitations to anger, fear (Rothbart) to fear, and persistence to the expression of interest.

According to Goldsmith and Campos (1982), temperament can be viewed as structures that organize the expression of emotion which, in turn, regulate parent–child social interactions. Expressive behaviors have social-communicative value, especially with respect to the issue of emotion socialization. Affective signals are salient and compelling elicitors of responses between caregiver and infant. Affective exchanges between caregivers and infants provide infants with one of the earliest occasions for the learning of display rules as well as individual-familial expressive patterns (Lewis & Saarni, 1985). It has been demonstrated that caregivers react in specific ways to their infants' expressions of emotions, and that these differentiated responses may affect subsequent emotional development (Brazelton, Koslowski, & Main, 1979; Malatesta & Haviland, 1982).

The responsiveness of caregivers to their infants and the type of emotion socialization in which they engage are not, of course, unrelated to infant characteristics. Temperamental characteristics can play an important role in shaping the child's social environment, including what materials and resources are available, what demands are placed upon him or her, what stresses are present, and what social behaviors are provided. The infant's temperament regulates and is regulated by the actions of others very early in life. The contingency or lack of contingency with which caregivers respond to infant signals has been of considerable interest to those studying emotion socialization. It is now understood that establishing synchrony in caregiver–infant interactions involves not only contingent responsiveness between infant and caregiver, but also the caregiver's tuning in to the infant's temperamental characteristics (Bornstein, 1989). Individual differences in temperament will influence dyadic interaction and regulation provided by the caregiver (Rothbart, 1984). It is easier to be sensitive, interactive, and accepting with infants who are easy to manage than it is with those who are difficult. Grossman, Grossman, Spangler, Suess, and Unzner (1985) demonstrated the way in which such infant temperament characteristics as ability to orient and ability to tolerate frustration affect the nature of the interactions that caregivers have with their infants. In this regard, research comparing the variability of temperamental characteristics among at-risk and normal infants is important for identifying individual differences that may be of consequence to the caregiver–infant relationship.

Pre- and Postnatal Risk Factors and Infant Temperament

Two types of clinical conditions can potentially influence the child's temperament. The first is established organic pathology such as genetic, chromosomal, and other congenital anomalies, and postnatal insults to the central nervous system. The other consists of risk factors such as prematurity or exposure to toxins, in which organic pathology may or may not be documented in the child. Studies with clinical samples that examine the relations between pre- and postnatal factors and behaviors conceptually related to temperament are relatively sparse.

In studies of infants with Down's syndrome, it has been found that they are rated lower on scales that measure smiling and laughter, activity level, and threshold for stimulation. Infants with Down's syndrome also have higher scores on scales that measure fear and startle behaviors (Bridges & Cicchetti, 1982; Gunn & Berry, 1985; Rothbart & Hanson, 1983). On the other hand, Greenberg and Field (1985) found that normal and infants with Down's syndrome were rated less difficult than infants who were delayed, had cerebral palsy, or had sensory impairments. Descriptive studies of infants with nonorganic failure to thrive reveal several temperamental characteristics such as low activity level and minimal smiling (Gaensbauer, 1982; Leonard, Rhymes, & Solnit, 1986; Powell & Low, 1983).

Several studies have examined the relation between prematurity and temperament. Parents of preterm infants tend to rate their infants' temperaments as more difficult during the first year of life (Field, Hallock, Dempsey, & Shulman, 1978; Schraeder & Medoff-Cooper, 1983; Spungen & Farran, 1986). Preterm infants are less rewarding initally because it takes them longer to show alerting behaviors, to regulate their sleep–waking patterns, and to respond socially (Field, Sostek, Goldberg, & Shuman, 1979). Their motor organization is poorer and their states of arousal are less well modulated.

In the preterm infant, the caregiver is faced with a less adept social partner, one at risk for subsequent interactive difficulty. In fact, research indicates that the dyadic relationship of preterms both begins and remains more disadvantaged than that of term infants (Field, 1987). Parents of preterm infants make less body contact with them, spend less time interacting with them in face-to-face play, smile at and touch them less, and appear to be emotionally withdrawn (Field, 1987; Goldberg, Brackfield, & DiVitto, 1980). Thus, individual differences in affective responsivity from birth suggest that prenatal and postnatal events can influence infants' emotional predispositions.

COCAINE EXPOSURE IN UTERO
AND EMOTIONAL BEHAVIOR

Studies have documented neurobehavioral problems in cocaine-exposed neonates that include hyperirritability, poor feeding patterns, and irregular sleeping patterns, which may be related to temperament (Doberczak, Shanzer, Senie, & Kandall, 1988; Fulroth, Phillips, & Durand, 1989; Oro & Dixon, 1987; Shih, Cone-Wesson, Reddix, & Wu, 1989). In studies using the Brazelton Scale, cocaine-exposed neonates showed diminished interactive behavior and poor state organization (Chasnoff, Burns, Schnoll, & Burns, 1985, 1986; Chasnoff & Griffith, 1991; Dixon, Coen, & Crutchfield, 1987). There are inconsistencies in the literature, however, and the pathogenesis of these observations is not clearly understood.

Reports of follow-up beyond the newborn period still are sparse due, in part, to methodological problems and sample selection, and in the identification and measurement of confounding variables. In a study of 1-month-old infants, Lester et al. (1991) found that both excitable and depressed cry characteristics were related to in utero cocaine exposure. Excitable cry characteristics (e.g., long duration, high fundamental and variable frequency) were directly related to cocaine exposure and may reflect withdrawal effects, whereas depressed cry characteristics (e.g., few utterances, low amplitude) were due to the indirect effects of cocaine secondary to low birth weight. According to Lester et al. (1991), the depressed cry characteristics suggest a decrease in functional activity or underaroused behavior that may reflect more chronic effects of early and prolonged cocaine exposure.

Schneider and Chasnoff (1987) found that cocaine-exposed toddlers performed adequately on cognitive measures, but had poor concentration, organizational, and motor skills. Similar findings were reported in a 2-year follow-up of a cohort of cocaine- or polydrug-exposed infants (Chasnoff, Griffith, Freier, & Murray, 1992). On the Bayley Scales of Infant Development, there was no difference in mean developmental scores between drug-exposed and control infants. The researchers concluded, however, that the highly structured tasks on the Bayley may have masked self-regulatory difficulties experienced by drug-exposed children (Chasnoff et al., 1992). Rodning, Beckwith, and Howard (1991) examined quality of attachment in children prenatally exposed to phencyclidine (PCP) and cocaine. They reported that the majority of drug-exposed infants were insecurely attached to their caregivers and that this did not differ in three caregiving environments in which the infants were being raised (e.g., mother care, kinship care, or foster care).

Taken together, these findings may be interpreted as indicating that cocaine exposure in utero may affect, among other things, infant temperament. For example, Alessandri, Sullivan, Imaizumi, and Lewis (1993) reported that infants exposed to cocaine showed less overall arousal in a learning situation and expressed less interest and joy during learning and anger when frustrated. Such deficiencies in arousal and emotional responsivity may be partly due to cocaine exposure.

TEMPERAMENT IN COCAINE-EXPOSED INFANTS

We recently collected data that examine the relations among temperament, learning, and emotional responsivity in cocaine-exposed infants. We selected the Rothbart (1978) Infant Behavior Questionnaire (IBQ) as the measure of temperament from among the two dozen or so instruments currently available (Bates, 1987). The IBQ was chosen because it purports to measure individual differences in reactivity and self-regulation that may have a constitutional base, such as activity and emotionality (Rothbart, 1986) and because a primary goal in its construction was to investigate both developmental continuity and change in infant behavior as observed by the caregiver in the home (Rothbart, 1981). Moreover, unlike other temperament scales, the IBQ does not ask for the mother's opinion of her infant or require her to make comparative judgments about the infant. Instead, the items refer to the presence of specific behaviors in specific situations. There are six scales on the IBQ: *activity level*—gross motor activity, including squirming and arm and leg movement; *smiling and laughter*—smiling or laughter in any situation; *fear*—distress and latency to approach a sudden or novel stimulus; *distress to limitations*—distress during caretaking procedures (e.g., waiting for food, getting dressed and undressed) or when prevented access to a goal; *soothability*—reduction of fussing and crying in response to soothing efforts; and, *duration of orienting*—vocalizing and looking at or interacting with an object for extended periods of time. Validational support for the use of the IBQ has been established in both home (Rothbart, 1986) and laboratory settings (Goldsmith & Campos, 1986).

Results indicated that cocaine-using mothers rated their infants on the IBQ lower in activity level, smiling and laughter, and distress to limitations compared to nonusing mothers who were equated in all respects except for cocaine use. Means and standard deviations for the six IBQ dimensions by group are presented in Table 14.1. Following Rothbart (1986), smiling and laughter and activity were collapsed into a factor that termed *positive reactivity*, and fear and distress to limits were collapsed into *negative reactivity*. Results indicated that cocaine-using, relative to nonusing mothers, rated their infants as lower in both positive reactivity and negative reactivity. Mothers' ratings of their infants' behavior were consistent with our behavioral observations of their infants in the laboratory. As reported by Alessandri et al. (1993), cocaine-exposed infants showed less overall arousal and activity during contingency learning and expressed fewer positive and negative emotions than infants not exposed to cocaine.

TABLE 14.1
Means and Standard Deviations for the IBQ Dimensions by Group

IBQ Dimension		Cocaine (n = 36)	Noncocaine (n = 36)	F (1,70)
Activity level	M	3.73	4.41	7.00**
	SD	.91	.72	
Smiling/laughter	M	3.72	4.96	11.02**
	SD	.85	1.03	
Distress to limits	M	3.15	3.62	5.10*
	SD	.70	.86	
Fear	M	2.76	2.99	1.46
	SD	.74	.72	
Soothability	M	4.93	5.38	2.04
	SD	.94	.93	
Duration of orienting	M	3.80	3.66	.76
	SD	.89	.70	
Positive reactivity	M	3.73	4.68	14.54**
	SD	.48	.62	
Negative reactivity	M	2.95	3.30	4.96*
	SD	.52	.66	

Note. IBQ = Infant Behavior Questionnaire.
*$p < .01$. **$p < .001$.

TEMPERAMENT AND CAREGIVER–INFANT INTERACTION

These data along with those of Alessandri et al. (1993) suggest that cocaine-exposed infants tend to be compromised in their capacities for participation in the subtle give-and-take of interaction, and communication about their states and needs through smiles, frowns, cries, and eye contact. Given the lower activity level and lower affective responsivity in cocaine-exposed infants, the caregiver is faced with a difficult task of modulating his or her stimulation to match the infant's arousal and stimulation needs. Such temperamental differences in cocaine-exposed infants may require parents to adapt their style to accommodate their infant's disposition toward lower activity and emotional inhibition. For example, the infant who responds less and expresses fewer affective behaviors may be unresponsive because of higher sensory thresholds or less developed arousal-modulation and information-processing skills. The caregiver who is sensitive to the need for higher levels of stimulation will attempt to modify the level and variety of stimulation to the infant. Caregivers must learn to understand the nature of their infants' needs and successfully adapt their caregiving behavior. The overly placid infant who, in the long run, may be in greater need of stimulation, may receive less by virtue of his or her calmness. Individual differences in infants, therefore, necessitate modifications by caregivers to achieve successful patterns of relatedness.

It is possible, however, for caregivers to have rewarding, reciprocal relationships with infants who manifest atypical patterns of development. For example, caregivers of preterm infants who exhibit less overall activity in response to stimulation and fewer positive responses are more likely to engage in more physical contact and to offer and demonstrate more toys to their infants (Field, 1977). These data suggest that caregivers can learn to make adjustments to their preterm infants by investing more effort in their interactions with their less responsive and less active infants. Caregivers must also employ compensatory mechanisms, such as substituting vocal contact for the missing visual channel in congenitally blind infants (Fraiberg, 1979). Mothers of deaf infants also compensate for their infants' diminished responsiveness and less active involvement by being more dominant (Meadow, Greenberg, & Erting, 1983). What may appear to be overstimulation to the observer may be the manifestation of a contingently responsive caregiver who, in making compensatory adjustments in their parenting style, encourage the adaptation of the infant.

Temperament differences in cocaine-exposed infants may influence the optimal level of caregiver stimulation and emphasize that the child needs to be taken into account in planning intervention programs. Caregivers of cocaine-exposed infants need to learn the way in which infant characteristics such as low activity level, lags in social smiling, and low frustration tolerance affect the nature of their interactions with their infants. Moreover, caregivers of cocaine-exposed infants may need to adopt their caregiving style to their infant's disposition in order to maximize their infant's development. That is, caregivers must play a more active role in helping cocaine-exposed infants generate enough affect to become emotionally engaged in social interaction. This is no easy task, however, because the parents of cocaine-exposed infants themselves often have past and/or present experiences that can compromise their ability to meet the needs of their infants. Factors such as poverty, a history of child abuse, family instability and violence, and a history of psychiatric illness can compromise a caregiver's ability to parent. Because of the highly addictive nature of cocaine, drug-abusing mothers are at risk for dysfunctional parenting and failure in meeting the special needs of their infants, which may significantly contribute to developmental morbidity. Some studies have found that mothers are less engaging with their infants if they are difficult or irritable (Crockenberg & Acredolo, 1983; Linn & Horowitz, 1983) and relations have been reported between early interactional disturbances and later, school-age behavioral and emotional problems including short attention span, hyperactivity, and disturbed social interactions (Bakeman & Brown, 1980; Field, 1984).

Thus, children who experience prenatal exposure to cocaine are even more at risk when they do not experience the consistent parenting children need to thrive, and may, therefore, be at greater risk for poorer developmental outcomes at later ages. Although resiliency and change are always possible for the child and for the adult, resiliency cannot be taken for granted. Interventions that provide education and support to the caregiver and take into consideration the cocaine-exposed child's needs are likely to be the most effective in promoting the child's future development. This approach recognizes that fetal exposure to cocaine compromises or jeopardizes developmental processes but that organismic and environmental factors can contribute to positive developmental outcomes. However, the mitigating influence of a positive childrearing environment on developmental outcomes for cocaine-exposed children is yet to be determined. In this chapter the question is raised as to whether the construct of temperament will facilitate understanding of individual differences in learning and emotional responsivity, particularly among cocaine-exposed infants. We observed that temperament is typically understood as behavioral differences in affective expressiveness, motor activity, stimulus sensitivity, and self-regulation. We examined the role of temperament in learning and emotional behavior in normal populations and, finally, we presented data representing our initial efforts toward a working assessment of the interplay among temperament, learning, and emotional responsivity in cocaine-exposed infants. Cocaine-using mothers rated their infants lower on the temperament dimensions of activity level, smiling and laughter, and distress to limitations. Our laboratory observations during a learning-contingent procedure confirmed a pattern of less engagement in the task among cocaine-exposed infants. The social communicative role of temperament, at least in terms of what the infant brings to the caregiver–infant relationship, has important clinical implications. Given that temperament is likely to influence the optimal level of caregiver stimulation suggests that the particular needs of the cocaine-exposed infant be taken into account in planning intervention programs. Caregivers of cocaine-exposed infants need to learn the ways in which temperamental characteristics such as low activity level, lags in social smiling, and limited emotional responsiveness affect the nature of their interaction with their infants. Teaching caregivers to adopt their caregiving style to meet the needs of their infants is likely to significantly contribute to positive short-term and, potentially, long-term developmental outcomes.

ACKNOWLEDGMENTS

Preparation of this chapter was supported by an MCP grant awarded to Steven M. Alessandri and a NIDA grant #RO1DA07109 awarded to Michael Lewis.

REFERENCES

Alessandri, S. M., Sullivan, M. W., Imaizumi, S., & Lewis, M. (1993). Learning and emotional responsivity in cocaine-exposed infants. *Developmental Psychology, 29*, 989–997.

Alessandri, S. M., Sullivan, M. W., & Lewis, M. (1990). Violation expectancy and frustration in early infancy. *Developmental Psychology, 26*, 738–744.

Bakeman, R., & Brown, J. V. (1980). Early interaction: Consequences for social and mental development at three years. *Child Development, 51,* 437–447.

Bates, J. E. (1987). Temperament in infancy. In J. D. Osofsky (Ed.), *Handbook of infant development* (2nd ed., pp. 1101–1149). New York: Wiley.

Bates, J. E. (1989). Concepts and measures of temperament. In G. A. Kohnstamn, J. E. Bates, & M. K. Roth (Eds.), *Temperament in childhood* (pp. 3–26). New York: Wiley.

Bornstein, M. H. (1989). *Maternal responsiveness characteristics and consequences.* San Francisco: Jossey-Bass.

Bornstein, M. H., Gaughran, J., & Homel, P. (1985). Infant temperament: Theory, tradition, critique, and new assessments. In C. E. Izard & P. B. Read (Eds.), *Measurement of emotions in infants and children* (Vol. 2, pp. 172–199). New York: Cambridge University Press.

Brazelton, T. B., Koslowski, B., & Main, M. (1979). The origins of reciprocity: The early mother/infant interaction. In M. Lewis & L. A. Rosenblum (Eds.), *The effect of the caregiver on the infant* (pp. 49–77). New York: Wiley.

Bridges, F. A., & Cicchetti, D. (1982). Mother's ratings of the temperament characteristics of Down's syndrome infants. *Developmental Psychology, 18,* 238–244.

Buss, A. H., & Plomin, R. (1984). *Temperament: Early developing personality traits.* Hillsdale, NJ: Lawrence Erlbaum Associates.

Campos, J. J., Barrett, K. C., Lamb, M. E., Goldsmith, H. H., & Stenberg, C. (1983). Socioemotional development. In M. M. Haith & J. J. Campos (Eds.), *Handbook of child psychology: Vol. 2. Infancy and developmental psychobiology* (pp. 783–915). New York: Wiley.

Carey, W. B., & McDevitt, S. C. (1978). Revision of the Infant Temperament Questionnaire. *Pediatrics, 61,* 735–739.

Chasnoff, I. J., Burns, W. J., Schnoll, S. H., & Burns, K. A. (1985). Cocaine use in pregnancy. *New England Journal of Medicine, 313,* 666–669.

Chasnoff, I. J., Burns, W. J., Schnoll, S. H., & Burns, K. A. (1986). Effects of cocaine on pregnancy outcome. *National Institute of Drug Abuse and Research Monograph Series, 7,* 335–341.

Chasnoff, I. J., & Griffith, D. R. (1991). Maternal cocaine use: Neonatal outcome. In H. Fitzgerald, B. M. Lester, & M. Yogman (Eds.), *Theory and research in behavioral pediatrics* (Vol. 5, pp. 1–17). New York: Plenum.

Chasnoff, I. J., Griffith, D. R., Freier, C., & Murray, J. (1992). Cocaine/polydrug use in pregnancy: Two-year follow-up. *Pediatrics, 89,* 284–289.

Crockenberg, S., & Acredolo, C. (1983). Infant Temperament Ratings: A function of infants, mother, or both. *Infant Behavior and Development, 6,* 61–72.

Derryberry, D., & Rothbart, M. K. (1984). Emotion, attention, and temperament. In C. E. Izard, J. Kogan, & R. Zajonc (Eds.), *Emotion, cognition, and behavior* (pp. 132–167). New York: Cambridge University Press.

Dixon, S. D., Coen, R. W., & Crutchfield, S. (1987). Visual dysfunction in cocaine-exposed infants. *Pediatric Research, 21,* 359A.

Doberczak, T. M., Shanzer, S., Senie, R. T., & Kandall, S. R. (1988). Neonatal neurologic and electroencephalographic effects of intrauterine cocaine exposure. *Journal of Pediatrics, 113,* 354–358.

Dunst, C. J., & Lingerfelt, B. (1985). Maternal ratings of temperament and operant learning in two-to-three-month-old infants. *Child Development, 56,* 555–563.

Ekman, P., & Friesen, W. (1975). *Unmasking the face: A guide to recognizing emotions from facial clues.* Englewood Cliffs, NJ: Prentice-Hall.

Fagen, J. W., & Ohr, P. S. (1985). Temperament and crying response to the violation of a learned expectancy in early infancy. *Infant Behavior and Development, 8,* 157–166.

Fagen, J. W., Ohr, P. S., Singer, J. M., & Fleckenstein, L. K. (1987). Infant temperament and subject loss due to crying during operant conditioning. *Child Development, 58,* 497–504.

Field, T. (1977). Effects of early separation, interactive deficits, and experimental manipulations on infant–mother face-to-face interaction. *Child Development, 48,* 763–771.

Field, T. (1984). Early interactions between infants and their postpartum depressed mothers. *Infant Behavior and Development, 7*, 527–532.

Field, T. (1987). Affective and interactive disturbances in infants. In J. Osofsky (Ed.), *Handbook of infant development* (2nd ed., pp. 972–1005). New York: Wiley.

Field, T., Hallock, N., Dempsey, J., & Shulman, H. H. (1978). Mother's assessments of term infants with respiratory distress syndrome: Reliability and predictive validity. *Child Psychiatry and Human Development, 9*, 75–85.

Field, T. M., Hallock, N., Ting, G., Dempsey, J., Dabiri, C., & Shulman, H. H. (1978). A first-year follow-up of high-risk infants: Formulating a cumulative risk index. *Child Development, 49*, 119–131.

Field, T. M., Sostek, A. M., Goldberg, S., & Shulman, H. H. (1979). *Infants born at risk: Behavior and development.* New York: Spectrum.

Fraiberg, S. (1979). Blind infants and their mothers: An examination of the sign system. In M. Bullowa (Ed.), *Before speech* (pp. 247–369). New York: Cambridge University Press.

Fulroth, R. F., Phillips, B., & Durand, D. J. (1989). Perinatal outcome of infants exposed to cocaine and/or heroin in utero. *American Journal of Diseases in Children, 143*, 905–910.

Gaensbauer, T. (1982). Regulation of emotional expression in infants from two contrasting caretaking environments. *Journal of the American Academy of Child Psychiatry, 21*, 163–171.

Garcia-Coll, C., Kagan, J., & Reznick, J. S. (1984). Behavioral inhibition in young children. *Child Development, 55*, 1005–1019.

Goldberg, S., Brackfield, S., & DiVitto, B. (1980). Feeding, fussing and playing parent–infant interaction in the first year as a function of prematurity and perinatal problems. In T. Field, S. Goldberg, D. Stern, & A. Sostek (Eds.), *High-risk infants and children: Adult and peer interactions* (pp. 120–145). New York: Academic.

Goldsmith, H. H., Buss, A. H., Plomin, R., Rothbart, M. K., Thomas, A., Chess, S., Hinde, R. A., & McCall, R. B. (1987). Roundtable: What is temperament? Four approaches. *Child Development, 58*, 505–529.

Goldsmith, H. H., & Campos, J. J. (1982). Toward a theory of infant temperament. In R. N. Emde & R. J. Harmon (Eds.), *The development of attachment and affiliative systems* (pp. 161–193). New York: Plenum.

Goldsmith, H. H., & Campos, J. J. (1986). Fundamental issues in the study of early temperament: The Denver Twin Temperament Study. In M. E. Lamb & A. Brown (Eds.), *Advances in developmental psychology* (pp. 231–283). Hillsdale, NJ: Lawrence Erlbaum Associates.

Greenberg, R., & Field, T. (1985). Temperament ratings of handicapped infants during classroom, mother, and teacher interactions. *Journal of Pediatric Psychology, 7*, 387–405.

Grossmann, K., Grossmann, K. E., Spangler, G., Suess, G., & Unzner, L. (1985). Maternal sensitivity and newborns' orientation responses as related to quality of attachment in Northern Germany. In I. Bretherton & E. Waters (Eds.), *Growing points of attachment theory and research* (pp. 233–256). *Monographs of the Society for Research in the Society for Research in Child Development, 50* (1–2, Serial No. 209).

Gunn, P., & Berry, P. (1985). Down syndrome temperament and maternal response to descriptions of child behavior. *Developmental Psychology, 21*, 842–847.

Izard, C. E. (1983). *The maximally discriminative facial coding system (MAX)* (Rev. ed.). Newark, DE: Instructional Resource Center, University of Delaware.

Izard, C. E., Hembree, E. A., Dougherty, L. M., & Spizzirri, C. L. (1983). Changes in facial expressions of 2 to 19 month old infants following acute pain. *Developmental Psychology, 19*, 418–426.

Izard, C. E., & Malatesta, C. Z. (1987). Perspectives on emotional development: Differential emotions theory of early emotional development. In J. D. Osofsky (Ed.), *Handbook of infant development* (2nd ed., pp. 494–554). New York: Wiley.

Kagan, J., Reznick, J. S., Clarke, C., Snidman, N., & Garcia-Coll, C. (1984). Behavioral inhibition to the unfamiliar. *Child Development, 55*, 2212–2225.

Keogh, B. (1982). Children's temperament and teachers' decisions. In R. Porter & G. Collins (Eds.), *Temperamental differences in infants and young children* (pp. 269–285). London: Pitman.

Krafchuk, E., Sameroff, A., & Barkow, H. (1976, April). *Newborn temperament and operant head turning*. Paper presented at the Southeast Regional Meeting of the Society of Research in Child Development, Nashville, TN.

Leonard, M. F., Rhymes, J. P., & Solnit, A. J. (1986). Failure to thrive in infants. *American Journal of Diseases in Children, 3,* 600–612.

Lester, B. M., Corwin, M. J., Sepkoski, C., Seifer, R., Peucker, M., McLaughlin, S., & Golub, H. (1991). Neurobehavioral syndromes in cocaine-exposed newborn infants. *Child Development, 62,* 694–705.

Lewis, M., & Saarni, C. (1985). Culture and emotions. In M. Lewis & C. Saarni (Eds.), *The socialization of emotions* (pp. 1–17). New York: Plenum.

Linn, P., & Horowitz, F. (1983). The relationship between infant individual differences and mother/infant interaction during the neonatal period. *Infant Behavior and Development, 6,* 415–427.

Malatesta, C. A., & Haviland, J. M. (1982). Learning display rules: The socialization of emotion expression in infancy. *Child Development, 53,* 991–1003.

Matheny, A. P., Dolan, A. B., & Wilson, R. S. (1974). Bayley's infant behavior record: Relations between behaviors and mental test scores. *Developmental Psychology, 10,* 696–702.

McDevitt, S. C., & Carey, W. B. (1981). Stability of ratings versus perceptions of temperament from early infancy to 1–3 years. *American Journal of Orthopsychiatry, 51*(2), 342–345.

Meadow, K. P., Greenberg, M., & Erting, C. (1983). Attachment behavior of deaf children with deaf parents. *Journal of American Academy of Psychiatry, 22,* 23–38.

Oro, A. S., & Dixon, S. D. (1987). Perinatal cocaine and methamphetamine exposure: Maternal and neonatal correlates. *Journal of Pediatrics, 3,* 571–578.

Peters-Martin, P., & Wachs, T. D. (1984). A longitudinal study of temperament and its correlates in the first 12 months. *Infant Behavior and Development, 7,* 285–298.

Powell, G. F., & Low, J. (1983). Behavior in nonorganic failure to thrive. *Journal of Developmental and Behavioral Pediatrics, 4*(1), 26–33.

Rodning, C., Beckwith, L., & Howard, J. (1991). Quality of attachment and home environments in children prenatally exposed to PCP and cocaine. *Development and Psychopathology, 3,* 351–366.

Rothbart, M. K. (1978). *Infant Behavior Questionnaire.* Unpublished manuscript, University of Oregon, Eugene, OR.

Rothbart, M. K. (1981). Measurement of temperament in infancy. *Child Development, 52,* 569–578.

Rothbart, M. K. (1984). Social development. In M. J. Hanson (Ed.), *Atypical infant development* (pp. 171–194). Baltimore, MD: University Park Press.

Rothbart, M. K. (1986). Longitudinal observation of infant temperament. *Developmental Psychology, 22,* 350–365.

Rothbart, M. K., & Derryberry, D. (1981). Development of individual differences in temperament. In M. E. Lamb & A. L. Brown (Eds.), *Advances in developmental psychology* (Vol. 1, pp. 37–86). Hillsdale, NJ: Lawrence Erlbaum Associates.

Rothbart, M. K., & Hanson, M. J. (1983). A caregiver report comparison of temperament characteristics of Down's syndrome and normal infants. *Developmental Psychology, 19,* 766–769.

Schneider, J. W., & Chasnoff, I. J. (1987). Cocaine abuse during pregnancy: Its effects on infant motor development. A clinical perspective. *Top Acute Care Rehabilitation, 2,* 59–69.

Schraeder, B., & Medoff-Cooper, B. (1983). Temperament and development in VLBW infants: The second year. *Nursing Research, 32,* 231–335.

Shih, L., Cone-Wesson, B., Reddix, B., & Wu, P. Y. K. (1989). Effect of maternal cocaine abuse on the neonatal auditory system. *Pediatric Research, 25,* 264A.

Sostek, A. M., & Anders, T. F. (1977). Relationships among the Brazelton Neonatal Scale, Bayley Infant Scale, and early temperament. *Child Development, 48,* 320–323.

Spungen, L. B., & Farran, A. C. (1986). Effect of intensive care unit exposure on temperament in low birth weight preterm infants. *Journal of Developmental and Behavioral Pediatrics, 7*, 288–292.

Thomas, A., & Chess, S. (1977). *Temperament and development.* New York: Brunner-Mazel.

Thomas, A., & Chess, S. (1980). *The dynamics of psychological development.* New York: Brunner-Mazel.

Thomas, A., & Chess, S. (1989). Temperament and personality. In G. A. Kohnstamn, J. E. Bates, & M. K. Rothbart (Eds.), *Temperament in childhood* (pp. 249–263). New York: Wiley.

15

▼▼▼▼▼▼▼

Attentional and Social Functioning of Preschool-Age Children Exposed to PCP and Cocaine in Utero

Leila Beckwith
University of California at Los Angeles

Senobia Crawford
University of Alabama at Birmingham

Jacqueline A. Moore
University of Texas Medical School at Houston

Judy Howard
University of California at Los Angeles

This chapter describes three interrelated research studies that examined the development of infants and young children from birth to preschool born to mothers who used phencyclidine (PCP) and cocaine during pregnancy. The first study, the basis of the other two, recruited neonates and their families and assessed cognition, play, and attachment in the first 2 years of life. The other two studies, with overlapping samples, including subjects from the original research, examined the children at preschool age. One research scrutinized cognitive and attentional processes, and the other investigated peer interaction.

There is a burgeoning research literature that indicates the association of prenatal exposure to substances of abuse and physical and behavioral alterations in the neonatal period (e.g., Chasnoff, Burns, & Burns, 1987; Hawley & Disney, 1992; MacGregor et al., 1987; Ryan, Ehrlich, & Finnegan, 1987; Zuckerman et al., 1989). The most consistent finding is decreased fetal growth, as shown by significant decreases in head circumference and weight at birth. Behavioral deviance during the neonatal period in the cry (Corwin et al., 1992) as well as state and orientation behaviors manifested by increased periods of apathy and irritability are also consistently reported.

There is, however, a paucity of information regarding the longer term impact of intrauterine exposure to drugs on cognition, attention, and social behavior at preschool (Hawley & Disney, 1992). It is unclear if the deviations in behavior during the neonatal period are a temporary manifestation of drug exposure or continue throughout development as a precursor to other cognitive or behavioral problems. Whereas several studies find that children with prenatal drug exposure, as a group, score within the average range on standardized tests that are highly structured and under adult supervision (Chasnoff, Griffith, Freier, & Murray, 1992), when presented with unstructured tasks or left to their own devices during play these children often appear less competent (Rodning, Beckwith, & Howard, 1989). There is limited information available describing these dimensions for preschool children.

To date, there is some support, but it is weak, as to whether prenatal drug exposure is—or is not—linked to later diminished cognitive performance. With reference to cocaine and polydrug exposure, one study concluded that drug exposure did have a direct and an indirect effect on cognitive ability at 3 years of age (Azuma & Chasnoff, 1993). However, the data from the study showed the effects to be subtle. Although mean IQ scores on the Stanford–Binet scale for two drug-exposed groups, polydrug with cocaine exposure, and polydrug without cocaine, were lower than the drug-free controls, all groups scored within the average range and the differences were not statistically significant. When the groups were combined, however, a correlation coefficient linking group membership to IQ became statistically significant. Further, a path analysis supported the notion that drug exposure was associated with decreased head circumferences and more negative home environments at age 3, which in turn were linked indirectly to lower IQ scores.

Particularly relevant to our study was the inclusion of a measure of attentional processes, perseverance, a sum of Stanford–Binet behavioral ratings of distractibility, activity, preference for easy tasks, and giving up easily (Azuma & Chasnoff, 1993). Poor perseverance co-occurred with lower IQ scores, and was more likely in children with smaller head circumference, which in turn was more likely with drug exposure.

A similar multirisk study of children born to methadone-maintained pregnant women or drug-free women had consistent findings (Johnson, Glassman, Fiks, & Rosen, 1987). At age 3, the two groups did not differ significantly in Merrill–Palmer IQ scores, although smaller head circumferences, below the third percentile, were more frequent in the methadone group. When the groups were merged, however, and multiple factors considered, then the adverse impact of drug abuse, as it co-occurred with social disorganization of the rearing environment, was associated with lower IQ performance.

In contrast, discrepant findings were shown when preschool children of untreated heroin addicts, women who received methadone therapy, and a drug-free comparison group were compared (Lifschitz, Wilson, Smith, & Desmond, 1985).

Again, the groups did not differ at age 3.4 years in level of cognitive functioning (i.e., McCarthy General Cognitive Indices), although performance in the mildly retarded range was more frequent in the heroin-exposed group. When the groups were combined, drug use by mothers was unrelated to intellectual level. Rather, more prenatal care, fewer perinatal medical risk factors, and better home environments predicted higher intellectual performance, regardless of exposure to heroin or methadone. The authors concluded that the outcome of children of substance-abusing women was less related to intrauterine chemical exposure than to environmental and health factors associated with maternal addiction.

Whereas there is some information about cognition and attention in prenatally drug-exposed children, albeit conflicting, there is no knowledge about peer relations (Hawley & Disney, 1992). The study described in this chapter is the first research to be completed examining the peer relations of prenatally drug-exposed children during the preschool period.

Existing studies of prenatally drug-exposed children in the first 2 years suggest potential effects on later peer relations. Peer play can be affected indirectly through mother–child interaction patterns and resulting quality of attachment (Cassidy, 1986; Sroufe, 1983; Waters, Wippman, & Sroufe, 1979). The child who has gained a sense of confidence through the caregiver–infant relationship and continues to receive support through the toddler years will be confident, skilled, and positive in dealing with peers. Children with insecure and disorganized attachments may be more prone to aggression with peers (Lyons-Ruth, Alpern, & Repacholi, 1993). Being perceived as aggressive by peers puts a child at risk for being rejected by peers. The present chapter provides evidence that infants exposed to drugs in utero and growing up with their substance-abusing mother or kinship caregivers have an increased occurrence of insecure and disorganized attachments, which may later be linked to deviance in peer play.

Peer play in this group might also be adversely influenced by lack of experience with peers due to the isolation of the drug culture. Cognitive, gross motor, or fine motor deficits related to in utero drug exposure may cause problems with manipulating toys, resulting in frustration and making it more difficult to engage in peer play.

The importance of peer contact increases as the child reaches the preschool years. Typically by preschool age, children have a general knowledge about the differences between friends and acquaintances and can interact across a variety of settings (Howes, 1987). As children develop, relationships with peers take on greater significance (Rubenstein & Howes, 1976). During the late toddler period children spend more time interacting with peers than adults. Peer relationships then become a viable mechanism in understanding such areas as social competence, self-organization, and social status (Kagan, 1981; Waters & Sroufe, 1983; Waters et al., 1979). For the preschool period, peer play becomes a good marker of social competence. Howes and Matheson (1992) suggested that for a child to be socially competent he or she must be able to enter ongoing play groups, appropriately respond to a peer's initiations, integrate affect and action, and resolve conflicts. The level of complexity of play and sustained interactions indicate the child's increasing ability to negotiate the environment (Cassidy, 1986).

STUDY 1

Sample

Development of the quality of attachment of the infant to its caregiver and the quality of spontaneous play was investigated in infants prenatally exposed to PCP and cocaine, and a comparison group of non-drug-exposed infants who came from families with similar ethnic, socioeconomic, and marital status, living in the same neighborhoods. The majority of subjects in both groups received their income from Aid to Families with Dependent Children, were single parents, African Americans, and lived in impoverished and often violent neighborhoods. Forty percent of the infants in the drug-exposed group were female; 44% were female in the comparison group. The groups did differ, however, in maternal education. The mean was 10.8 years for the substance-abusing biological mothers and 12.2 years for the comparison mothers.

Recruitment of 46 drug-exposed newborns of English-speaking women who were not teenagers was done in a county hospital in the inner-city area of Los Angeles. At the time of recruitment in 1981, because PCP was the most accessible and affordable drug of choice for women living in the inner city of Los Angeles, the presence of PCP in the infant's urine after birth was used as a selection criterion for this study. By the close of the study, crack cocaine became readily available and inexpensive in the Los Angeles area, and eventually replaced PCP as the most widely used drug in the inner city. In fact, the majority of infants recruited also had evidence of cocaine exposure in the urine although they were identified on the basis of positive urine toxicology screens for PCP. Thirty-nine were assessed at 15 months, and 31 at 24 months.

Recruitment of 39 comparison newborns of English-speaking, nonadolescent mothers took place in the same hospital and other hospitals in the geographical area. Twenty-five were assessed at 15 months, and 21 at 24 months. The comparison mothers showed no signs of PCP, cocaine, or heroin use at birth or over the course of the study, as shown by repeated interviews, contacts, and observations. Some mothers, however, did use nicotine and alcohol.

Whereas all comparison children lived continuously with the biological mothers for the course of the study, that was not so for the drug-exposed group. At birth, 15 prenatally exposed infants were with their biological mothers, 16 were with extended family members, and 13 in professional foster care. By the second year of life, 13 children had experienced one to three changes in caregivers, with

20 children now in the daily care of their biological mothers, and 18 children cared for by others.

Poignant glimpses of the difficult lives that the children experienced were seen in the laboratory assessments, in which it was not uncommon for children to arrive hungry. Many babies came to the testing sessions with empty bottles. The staff learned to always have food, formula, and diapers on hand.

Measures

Although the importance of the postnatal rearing environment is recognized for children exposed prenatally to drugs, there is a paucity of data—particularly observational—about the quality of the relationship that develops over time between the children and their caregivers. Our study (Rodning, Beckwith, & Howard, 1991) assessed quality of attachment in the laboratory at 15 months of age, using the standard eight-episode Ainsworth Strange Situation procedure (Ainsworth, Blehar, Waters, & Wall, 1978). Additionally, the rearing environments and caregiver behaviors experienced by the infants in the two groups were assessed by naturalistic observations at home at 3 and 9 months, using the Ainsworth (1976) system for rating maternal-care behavior. Seven 9-point scales were selected for the study: acceptance/rejection, accessibility/ignoring, cooperation/interference, sensitivity/insensitivity, amount of physical contact, quality of physical contact, and responsiveness/effectiveness of soothing.

Spontaneous play was assessed at 24 months in the laboratory during 16 videotaped minutes with a prescribed set of age-appropriate toys (Beckwith et al., 1994). The caregiver, although present in the room, was instructed to allow the child to play on his or her own. Play behavior was measured by frequency counts every 15 seconds of manipulative, functional, and symbolic acts, as well as by ratings of the quality of play.

Results

As shown in Table 15.1, the distribution of attachment classifications within the comparison group was consistent with rates of security found in other studies of low-income, non-drug-abusing populations (Waters, Vaughn, & Egeland, 1980), with the majority (64%) being secure. In contrast, the distribution of attachment classifications within the drug-exposed group was very deviant. Only 18% were judged secure, and the majority (68%) were judged to be disorganized.

Chi-square analyses indicated that within the drug-exposed group, quality of attachment was not affected by number of changes in primary caregiver, nor by whether the child was being reared by the biological mother, foster parents, or kinship caregivers. For those children residing with their biological mothers, however, maternal abstinence after birth was a significant factor. Only children

TABLE 15.1
Attachment Classifications at 15 Months

Group	(A) Avoidant	(B) Secure	(C) Ambivalent	(D) Disorganized
Drug exposed N = 38	15 (39%)	7 (18%)	16 (42%)	26 (68%)
Comparison N = 25	4 (16%)	16 (64%)	5 (20%)	3 (12%)

with mothers who reported being abstinent during their infant's first 15 months of life showed secure attachment, whereas all children living with mothers who continued to use drugs were insecurely attached.

In understanding how the attachment relationships developed, we considered it important to have direct observations of the infants' home environments. Home observations during the first year of life showed that there were significant differences among the caregiving environments provided by the biological substance-abusing mothers and the mothers in non-drug-abusing homes. Two multivariate analyses of variance (MANOVAs) were conducted for the 3- and 9-month observations. At 3 months, univariate analyses of variance (ANOVAs) were significant for acceptance, accessibility, cooperation, sensitivity, quality of physical contact, and effectiveness of mother's response to baby's crying. Mothers caring for their prenatally drug-exposed children were less responsive to their infants than the comparison mothers. By 9 months, the overall MANOVA was significant, Wilks's lambda $F(21, 98) = 2.3$, $p < .01$. Children growing up with substance-abusing mothers experienced more rejection, neglect, interference, and insensitivity to their communications; less response to their distress; and they had less physical contact of poorer quality than comparison children.

By 24 months, a series of 2 (Group) × 2 (Gender) ANOVAs indicated that the play of the majority of the prenatally drug-exposed children differed from the comparison group by demonstrating significantly more immature play strategies, less sustained attention, more deviant behaviors, and fewer positive social interactions with their caregivers (see Table 15.2). A subgroup within the prenatally exposed group, however, was indistinguishable in play from the control group. Comparisons of the two subgroups within the drug-exposed group, by a series of t tests, indicated that those children who showed deviant play as compared to those who showed play more similar to the controls were not more likely to have suffered fetal growth impairment, but they were more likely to have been classified as disorganized in attachment, to have significantly lower developmental (DQ) scores at 15 and 24 months, to be born to mothers with less education, and to have received less sensitive, responsive caregiving during the first year of life.

TABLE 15.2
Means and Standard Deviations (in parentheses) of Frequency Counts and
Ratings for Play by Group and Gender

	Drug Exposed				Comparison				
	Boys n = 19		Girls n = 12		Boys n = 12		Girls n = 7		Significant Contrasts
Manipulative*	6.2	(9.2)	3.7	(5.0)	1.7	(2.0)	1.1	(1.1)	D > C
Functional*	22.0	(6.7)	32.5	(15.1)	19.0	(10.1)	17.1	(10.4)	D > C
Symbolic	3.4	(4.3)	7.7	(9.1)	4.2	(6.4)	4.6	(5.3)	
Combine objects**	2.1	(1.0)	3.3	(1.5)	4.0	(1.0)	4.4	(1.1)	C > D; G > B
Expand theme**	2.7	(1.0)	3.8	(1.1)	4.2	(0.8)	4.0	(1.2)	DB < CB, CG,DG
Selection strategy**	2.3	(1.0)	3.1	(1.3)	4.1	(0.8)	4.3	(1.5)	C > D
Absorbed**	1.9	(0.9)	2.5	(1.3)	3.4	(0.9)	4.0	(1.2)	C > D
No deviances	2.3	(1.2)	3.2	(1.6)	4.3	(0.9)	4.0	(1.2)	C > D
Positive interaction with caregiver	2.6	(1.2)	3.3	(1.1)	4.1	(1.2)	3.3	(1.3)	CB > DB

Note. C = Control Group, D = Drug-exposed group, G = Girls, B = Boys.
*$p < .05$. **$p < .01$.

STUDY 2

Sample

Seventeen children age 3½ to 4½ from the original study participated in the follow-up assessment (13 with prenatal drug exposure and 4 without prenatal drug exposure). Twenty-four children of the original longitudinal sample could not be located, although postcards, telephone calls, and home visits were made to the last known addresses as well as to extended family members and neighbors. Further, two children moved out of state, two children did not participate due to repeated scheduling conflicts, and two families refused. Additionally, four children were excluded because they were too young at the time of testing, and three White and two Hispanic children were also excluded to maintain a homogeneous African-American sample in order to control for cultural differences.

In order to determine whether the 13 drug-exposed children differed systematically from the original sample, a series of *t* tests, comparing the follow-up and non-follow-up subjects, were conducted for ethnic status, marital status, maternal education, socioeconomic status (SES), and children's Gesell developmental quotients at 6, 15, and 24 months. There were no significant differences. To increase the size of the drug-exposed group, 3 additional children were added to constitute a follow-up sample of 16 children (10 boys and 6 girls) with a mean age of 4.3 years.

The control sample of 18 children (8 boys and 10 girls) was composed of 4 children from the original sample, plus 14 additional subjects recruited from a neighborhood preschool program. These children were African-American, aged 3½ to 4½, with a mean age of 4.4 years, equivalent to the drug-exposed group on SES, age, ethnic group, and neighborhood of residence. Health and medical records were available for review, indicating no evidence of prenatal drug exposure, and the staff members were familiar with the families and provided information on family composition, background, and stability.

All children in the comparison group had lived continuously with their biological mothers, whereas many within the drug-exposed group had experienced one or more shifts in primary caregiver, and at the time of testing 53% of the children resided with individuals other than their biological mothers.

Measures

Children were assessed using a standardized test of verbal, perceptual, quantitative, memory, and cognitive abilities (McCarthy Scales of Children's Abilities) to obtain a measure of each child's overall abilities and performance under very structured circumstances. A structured delay task, the Cookie Delay Task, was administered to assess impulsivity (Campbell, Szumowski, Ewing, Gluck, & Breau, 1982; Golden, Montare, & Bridger, 1977). A free play situation, in which the children played for 10 min with nine toys, similar to that used by Campbell et al. (1982), was also used to observe play behaviors under unstructured situations.

During the structured tasks, trained student observers coded activity and attention to task, quantifying every 10 sec: (a) out of seat, (b) off task (i.e., refused, stared into space, ignored directions, and/or attention to activities that are not task relevant), and (c) transitional behaviors (i.e., accepts, coaxing, refusal, tantrum, crying). During the unstructured free play, observers quantified every 10 sec over a 10-min period: (a) the number of activity shifts, (b) duration of activity, and (c) involvement in nontoy activity (Campbell et al., 1982). Additionally, the observers made clinical ratings of the children's behavior (Campbell, 1988), based on the entire laboratory session, according to the following dimensions: cooperation/compliance, irritability, restlessness, attentional focus, task involvement, out of seat, attempts to distract experimenter, task persistence, sociability, language, affect, and overall global rating. The ratings were on a 5-point scale from rare occurrence to frequent occurrence. The observers were blind to group membership of the children and were hidden from the children by a curtain during the entire laboratory session. The session was videotaped and tapes were used for reliability testing.

Additionally, parents were interviewed to obtain information on the youngster's temperament (Keogh, Pullis, & Caldwell, 1982), problem behavior (Behar, 1977), and general background information.

Results

In this study, the children with prenatal drug exposure performed significantly worse on each subscale of the McCarthy Scales of Children's Abilities and the General Cognitive Index (GCI) as compared to peers or a normative sample (see Table 15.3). Children with a history of prenatal drug exposure performed within the borderline range for cognitive deficits. In contrast, the comparison group performance clustered slightly below the mean in all areas with an overall GCI in the average range. This finding is consistent with the test results of the normative sample that found African-American preschool youngsters between the ages of 2½ to 5½ to obtain an average GCI of 96, not substantially different from the designated mean of 100 (A. S. Kaufman & N. L. Kaufman, 1977). The finding of borderline cognitive deficits among children with a history of prenatal drug exposure at age 4 is inconsistent with current literature suggesting that prenatal exposure to drugs does not seriously affect IQ. Moreover, the poor performance was particularly startling, because these specific children had had mean scores of 100.2 ($SD = 12.9$) at 6 months, 98.5 ($SD = 12.0$) at 15 months, and 89.0 ($SD = 15.3$) at 24 months on the Bayley Mental Development Index (MDI), within the average range of functioning.

As shown in Table 15.4, during administration of the McCarthy Scales, children with prenatal drug exposure were more frequently out of their seat (i.e., dropping to the floor, standing, moving about) than the comparison group. They were also more likely to refuse a task or require coaxing to transition from one activity to another, but the overall frequency of refusals and assisted transitions was a rare occurrence for both groups. The groups did not differ during the Cookie Delay Task; children with prenatal drug exposure were just as likely to delay their responses as the comparison group. Moreover, in contrast to reports of increased activity or withdrawal during unstructured activity, our laboratory observations found the exploration and manipulation of varied toys similar among both groups of children. The quality of play manipulations was not assessed.

In contrast, observer ratings of child behavior throughout the laboratory session described children with prenatal drug exposure as significantly less compliant,

TABLE 15.3
Means and Standard Deviations (in parentheses) for McCarthy Scales
of Children's Abilities

McCarthy Subscale	Drug Exposed $n = 16$		Comparison $n = 18$		Significance of F Test
Verbal	35.50	(9.90)	48.38	(9.27)	14.044**
Perceptual	35.56	(10.05)	46.50	(11.25)	8.719*
Quantitative	32.87	(8.49)	44.55	(9.35)	12.919**
Memory	36.06	(9.76)	48.83	(8.17)	17.942**
General Cognitive Index	70.25	(18.25)	95.11	(15.22)	15.667**

$df = (1,30)$.
*$p < .01$. **$p < .001$.

TABLE 15.4
Means and Standard Deviations (in parentheses) for Activity
and Attention During Structured Task

Variable	Drug Exposed n = 16		Comparison n = 18		Significance of F Test
Total time on task	46.00	(14.12)	48.33	(8.27)	.183
Total time out of seat	13.94	(11.16)	3.33	(4.14)	14.664***
Off task refuse task	2.12	(1.83)	0.66	(1.33)	6.187*
Off task ignore direction	1.50	(1.86)	0.83	(2.57)	1.157
Off task stare into space	0.94	(2.62)	0.28	(0.75)	0.558
Off task inattentive	6.00	(6.08)	3.56	(3.54)	2.825
Transition accepts	10.13	(3.50)	12.94	(3.30)	7.874
Transition coaxing	2.44	(2.31)	0.22	(0.65)	18.719***
Transition refused	0.63	(1.15)	0.00	(0.00)	12.597**
Transition tantrum crying	0.25	(0.77)	0.00	(0.00)	2.615

$df = (1,30)$.
*$p < .05$. **$p < .01$. ***$p < .001$.

less persistent, more irritable, and requiring more verbal cues or coaxing to maintain active involvement with an activity than the comparison children. The strong differentiation of the drug-exposed from the comparison children by observer ratings was not obvious from the objective scoring of activity and attention during the structured and unstructured tasks. This finding suggests that more qualitative assessment of behavior may be warranted to identify some behavioral characteristics.

The pattern of associations between the clinical ratings and the more objective measures indicated that ratings of noncompliance, inattentive, and restless behaviors were negatively associated with the GCI and positively associated with off-task behaviors, poor transitional skills, frequency of activity shifts, and duration of play activity lasting 30 seconds or less.

Whereas increased activity, inattentiveness, and impulsivity may be used to describe children who are difficult to handle or require extraordinary behavior management, these issues were not reflected in parent ratings of children with prenatal drug exposure. Parents in both groups reported average temperamental dimensions and did not differ significantly in their ratings of problem behaviors. Parents may tolerate certain types of behaviors in the home that observers find inappropriate or intolerable in a more structured setting (e.g., laboratory or school).

Parent ratings of temperament were unrelated to laboratory measures, with the exception of the dimensions of frustration threshold and persistence. Threshold and persistence displayed weak but significant correlations with the GCI, total time on task, and free play activity lasting 120 sec or more. Parental ratings of problem behaviors were more strongly related to laboratory behaviors than were ratings of temperament. Increased numbers of problem behaviors reported by the parent were associated with less total time on task, poor transitional skills, more activity shifts during free play, more brief activities lasting 20 sec or less, and less play activities lasting 120 sec or more. Moreover, parental report of disturbed behavior—hostile aggressive and hyperactive distractible—was positively correlated with observers' clinical ratings of restless and out-of-seat behaviors.

STUDY 3

Sample

The drug-exposed sample is described in Study 2, as 14 children from the longitudinal sample.

Given that only four children were available from the longitudinal sample for the comparison group, additional children were recruited separately from Study 2 in order to equate the drug-exposed and the comparison groups in lack of day-care experience. They were identified by a community worker who resided in the same neighborhood as the children in the drug-exposed group. The community worker had known all of the families since before the births of the children and could vouch for the accuracy of the mothers' statements that they had not used drugs during their pregnancy.

All of the comparison group children had lived continuously with their mothers, in contrast to the prenatally drug-exposed children.

The average age for the sample was 46.2 months (SD = 5.8 months), and there were six girls and eight boys in each group.

Procedure and Measures

The 28 children were assembled into seven same-gender play groups with unfamiliar peers by assigning two prenatally drug-exposed children and two comparison children to each group. Transportation to the laboratory at UCLA was provided for each group of children and their caregivers. In the laboratory, the preschoolers were videotaped playing together during 40 minutes of structured and unstructured tasks, while the caregivers were interviewed in a separate room.

The tasks began with the presentation of paper and markers at a table, and a request for the children "to draw a present for someone special." The duration of the coloring task was 7 min, and was considered the structured activity. At the end of the coloring task, the children were asked to give their pictures to the tester, to put away the markers, and to assist in getting toys off the shelves for free play. The transition from the coloring task to the free play took approximately 3 min. The children were then told that they could play with any of the toys in the room. They were allowed free play for 20 min, with the tester seated in the background. At the end of the 20 min, the tester imposed a compliance task, asking the children to assist her in picking up the toys to get ready for a snack. The children were then given a snack and reunited with their caregivers.

Videotapes were coded by the third author who was blind to the group assignment of the children. Each child's behavior was coded every 20 sec. The codes were derived from the Howes Peer Play Scale (Howes, 1987). The scale ranges from solitary play through parallel play (engaged in same activity as peer without awareness of peer) to simple social (play with turntaking structure) and complementary (action reversals and reciprocal play). The scale also allows for coding of affect and aggressive behavior in initiations and responses to initiations. Also included was the Howes Social Pretend Play Scale, which measures the increasing complexity of a child's symbolic actions across eight levels.

Additional codes during the coloring task were imitating peers' work, intentional destruction of peers' work, seeking adult assistance, and seeking adult praise. Additional categories during the transitional period were verbal or physical resistance to change from one activity to another, and off-task behavior. The compliance task added codes of number of toys picked up, number of redirects back to task, off task, conflict resolution with peers, and insensitivity to peers.

Results

A series of 2 (Group) × 2 (Gender) MANOVAs were conducted for the following groups of behaviors: (a) entry behavior, which included the codes for amount and style of initiations by the target child to others and his or her response to other's initiations; (b) conflict resolution, which included questions, negotiates, and directives; (c) off-task behavior, coding solitary, onlooker, and parallel; (d) use of adults; (e) level and frequency of interactional play with peers; (f) compliance scored by redirects and number of toys put away; (g) affect; and (h) insensitivity coded by categories of intentional destruction, forced interactions, and intruding.

There were no significant multivariate main effects, and prenatally drug-exposed children did not appear to differ from comparison children in the areas of entry behavior, conflict resolution, off-task behavior, use of adults, level of play with peers, and affect. However, univariate ANOVAs indicated that drug-exposed children made more agonistic and forced initiations in their entry behavior (see Table 15.5).

The overall MANOVA was significant, however, concerning compliance, $F(2,23) = 3.3$, $p < .05$. Children who were prenatally exposed to drugs were more noncompliant than comparison children.

Differences were also found concerning insensitivity. Prenatally drug-exposed children were found to be more insensitive to peers than comparison children, $F(1,26) = 4.2$, $p < .05$. This result suggests that the prenatally drug-exposed children, in comparison to their peers, made overtures and responses that were either aggressive in nature or very inappropriate. The potential problem for prenatally drug-exposed children in their interactions with peers may therefore be in their style and ability to effectively initiate and sustain play so that they are seen as desirable companions.

TABLE 15.5
Means and Standard Deviations (in parentheses) for Play Behaviors
by Group and Gender

	Drug Exposed				Comparison				
	Girls		Boys		Girls		Boys		F Value for
Variable	n = 6		n = 8		n = 6		n = 8		Group
Entry									
Positive initiations	8.3	(6.3)	4.9	(3.6)	6.0	(3.3)	3.3	(4.2)	1.3
Agonistic initiations	6.2	(7.1)	3.0	(3.5)	0.3	(0.5)	2.6	(2.7)	4.1*
Forced interactions	3.7	(6.2)	1.9	(2.7)	0.2	(0.4)	0.3	(0.5)	4.2*
Positive responses	3.3	(2.0)	3.0	(2.7)	4.7	(2.6)	2.6	(2.0)	0.2
Aggressive responses	0.5	(0.6)	1.8	(2.3)	1.0	(1.3)	2.1	(2.4)	0.4
Rejection of initiations	10.2	(20.0)	1.8	(1.8)	1.2	(0.8)	1.0	(1.3)	1.5
Compliance									
# Toys picked-up	7.2	(6.5)	12.0	(8.1)	5.5	(4.2)	18.0	(4.0)	0.9
# Redirects	1.3	(1.4)	1.8	(2.3)	0.0	(0.0)	0.3	(0.5)	7.6**

*p < .05. **p < .01

There was no evidence from a repeated-measures 2 (Group) × 2 (Gender) × 2 (Structured vs. Unstructured Task) MANOVA that the behavior of prenatally drug-exposed children was more or less competent on a structured task than on an unstructured task.

In addition to describing each child's behaviors in each situation by use of frequency counts, each child was classified as solitary, complementary, or intrusive or rejected based on their entry behavior, levels of interaction, and aggression across all of the tasks. The children classified as intrusive or rejected had more agonistic initiations, forced interactions, and rejected initiations than children classified as either solitary or complementary. Children classified as solitary engaged in more noninteractive play than the other children. Children classified as complementary used conflict resolution as a method of settling disputes more than children classified as solitary or intrusive or rejected. Prenatally drug-exposed children were more likely to be classified as solitary or intrusive or rejected than complementary, $\chi^2 = 6.3$, $p < .05$.

DISCUSSION

These three interrelated studies have addressed aspects of development of young children exposed in utero to drugs that heretofore have barely been investigated by research studies. These domains—quality of attachment and quality of play during infancy, attention, cooperation to a strange adult, and quality of peer interaction during preschool—are significant developmental tasks that represent the child's evolving abilities in social relationships and self-organization.

The studies have found that children exposed prenatally to drugs, as a group, differ from their peers in several ways. As infants, they are much more likely to show insecure, disorganized attachments to their primary caregiver. They are more likely to be restless, aggressive, and show regressive play as toddlers. At preschool, they continue to be more inattentive and restless, require more adult direction to cooperate, and are less sensitive with peers.

The group differences suggest that the prenatally drug-exposed children struggle with tasks that require self-organization. The difficulties found with this sample at the toddler period in Study 1 with organizing and sustaining spontaneous play seem to continue into the preschool period. In both Study 2 and Study 3, the prenatally drug-exposed children were found to be more noncompliant. They needed more adult assistance in the form of coaxing or redirection to maintain their attention to the specified task. These findings suggest that difficulty in sustaining attention to a task may be a factor in their noncompliance. Their significantly lowered IQ scores at preschool may also be related to their inattentiveness and restlessness, suggesting that the scores may represent performance, but not cognitive ability.

Another important continuum of behavior from infancy to preschool concerns the alterations in social behaviors of the prenatally drug-exposed children. Study 1 and Study 3 both found that prenatally drug-exposed children have problems with social skills with both caregivers and peers. In Study 1, the prenatally drug-exposed children at 15 months were more insecure in attachment, and at 24 months they made fewer positive social bids and showed more deviant behaviors with their caregivers. Study 1 posited that if these behaviors continued past the toddler period, difficulties with relationships and interactions in settings other than those with the caregiver would occur. Study 3 substantiated and furthered the results of Study 1 by examining prenatally drug-exposed interactions with peers at preschool age. Study 3 found that prenatally drug-exposed children were more inappropriate in their overtures to peers, which made them appear insensitive. For instance, one child's strategy to initiate play was to repeatedly stick a toy telephone in the face of another child already engaged in play and continuously say "look at this." The child was forcing his presence on another child without realizing the ineffectiveness of his overture. Behavior such as this usually resulted in the initiator being ignored or rejected. The inappropriateness of these children's overtures suggests that they are less likely to survey the context of the setting and tune into social cues before attempting to engage in play with a peer. The prenatally drug-exposed children's insensitivity may further suggest that they have a limited repertoire of behaviors from which to choose when engaging in play with a peer, thereby making them appear insensitive and inexperienced when attempting to be sociable with a peer. Dodge (1985) suggested that children who have trouble initiating to peers may be at risk for being rejected or neglected. Further research is needed to determine whether the deficits in social competence observed in the toddler and preschool period carry over to kindergarten age as well.

It must be remembered, however, that variability existed within the drug-exposed group so that there were some children who were securely attached, were attentive and cooperative with adults, and did play sensitively with peers. Moreover, the findings about group differences must be accepted with caution. All three studies were subject to the methodological problems that vex the investigation of in utero drug exposure in humans. The drug-exposed samples were biased by the nature of the recruitment of minority subjects living in poverty, whose mothers were chronic and heavy drug users. The majority of mothers used both PCP and cocaine, as well as nicotine, marijuana, and alcohol. Our small samples meant that we could not statistically differentiate the effects of single drugs, so that the findings refer only to polydrug exposure. Also, the initial samples were subject to high rates of attrition that required additional subjects to be added to the studies during preschool. Moreover, the comparison samples, although also minority subjects living in poverty in the same geographical areas most of whom received their income from Aid to Families with Dependent Children and were single parents, did differ in significant ways from the drug-exposed group. Additionally, children in the comparison samples did not suffer loss or changes in the primary attachment figure, whereas the drug-exposed children did. Thus, our tentative findings require confirmation from other laboratories.

Finally, it is important to note that referring to these children as prenatally drug exposed is shorthand for a complex of co-occuring risk factors that begin during pregnancy and continue after birth. It is not only the biological effects that occur to the fetus, but the continuing adversities in experience, growing up in poverty, living in a drug-centered environment, or experiencing inadequate nurturing, loss, and/or changes in the primary adult caregiver, that place most of these children in double jeopardy. We do not yet know about compensatory or protective factors that might be seen in the development of prenatally drug-exposed children who grow up in stable, responsive homes; nor do we have information about children reared by substance-abusing mothers who did not use drugs during pregnancy. For the children in our study, the interactions between organic effects of prenatal drug exposure and continuing adversities in the rearing environment may serve to exponentially increase the risk of the factors considered singularly. Future studies will need to explore the trajectories of these children across developmental points to ascertain what factors or combination of factors causes vulnerabilities and resilience in these children.

ACKNOWLEDGMENTS

This work was supported by grants from the National Institute on Drug Abuse (#5R01DA04139 and #5R18DA6380) to Judy Howard. Study 2 was conducted at the University of California at Los Angeles by the second author in partial fulfillment of the requirements for the degree of Doctor of Philosophy. Study 3 was conducted at the University of California at Los Angeles by the third author in partial fulfillment of the requirements for the degree of Doctor of Philosophy. The authors wish to thank Clementine Royston for her dedication to the families and assistance with the research.

REFERENCES

Ainsworth, M. D. S. (1976). *System for rating maternal-care behavior*. Princeton, NJ: Educational Testing Service.

Ainsworth, M. D. S., Blehar, M. C., Waters, E., & Wall, S. (1978). Patterns of attachment: A psychological study of the strange situation. Hillsdale, NJ: Lawrence Erlbaum Associates.

Azuma, S., & Chasnoff, I. (1993). Outcome of children prenatally exposed to cocaine and other drugs: A path analysis of three-year data. *Pediatrics, 92*(3), 396–402.

Beckwith, L., Rodning, C., Norris, D., Phillipsen, L., Khandabi, P., & Howard, J. (1994). Spontaneous play in two-year-olds born to substance-abusing mothers. *Infant Mental Health Journal, 15*, 189–201.

Behar, L. B. (1977). The preschool behavior questionnaire. *Journal of Abnormal Child Psychology, 5*(3), 265–276.

Campbell, S. (1988, October). *Longitudinal studies of active and aggressive preschoolers: Individual differences in early behavior and in outcome*. Paper presented at the Second Rochester Symposium on Developmental Psychopathology, Rochester, NY.

Campbell, S. B., Szumowski, E. K., Ewing, L. J., Gluck, D. S., & Breau, A. M. (1982). A multidimensional assessment of parent-identified behavior problem toddlers. *Journal of Abnormal Child Psychology, 10*(4), 592–599.

Cassidy, J. (1986). The ability to negotiate the environment: An aspect of infant competence as related to quality of attachment. *Child Development, 57*, 331–337.

Chasnoff, I., Burns, K. A., & Burns, W. J. (1987). Cocaine use in pregnancy: Perinatal morbidity and mortality. *Neurobehavioral Toxicology and Teratology, 9*, 291–293.

Chasnoff, I., Griffith, D. R., Freier, C., & Murray, J. (1992). Cocaine/polydrug use in pregnancy: Two-year follow-up. *Pediatrics, 89*, 284–289.

Corwin, M. J., Lester, B. M., Sepkoski, C., McLaughlin, S., Kayne, H., & Golub, H. L. (1992). Effects of in utero cocaine exposure on newborn acoustical cry characteristics. *Pediatrics, 89*(6), 1199–1203.

Dodge, K. (1985). Facets of social interaction and the assessment of social competence in children. In B. Schneider, K. Rubin, & S. Ledingham (Eds.), *Children's peer relations: Issues in assessment and intervention* (pp. 3–22). New York: Springer-Verlag.

Golden, M., Montare, A., & Bridger, W. (1977). Verbal control of delay behavior in two-year-old boys as a function of social class. *Child Development, 48*, 1107–1111.

Hawley, T. L., & Disney, E. R. (1992, Winter). Crack's children: The consequences of maternal cocaine abuse. *Social Policy Report of the Society for Research in Child Development, 6*(4), 1–23.

Howes, C. (1987). Social competence with peers in young children: Developmental sequences. *Developmental Review, 7*, 252–272.

Howes, C., & Matheson, C. C. (1992). Sequences in the development of competent play with peers: Social and social pretend play. *Developmental Psychology, 28*(5), 961–974.

Johnson, H. L., Glassman, M. B., Fiks, K. B., & Rosen, T. S. (1987). Path analysis of variables affecting 36-month outcome in a population of multi-risk children. *Infant Behavior and Development, 10*, 451–465.

Kagan, J. (1981). *Second year: The emergence of self-awareness.* Cambridge, MA: Harvard University Press.

Kaufman, A. S., & Kaufman, N. L. (1977). *Clinical evaluation of young children with the McCarthy Scales.* New York: Grune & Stratton.

Keogh, B. K., Pullis, M. E., & Caldwell, J. (1982). A short form of the Teacher Temperament Questionnaire. *Journal of Educational Measurement, 19*(4), 323–329.

Lifschitz, M. H., Wilson, G. S., Smith, E., & Desmond, M. M. (1985). *The Journal of Pediatrics, 102*, 686–691.

Lyons-Ruth, K., Alpern, L., & Repacholi, B. (1993). Disorganized infant attachment classification and maternal psychosocial problems as predictors of hostile-aggressive behavior in the pre-school classroom. *Child Development, 64*, 572–585.

MacGregor, S. N., Keith, L. G., Chasnoff, I., Rosner, M. A., Chisum, G. M., Shaw, P., & Minogue, J. P. (1987). Cocaine use during pregnancy: Adverse perinatal outcome. *American Journal of Obstetrics and Gynecology, 157*, 686–690.

Rodning, C., Beckwith, L., & Howard, J. (1989). Characteristics of attachment organization and play organization in prenatally drug-exposed toddlers. *Development and Psychopathology, 1*, 277–289.

Rodning, C., Beckwith, L., & Howard, J. (1991). Quality of attachment and home environment in children prenatally exposed to PCP and cocaine. *Development and Psychopathology, 3*, 351–366.

Rubenstein, J., & Howes, C. (1976). The effects of peers on toddler interaction with mother and toys. *Child Development, 47*, 597–605.

Ryan, L., Ehrlich, S., & Finnegan, L. (1987). Cocaine abuse in pregnancy: Effects on the fetus and the newborn. *Neurotoxicology and Teratology, 9*, 295–299.

Sroufe, L. A. (1983). Infant–caregiver attachment and patterns of adaptation in preschool: The roots of maladaption and competence. In M. Perlmutter (Ed.), *Minnesota symposium in child psychology* (Vol. 16, pp. 41–81). Hillsdale, NJ: Lawrence Erlbaum Associates.

Waters, E., & Sroufe, L. A. (1983). Social competence as a developmental construct. *Developmental Review, 3*, 79–97.

Waters, E., Vaughn, B., & Egeland, B. (1980). Individual differences at age one: Antecedents in neonatal behavior in an urban, economically disadvantaged sample. *Child Development, 51*, 208–216.

Waters, E., Wippman, J., & Sroufe, L. A. (1979). Attachment, positive affect, and competence in the peer group: Two studies in construct validation. *Child Development, 50*, 821–829.

Zuckerman, B., Frank, D. A., Hingson, R., Amaro, H., Levenson, S. M., Kayne, H., Parker, S., Vinci, R., Aboagye, K., Fried, L. E., Cabral, H., Timperi, R., & Bauchner, H. (1989). Effects of maternal marijuana and cocaine use on fetal growth. *The New England Journal of Medicine, 320*(12), 762–768.

16
▼▼▼▼▼▼▼

Cocaine Use Among
Pregnant Women:
Socioeconomic, Obstetrical,
and Psychological Issues

Nanci Stewart Woods
Austin Peay State University

Marylou Behnke
Fonda Davis Eyler
Michael Conlon
Kathleen Wobie
University of Florida College of Medicine

To date, research on the effects of prenatal substance use has focused almost exclusively on the offspring of women of low socioeconomic status (SES). The majority of studies have been conducted at large teaching hospitals, which provide primarily indigent and high-risk medical care. Ideally, research should investigate the effects of drug use by all pregnant women. Currently, it can be difficult to interpret the results of prenatal drug use research conducted exclusively on women of low SES due to a variety of confounding sociodemographic and lifestyle factors. These factors include, but are not limited to poorer general health and nutrition, less than optimal general life circumstances, and greater use of multiple substances during pregnancy.

Research on substance use in low-SES pregnant women indicates that they differ on sociodemographic and lifestyle variables not only from middle-class pregnant nonusers, but also from low-SES pregnant nonusers (Finnegan, Oehlberg, Regan, & Rudraveff, 1981; Frank et al., 1988; Hans, 1989; Neuspiel & Hamel, 1991; Parker, Greer, & Zuckerman, 1988; Zuckerman & Bresnahan, 1991). For example, published studies examining the effects of prenatal cocaine exposure on infant outcome using the Brazelton Neonatal Behavioral Assessment Scale (NBAS; Brazelton, 1984) have evaluated the infants of predominantly low-SES women (Chasnoff, Burns, Schnoll, & Burns, 1985; Chasnoff, Griffith, MacGregor, Dirkes, & Burns, 1989; Coles, Platzman, Smith, James, & Falek,

1992; Eisen et al., 1991; Neuspiel, Hamel, Hochberg, Greene, & Campbell, 1991; Richardson & Day, 1994; Woods, Eyler, Behnke, & Conlon, 1993). In all but one of these studies (Chasnoff et al., 1985) the cocaine-using women had higher rates of alcohol, tobacco, and marijuana use than did the nonusing women. As another example, even though the samples are predominantly comprised of low-SES subjects, cocaine-using women receive significantly less and later prenatal care (Eyler, Behnke, Conlon, Woods, & Frentzen, 1994; MacGregor, Keith, Bachicha, & Chasnoff, 1989; MacGregor et al., 1987; McCalla et al., 1991; Neuspiel et al., 1991; Richardson & Day, 1994; Woods et al., 1993; Zuckerman, Frank, et al., 1989) than nonusing women.

In addition to the narrow study population already discussed, the majority of research on prenatal cocaine use has focused exclusively or primarily on infant effects. Given that the mother is one of the most important influences on infant development, this infant-focused approach is undoubtedly short sighted (Sameroff & Chandler, 1975). Research on the importance of mother–infant interaction for optimal infant development suggests that the impact of drug abuse on the psychosocial functioning of mothers, the home environment, and parenting skills should be examined (Cohn, Matis, Tronick, Connell, & Lyons-Ruth, 1986; Field et al., 1988). If one of our goals is to improve outcome for the infants of pregnant drug users, then it is vital that we examine the effects of cocaine use on both the mother and the child.

The goal of this chapter is to discuss the relationship of prenatal cocaine use to the psychosocial functioning and obstetrical problems of pregnant women. Because the majority of research has been conducted with low-SES women, and there are population-based differences in other predictors of poor obstetrical and psychosocial functioning, the studies reviewed and new data presented in this chapter may not be generalizable to all pregnant women who use cocaine.

This chapter is organized in the following manner. First, we review the epidemiology of prenatal cocaine use and the sociodemographic and lifestyle issues that are involved. We discuss the ways in which cocaine users differ from nonusers in available studies. Second, we review the current literature on the perinatal problems of prenatal cocaine users. Third, we present data on a large sample of low-SES, rural women who used cocaine during pregnancy. The sample was collected for the purpose of comparing the perinatal outcome of their infants to the infants of a nonusing sample matched on potentially confounding factors. Fourth, we describe our ongoing, prospective, longitudinal study that is designed to determine the effects of prenatal crack and cocaine use on the psychosocial functioning of low-SES women and the medical and neurodevelopmental outcome of their infants. Finally, we review the limited published data and present preliminary data from our prospective study on the psychosocial functioning of women who use cocaine during pregnancy and discuss its potential influences on infant outcome.

EPIDEMIOLOGY OF PRENATAL COCAINE USE: WOMEN'S ISSUES

Prevalence

The United States is currently experiencing the fifth epidemic of stimulant use since 1890 (Farrar & Kearns, 1989). Today cocaine exposure is found throughout all age groups and socioeconomic classes in our society (Chasnoff, Keith, & Schnoll, 1986; O'Malley, Bachman, & Johnston, 1988). Of particular concern are the use of cocaine by women of childbearing age and the effects of cocaine exposure on the fetus, infant, and developing child. Studies across the country from large cities, suburban communities, the urban and rural South, and public and private health-care facilities have used various techniques to document the prevalence of prenatal cocaine use. These techniques have included maternal history, maternal urine screening, infant urine screening, and infant meconium screening either singly or in combination at various times throughout pregnancy and at delivery. Variability in populations studied and in the techniques used for screening have led to prevalence rates ranging from 1% to 30% (Behnke, Eyler, Conlon, Woods, & Casanova, 1994; Chasnoff, Landress, & Barrett, 1990; George, Price, Hauth, Barnette, & Preston, 1991; Gillogley, Evans, Hansen, Samuels, & Batra, 1990; Hollinshead et al., 1990; Little, Snell, Palmore, & Gilstrap, 1988; Matera, Warren, Moomjy, Fink, & Fox, 1990; McCalla et al., 1991; Neerhof, MacGregor, Retzky, & Sullivan, 1989; Ostrea, Brady, Gause, Raymundo, & Stevens, 1992; Schutzman, Frankenfield-Chernicoff, Clatterbaugh, & Singer, 1991; Sloan, Gay, Snyder, & Bales, 1992; Streissguth et al., 1991; Vega, Kolody, Hwang, & Noble, 1993; Weathers, Crane, Sauvain, & Blackhurst, 1993; Zuckerman, Frank et al., 1989).

Sociodemographic and Lifestyle Differences

Sociodemographic and lifestyle differences have been identified between prenatal cocaine users and nonusers in a number of studies published between 1985 and 1994. Although methodological differences exist among virtually all of these studies, the results of a representative sample of available studies are summarized in Table 16.1.

Age. The studies available are split on findings of age differences between users and nonusers. However, the majority of studies show that prenatal cocaine users are significantly older than nonusers (Behnke et al., 1994, Cartwright, Schorge, & McLaughlin, 1991; Coles et al., 1992; Dombrowski, Wolfe, Welch, & Evans, 1991; Eyler et al., 1994; George et al., 1991; Gillogley et al., 1990;

TABLE 16.1
Sociodemographic and Lifestyle Differences in Prenatal Cocaine Users Compared to Nonusers

Sociodemographic and Lifestyle Outcomes[a]

Author[b]	Year	Age	Education	Black Race	Single	SES	Alc	MJ	TOB	Gravidity	Parity	Induced Abs	Prenatal Care	Weight Gain	STD	Paternal Drug Use
Bingol	1987	no ▲	-	no ▲	-	no ▲	-	-	no ▲	↑	-	-	-	-	-	-
MacGregor	1987	-	-	-	-	-	↑	-	-	↑	↑	↑	↓	no ↑	-	-
Frank	1988	no ▲	no ▲	↑	↑	no ▲	↑	↑	↑	no ▲	no ▲	↑	↓	↓	↑	↑
Hadeed	1989	no ▲	-	no ▲	-	no ▲	-	-	no ▲	-	no ▲	-	-	-	-	-
Little	1989	↑	-	↑	-	-	↑	-	↑	-	↑	-	-	-	no ▲	-
MacGregor	1989	↑	-	-	-	-	↑	↑	↑	↑	↑	↑	↓	-	-	-
Neerhof	1989	↑	-	no ▲	↑	-	↑	-	-	↑	↑	-	↓	-	↑	-
Zuckerman	1989	no ▲	-	-	-	-	↑	↑	↑	↑	↑	↑	↓	no ▲	-	-
Gillogley	1990	↑	-	-	↑	↓	↑	↑	↑	↑	↑	↑	↓	-	↑	↑
Hollinshead	1990	no ▲	-	↑	-	-	-	-	↑	-	↑	↑	-	-	-	-
Matera	1990	no ▲	-	no ▲	↑	no ▲	↑	-	↑	↑	no ▲	-	↓	-	no ▲	-
Cartwright	1991	↑	no ▲	↑	no ▲	-	↑	↑	↑	↑	↑	↑	-	-	-	-
Coles	1991	↑	no ▲	no ▲	↑	no ▲	↑	↑	↑	-	-	-	-	-	-	-
George	1991	↑	-	↑	↑	-	↑	-	↑	-	no ▲	↑	↓	-	-	-
Handler	1991	-	-	↑	↑	-	-	↑	↑	-	no ▲	-	↓	-	-	-
McCalla	1991	↑	-	↑	-	-	↑	no ▲	-	-	-	-	↓	-	-	-
Neuspiel	1991	no ▲	no ▲	no ▲	↑	-	↑	↑	↑	↑	↑	↑	↓	↓	-	-
Richardson	1991	no ▲	no ▲	↑	no ▲	no ▲	↑	↑	↑	no ▲	↑	-	↓	↓	-	-
Ostrea	1992	-	-	↑	↑	↓	↑	↑	-	↑	↑	-	↓	-	-	-
Behnke	1994	↑	-	↑	↑	-	-	↑	↑	-	↑	-	↓	-	-	-
Eyler	1994	↑	no ▲	↑	-	-	↑	↑	↑	-	↑	-	↓	-	-	-
Richardson	1994	↑	no ▲	↑	↓	↓	↑	↑	↑	↑	↑	-	↓	no ▲	-	-

[a]Comparison of cocaine users to drug-free control groups; ↑ = increase; ↓ = decrease; ▲ = no difference between groups; no = groups matched on this variable; SES = socioeconomic status; Alc = alcohol; MJ = marijuana; TOB = tobacco; Abs = abortions; STD = sexually transmitted diseases.
[b]Studies listed by first author and year published.

Little & Snell, 1991; Little, Snell, Klein, & Gilstrap, 1989; McCalla et al., 1991; Neerhof et al., 1989; Richardson & Day, 1994).

Education. Most studies do not evaluate the educational status of users versus nonusers. However, of the several that do, there is no significant difference in educational status between using and nonusing women (Cartwright et al., 1991; Coles et al., 1992; Eyler et al., 1994; Frank et al., 1988; Neuspiel et al., 1991; Richardson & Day, 1991, 1994).

Race. Only one study has demonstrated that prenatal cocaine users are more likely than nonusers to be White (Richardson & Day, 1991). Although several studies show no racial differences between users and nonusers (Bingol, Fuchs, Diaz, Stone, & Gromisch, 1987; Chasnoff et al., 1985; Coles et al., 1992; Hadeed & Siegel, 1989; Matera et al., 1990; Neerhof et al., 1989; Neuspiel et al., 1991; Ostrea et al., 1992), the majority of studies indicate that prenatal cocaine users are more likely to be African-American or non-White (Behnke et al., 1994; Cartwright et al., 1991; Eyler et al., 1994; Frank et al., 1988; George et al., 1991; Handler, Kistin, Davis, & Ferré, 1991; Hollinshead et al., 1990; Little et al., 1989; McCalla et al., 1991; Richardson & Day, 1994; Vega et al., 1993).

Marital Status. Only a few studies have examined marital status differences between users and nonusers. Two studies indicate no differences (Coles et al., 1992; Richardson & Day, 1991). The remaining studies reveal that users are more likely than nonusers to be classified as single or unmarried (Behnke et al., 1994; Cartwright et al., 1991; Eyler et al., 1994; Frank et al., 1988; George et al., 1991; Gillogley et al., 1990; Neuspiel et al., 1991; Ostrea et al., 1992; Richardson & Day, 1994).

Socioeconomic Status. Only a few studies have examined socioeconomic status. Some of the studies show no difference (Bingol et al., 1987; Coles et al., 1992; Frank et al., 1988; Hadeed & Siegel, 1989; Richardson & Day, 1991; Woods et al., 1993), although over half indicate that users are of lower socioeconomic status than nonusers (Hollinshead et al., 1990; Matera et al., 1990; Ostrea et al., 1992; Richardson & Day, 1994).

Other Drug Use. The preponderance of studies have demonstrated that prenatal cocaine users are more likely than nonusers to use other drugs. Specifically they have been shown to be more likely to use tobacco, alcohol, and marijuana (Behnke et al., 1994; Coles et al., 1992; Eyler et al., 1994; Frank et al., 1988; Gillogley et al., 1990; Handler et al., 1991; Little et al., 1989; MacGregor et al., 1987; MacGregor et al., 1989; Matera et al., 1990; Neuspiel et al., 1991; Richardson & Day, 1991, 1994; Vega et al., 1993; Zuckerman, Frank, et al., 1989). Only Chasnoff et al. (1985) reported no differences in usage patterns for marijuana between groups, and two studies showed no difference in tobacco usage (Bingol et al., 1987; Hadeed & Siegel, 1989). Additionally, one study had mixed results; McCalla et al. (1991) showed increased tobacco use but no differences in marijuana use between groups.

Gravidity/Parity. The vast majority of studies indicate there is increased gravidity (Bingol et al., 1987; Cartwright et al., 1991; Dombrowski et al., 1991; Gillogley et al., 1990; Handler et al., 1991; Keith et al., 1989; MacGregor et al., 1987; MacGregor et al., 1989; Neerhof et al., 1989; Neuspiel et al., 1991; Ostrea et al., 1992; Richardson & Day, 1994) as well as increased parity in users compared to nonusers (Behnke et al., 1994; Cartwright et al., 1991; Dombrowski et al., 1991; Gillogley et al., 1990; Eyler et al., 1994; Hollinshead et al., 1990; McCalla et al., 1991; Neerhof et al., 1989; Ostrea et al., 1992, Richardson & Day, 1994; Zuckerman, Frank, et al., 1989). Only one study demonstrated decreased parity among users (Richardson & Day, 1991) and only a few studies have shown no difference in gravidity (Frank et al., 1988; Richardson & Day, 1991) or parity (Frank et al., 1988; George et al., 1991; Hadeed & Siegel, 1989; Little & Snell, 1991; Little et al., 1989; Matera et al., 1990; Neuspiel et al., 1991).

Elective Abortions. Closely related to gravidity and parity is the number of elective abortions. Although a number of studies have evaluated differences in total number of abortions between cocaine-using and nonusing women, only a few have specifically examined elective abortions. All show an increase in the number of elective abortions among users compared to nonusers (Frank et al., 1988; Gillogley et al., 1990; Matera et al., 1990; Neuspiel et al., 1991).

Prenatal Care. In the studies that have investigated prenatal care, all have documented a reduced amount of prenatal care among users. This is reflected either as fewer total visits, entry into the prenatal care system later in pregnancy, or a higher percentage of users with no prenatal care compared to nonusers (Behnke et al., 1994; Eyler et al., 1994; Gillogley et al., 1990; Handler et al., 1991; Keith et al., 1989; MacGregor et al., 1987; MacGregor et al., 1989; Matera et al., 1990; McCalla et al., 1991; Neuspiel et al., 1991; Ostrea et al., 1992; Richardson & Day, 1994; Vega et al., 1993; Woods et al., 1993; Zuckerman, Frank, et al., 1989).

Weight Gain. Although cocaine is an appetite suppressant and generally is associated with weight loss in users, only a few studies have looked at weight gain of users during pregnancy. Only two studies document less weight gain in users (Frank et al., 1988; Neuspiel et al., 1991), whereas one study shows more weight gain (Richardson & Day, 1991) and several studies show no difference (MacGregor et al., 1987; Richardson & Day, 1994; Zuckerman, Frank, et al., 1989).

Sexually Transmitted Diseases. Because many female cocaine users trade sex for drugs and engage in prostitution, there has been a concern about the prevalence of sexually transmitted diseases among prenatal cocaine users. Few studies are available in this area. Two studies have shown no differences between users and nonusers (Little et al., 1989; Matera et al., 1990) and several studies have demonstrated an increase in sexually transmitted diseases among users (Frank et al., 1988; Zuckerman, Frank et al., 1989). Recent reports of increased rates of syphilis and HIV infections among users include the disturbing addendum that these women were the least likely to seek prenatal care and thus treatment for themselves and their fetuses (Minkoff et al., 1990; Nanda, Feldman, Delke, Chintalapally, & Minkoff, 1990; Rolfs, Goldberg, & Sharrar, 1990; Webber, Lambert, Bateman, & Hauser, 1993).

Paternal Drug Use. In this important area only one study was found. It documents an increased incidence of drug use by the fathers of the babies of women who are prenatal cocaine users (Frank et al., 1988).

PERINATAL PROBLEMS
OF PRENATAL COCAINE USERS

A number of studies are available that address the perinatal outcome of women who use cocaine during pregnancy. A consistent pattern of perinatal problems related to prenatal cocaine use has not been identified. Even in studies performed by the same research group results are sometimes widely disparate.

Inconsistency among published studies can be attributed to methodological issues including: (a) many of the earlier studies investigated outcome in a group of users who were enrolled in drug rehabilitation and received prenatal care (Chasnoff, 1989; Chasnoff et al., 1985; Keith et al., 1989; MacGregor et al., 1987; MacGregor et al., 1989), whereas later studies included women with little access to drug rehabilitation or prenatal care; (b) the majority of the studies have included women from poor, urban settings with few studies investigating outcome in rural populations (Behnke et al., 1994; Eyler et al., 1994) or in populations with higher socioeconomic status (Streissguth et al., 1991); and (c) the comparison groups vary from unmatched drug-free groups to matched drug-free groups (Chasnoff et al., 1985; Cherukuri, Minkoff, Feldman, Parekh, & Glass, 1988; Eyler et al., 1994; Gillogley et al., 1990; Keith et al., 1989; MacGregor et al., 1987; MacGregor et al., 1989) or use of statistical covariates (Coles et al., 1992; Eyler et al., 1994; Gillogley et al., 1990; Handler et al., 1991; McCalla et al., 1991; Richardson & Day, 1991, 1994; Zuckerman, Frank, et al., 1989) to control for numerous confounding variables.

The importance of an appropriate comparison group against which to evaluate outcome can not be overstated. Many studies have investigated the impact of sociodemographic and lifestyle variables on perinatal outcome and have shown a negative impact on outcome even where there was no drug use identified

(Golding & Butler, 1984; Kessel, Kleinman, Koontz, Hogue, & Berendes, 1988; National Institute of Medicine, 1985; Shiono & Klebanoff, 1993).

For example, socioeconomic status has been strongly associated with perinatal mortality and morbidity. SES also tends to be related to race, level of education, other drug use, nutritional and health status, number of pregnancies, and means of contraception. It has been shown that women in lower socioeconomic classes are more likely to be African-American, to be single, to have less education, to use other drugs, to have poor nutritional status, to be younger at the time of first pregnancy, and thus to have more children, to have less prenatal care, and to have more health problems, including sexually transmitted diseases, than women in higher socioeconomic classes (Chasnoff et al., 1990; Golding & Butler, 1984; Streissguth et al., 1991). Because each of these variables is independently related to perinatal outcome or is a risk factor for a more problematic pregnancy outcome independent of drug use, each should be taken into account when analyzing perinatal outcomes of drug-using women.

Increases in perinatal problems such as previous abortions, preterm labor and delivery, younger gestational age, smaller infant size at birth, and small-for-gestational-age infants have been documented among prenatal cocaine users (Behnke et al., 1994; Bingol et al., 1987; Chasnoff, 1989; Chasnoff et al., 1985; Cherukuri et al., 1988; Coles et al., 1992; Dombrowski et al., 1991; Eyler et al., 1994; Frank et al., 1988; Gillogley et al., 1990; Hadeed & Siegel, 1989; Handler et al., 1991; Keith et al., 1989; Little & Snell, 1991; Little et al., 1989; MacGregor et al., 1987; MacGregor et al., 1989; Matera et al., 1990; Neerhof et al., 1989; Ostrea et al., 1992; Richardson & Day, 1991, 1994; Woods et al., 1993; Zuckerman, Frank, et al., 1989). Notable exceptions to these general findings include reports of no differences between users and nonusers for number of previous abortions (Behnke et al., 1994; Bingol et al., 1987; Gillogley et al., 1990), incidence of preterm labor (Eyler et al., 1994; Hume, O'Donnell, Stanger, Killam, & Gingras, 1989), incidence of preterm delivery (Hadeed & Siegel, 1989; Hume et al., 1989; Keith et al., 1989; Matera et al., 1990), gestational age (Chasnoff et al., 1985; Little & Snell, 1991; Little et al., 1989; Richardson & Day, 1991, 1994), infant size at birth (Chasnoff et al., 1985; Richardson & Day, 1991, 1994), and small-for-gestational-age infants (Hume et al., 1989; MacGregor et al., 1989; Richardson & Day, 1991; Woods et al., 1993). Additionally, some studies have documented an increase in abruptio placentae (Bingol et al., 1987; Chasnoff et al., 1985; Chasnoff, 1989; Dombrowski et al., 1991; Hadeed & Siegel, 1989; Handler et al., 1991), meconium-stained amniotic fluid (Chasnoff, 1989; Hadeed & Siegel, 1989; Ostrea et al., 1992), and fetal distress (Chasnoff, 1989) and a decrease in Apgar scores (Keith et al., 1989; Little et al., 1989; McCalla et al., 1991). However, the majority of studies have found no differences in these problems between users and nonusers. Table 16.2 summarizes representative studies.

If an examination is made of just the studies that provide either subject matching or statistical control for sociodemographic and lifestyle variables (Chasnoff et al.,

1985; Coles et al., 1992; Eyler et al., 1994; McCalla et al., 1991; Richardson & Day, 1991, 1994; Zuckerman, Frank, et al., 1989), outcomes remain inconsistent and complicated. Few studies either match, control, or have no group differences for alcohol use, tobacco use, and race (Chasnoff et al., 1985; Coles et al., 1992; Eyler et al., 1994; Richardson & Day, 1991, 1994; Zuckerman, Frank, et al., 1989). Of this group of studies, four show no difference in infant size at birth or gestational age (see Table 16.2), and two continue to show that even after careful consideration of confounding variables, there remains evidence that cocaine-exposed infants are younger gestationally and smaller at birth. Those remaining inconsistencies may well be related to other differences in study design as well as relatively unexplored issues such as amount of cocaine use and gestational timing of use.

PERINATAL OUTCOME IN A MATCHED SAMPLE

Prior to initiation of the prospective, longitudinal study described in the next section, we conducted several preliminary studies on prenatal cocaine use in a rural population. Part of the importance of the study described in this section is that it further emphasizes the importance of matching for potentially confounding variables when evaluating perinatal outcome. Additionally, it includes a large sample from a growing population of women rarely represented in the scientific literature (Eyler et al., 1994). Most of the information on the effects of prenatal drug use has come from large city hospitals or programs for the perinatal care and drug treatment of pregnant women, many of whom are suffering from poly-drug addiction. The studies of our population of rural women are useful in describing the effects of cocaine separate from other illicit drugs commonly found in inner-city populations. Fewer than 6% of the target sample in this particular study used any illicit drug other than cocaine. In every case where maternal histories reflected route of drug administration, use of crack was reported.

Our regional hospital is a referral center for pregnancies with complications, and it draws patients from a 16-county, predominately rural district served by public health units. In addition to referred patients, all women receiving prenatal care at the local health department deliver at our institution. The majority of women using the public health departments are Medicaid eligible with relatively low incomes. During the time of this study there were few inpatient beds for drug treatment of pregnant women in the community. As routine practice at our hospital, the charts of each mother and infant are carefully reviewed by an experienced research nurse following delivery, and extensive prenatal and peri-natal histories of the pair are entered into a computerized data set.

Of the 7,250 women delivering over the 2-year period of this study, we identified 172 women who used cocaine prenatally. Using the hospital's computerized data set and an automated procedure, we were able to match 168 of those users to nonusers on six variables known to affect pregnancy outcome: African-American versus non-African-American; maternal age less than 18 years versus more than

TABLE 16.2
Prenatal Cocaine Use and Perinatal Outcome

Author[b]	Year	Maternal						Outcome[a]					
								Offspring					
		Abs	Abruptio Placenta	Preterm Labor	Preterm Delivery	MSF	Fetal Distress	GA	BW	LT	HC	SGA	Apgar Scores
Chasnoff	1985	↑	↑	-	-	-	-	no▲	no▲	no▲	no▲	-	-
Bingol	1987	no▲	↑	-	-	-	-	↓	↓	↓	no→	-	▲
MacGregor	1987	-	no▲	-	↑	-	-	→	→	▲	→	↑	no▲
Cherukuri	1988	↑	-	-	-	no▲	no▲	→	→	no▲	-	-	-
Frank	1988	-	↑	↑	-	↑	↑	→	→	→	→	↑↓	no▲
Chasnoff	1989	↑	↑	-	no▲	↑	no▲	-	-	▲	-	no↑	-
Hadeed	1989	-	no▲	no▲	no▲	-	no▲	→	→	→	→	no▲	no▲
Hume	1989	-	no▲	-	no▲	no▲	no▲	no→	-	→	-	-	-
Keith	1989	↑	↑	-	↑	-	-	→	→	▲	→	-	▲
Little	1989	-	-	-	↑	-	-	→	-	→	→	↑	-
MacGregor	1989	↑	no▲	-	↑	-	-	→	-	-	-	no▲	no▲
Neerhof	1989	-	no▲	-	-	-	-	-	→	→	→	↑	no▲
Zuckerman	1989	-	-	-	↑	-	-	no→	no▲	→	-	-	-
Gillogley	1990	no▲	no▲	-	no▲	-	-	→	-	▲	→	-	▲
Matera	1990	-	no▲	↑	-	-	-	→	-	→	-	-	-
Coles	1991	-	-	-	-	-	-	-	-	-	-	-	-
Dombrowski	1991	-	↑	-	↑	-	-	-	→	→	→	-	no▲
Handler	1991	-	↑	-	↑	-	-	→	-	-	-	↑	-
Little	1991	-	-	-	-	-	-	-	-	-	-	-	↑
McCalla	1991	-	no▲	-	-	no▲	no▲	no→	→	no▲	no▲	no▲	no▲
Richardson	1991	↑	no▲	no▲	-	no▲	no▲	→	→	→	→	↑	-
Ostrea	1992	-	no▲	-	-	↑	-	→	→	-	no▲	no↑	no▲
Woods	1993	-	-	-	-	▲	-	-	-	-	-	-	-
Behnke	1994	no▲	no▲	-	↑	no▲	no▲	no→	no▲	no→	no▲	-	no▲
Eyler	1994	-	no▲	no▲	↑	-	-	→	→	-	-	-	no▲
Richardson	1994	↑	-	-	-	-	-	no→	→	▲	no▲	-	no▲

[a]Comparison of cocaine users to drug-free control group; ↑ = increase; ↓ = decrease; no ▲ = no difference between groups; MSF = meconium-stained fluid; GA = gestational age; BW = birth weight; LT = length; HC = head circumference; SGA = small for gestational age.
[b]Studies listed by first author and year published.

18 years; first versus subsequent pregnancies; gestational age at entry into prenatal care system, less than 20 weeks versus more than 20 weeks; and the use of alcohol or nicotine. To avoid chance findings, these variables were chosen a priori, as were the outcome variables. The outcome variables chosen were those from the literature that were most commonly associated with prenatal cocaine exposure: abruptio placenta, premature labor, gestational age less than 37 weeks, birth weight less than 2,500 grams, birth weight less than 1,500 grams, 5-min Apgar less than or equal to 7, resuscitation at delivery, infant remained in hospital beyond the mother's discharge, congenital anomalies, and perinatal death.

Table 16.3 presents the percentage of the cocaine-exposed, matched control, and remaining delivery groups experiencing each of the adverse perinatal events. Cocaine-exposed neonates experience significantly more of the adverse events than the matched controls and are more likely to be preterm, of low birth weight, resuscitated at birth, and in the hospital after their mothers are discharged. The matched group is more likely to experience fetal or neonatal death.

Although the cocaine users entered the prenatal care system about the same time as matched controls, their prepregnancy weight was approximately 15 pounds less on average, and they continued to gain weight at a lower rate, so that their mean weight at delivery was significantly less than the matched controls. The users were also more than twice as likely as the nonusers to have sexually transmitted infections in the prenatal period.

Of equal interest to drug-related outcomes are the data describing cocaine users and their matched controls compared to the remaining sample of deliveries. Both study groups significantly differ from the remaining sample on all matching variables, supporting our use of one-to-one matching on the six variables chosen a priori. Cocaine users and controls compared to the remaining women delivering

TABLE 16.3
Percentage of Women With Each Outcome Variable

Outcome Variables	Cocaine Exposed (n = 168)	Matched Controls (n = 168)	Remaining Sample (n = 6914)
No adverse events	19.6*†	38.1†	48.5
Congenital anomalies	7.7	5.4	4.4
Abruptio placenta	1.8	0.6	1.0
Premature labor	39.9†	33.9†	22.6
Gestational age ≤ 37 weeks	43.4*†	31.5†	22.9
Birth weight ≤ 2,500 gms	28.0*†	17.9	13.2
Birth weight ≤ 1,500 gms	8.9†	4.8	3.8
5-min Apgars ≤ 7	16.1†	9.5	7.4
Resuscitation	33.9*†	18.4	22.5
Remained in nursery	32.1*†	16.1	15.5
Fetal/neonatal death	1.8*	4.2†	2.0

*$p < .05$, comparison with matched controls.
†$p < .05$; comparison with remaining sample.

are: more likely to be African-American (81% vs. 40%), older (4% vs. 21% less than 18 years old with mean ages of 25 versus 23 years), are less likely to have given birth to their first child (18% vs. 39%), and are more likely to have entered the prenatal care system after 20 weeks gestation (68% vs. 41% with a mean week of entry of 18 versus 17 weeks). Cocaine users and matched controls are also more likely than remaining mothers delivering to have used alcohol (34% vs. 6%) and tobacco (58% vs. 32%).

It is of interest that the matched controls also differ from the remaining deliveries on several outcome measures (Table 16.3). When the matched controls are compared to the remaining sample of all deliveries during the 2-year period, they are significantly less likely to have no adverse events (38% vs. 48%) and more likely to have premature labor (34% vs. 23%), as well as gestational age less than 37 weeks (32% vs. 23%).

These findings substantiate the need to match subjects and controls for confounding factors before evaluating outcome. Ignoring these risk factors may misattribute poor outcome to drug use alone. Also, drug effects may be obscured by not carefully considering the effect risk variables have on the control group.

COCAINE ABUSE IN THE RURAL ENVIRONMENT: A LONGITUDINAL INVESTIGATION

We are currently conducting a 5-year longitudinal research project funded by the National Institute on Drug Abuse. The goal of this study is to investigate and evaluate how cocaine use during pregnancy, maternal psychosocial functioning, and the caregiving environment interact with and impact upon infant medical and developmental outcome during the first 3 years of life. Our population of interest is women who live in the rural South and receive their prenatal care at county public health departments. The vast majority of research on the effects of cocaine use during pregnancy has been conducted with lower SES, urban, polydrug-using women. The rural women followed in this study do not have ready access to drug rehabilitation and use crack cocaine as their primary illicit drug (Eyler et al., 1994; Woods et al., 1993).

Subjects for this longitudinal project were recruited from among: (a) women who received their prenatal care at public health departments primarily located in two rural counties in north central Florida, and (b) women who received no prenatal care but delivered at our hospital. Excluded from the study were women less than 18 years old and women who had a chronic illness that might affect outcome diagnosed prior to the study pregnancy (e.g., diabetes, chronic hypertension, immune complex disease, seizure disorder, mental illness, or retardation). All eligible pregnant women were approached as soon as possible after they began prenatal care or at the time of delivery (if they received no prenatal care). Following consent, each woman was interviewed about her substance use history. Information was collected regarding prescription, over-the-counter, legal, and illegal substance use. In addition, information about factors such as health history, nutrition, physical injuries, and hospitalizations was obtained.

Potential subjects were not aware that they would be approached for participation in this study. If a woman consented to participate she was required to provide a urine sample the same day. If a urine sample could not be obtained she became permanently ineligible for this study. In addition to this unexpected urine sampling, a second urine screen was conducted at the time of delivery. Given that women cannot predict exactly when delivery will occur, this provided a second unpredictable testing time. Urine was screened for propoxyphene, phencyclidine, methaqualone, barbiturates, amphetamines, benzodiazepenes, opiates, cocaine, and cannabinoid metabolites by fluorescence polarization immunoassay methods (Mule & Casella, 1988). Positive toxicology screens were confirmed by gas chromatography/mass spectrometry.

During the 2½-year enrollment period, over 2,000 women were approached for informed consent. Of those, 82% were interviewed and the remainder refused to participate. One hundred fifty-one women who admitted prenatal cocaine use during pregnancy or tested positive for cocaine metabolites and for whom there was no evidence of other illicit drug use except marijuana were identified. Also enrolled were 150 control subjects who showed no evidence of prenatal cocaine use using the same entry and exclusion criteria. Control subjects were matched to targets on the county where they received prenatal care, African-American versus non-African-American, null versus multiparity, and level of socioeconomic status.

Eighty percent of the final 301 subjects were African-American and 20% were non-African-American (3 were of Hispanic background), 87% were multiparous, and 76% scored in the lowest Hollingshead category (Hollingshead, 1975). Subjects from the cocaine-exposed group were significantly more likely to have received no prenatal care (9% vs. 3%), to drink alcohol (38% vs. 14% at > 1–2 drinks per week), and to smoke (69% vs. 14%) than the nonusing group. Cocaine users did not differ significantly from nonusers in marijuana use (10% vs. 7%), and there was no other illicit drug use in either group.

At each interview women reported on their drug use patterns during the previous trimester. It has been established that better information is obtained if questions are asked about drug use in the recent past, but not about current use, which is likely to be more threatening and therefore more inaccurate (Day, Wagener, & Taylor, 1985). Subjects were asked about the timing of their conception, first recognition of pregnancy, and initial confirmation of their pregnancy. Drug use questions were asked using these important markers rather than simply asking questions about first trimester use. These events represent important biological or psychological timepoints in early pregnancy. A woman is unlikely to change her normal drug use patterns if she does not suspect that she is pregnant.

Most subjects were interviewed about prepregnancy and first trimester substance use during their fourth month. Second trimester use was evaluated during their seventh month and third trimester use after delivery. If a subject received no prenatal care and was not enrolled until delivery, she was interviewed at that time about drug use throughout her pregnancy. After delivery all subjects were administered a battery of psychosocial assessments including the following scales: Center for Epidemiological Studies-Depression Scale (Radloff, 1977), Levenson Locus of Control Scale (Levenson, 1974), Rosenberg Self-Esteem Scale (Rosenberg, 1965), Family Support Scale (Dunst, Jenkins, & Trivette, 1984), Life Experiences Survey (Sarason, Johnson, & Siegal, 1978), Family Adaptability and Cohesion Scales (Olson, Portner, & Lavee, 1985), Concepts of Development Questionnaire (Sameroff & Feil, 1984), Parenting Sense of Competence Scale (Gilbaud-Wallston & Wandersman, 1978). This chapter presents the results from the preliminary analyses on the first five of these psychosocial instruments.

At the time of delivery, fetal and neonatal complications were recorded and parent report inventories completed. Newborn measures include urine drug screens, cranial ultrasounds, cry recordings, medical/neurologic, and developmental evaluations. At 1, 12, and 24 months offspring age, maternal psychosocial functioning and the caregiving environment are assessed during home visits. At 6, 18, and 36 months offspring age, in addition to maternal measures, language, developmental, and behavioral assessments of the child are conducted in clinic settings. At all data collection timepoints mothers are interviewed about their substance use patterns since the previous interview.

The major goals of this project include: (a) evaluation of the separate and combined effects on the developing child of crack or cocaine use, maternal and neonatal health status, infant neurobehavioral status and temperament, maternal psychosocial functioning and the caregiving environment; (b) determination of the effects of the amount and timing of prenatal crack or cocaine use, separate from other infant, maternal, and caregiving risk factors, on medical/neurologic status and behavioral/developmental outcome; (c) determination of the relationship of cocaine metabolites in infant urine specimens to early neurobehavioral outcome and their relationship to sequelae.

One of the strengths of this longitudinal project is the prenatal and the 3-year postnatal monitoring of a variety of measures of the mothers' psychosocial functioning. The next section discusses our preliminary findings and the current literature regarding the relationship of cocaine use during pregnancy to self-reported depression, locus of control, self-esteem, social support, and stressful life events at the time of delivery.

PSYCHOSOCIAL EFFECTS ASSOCIATED WITH COCAINE USE IN PREGNANT WOMEN

Depression

In general, women appear to be at greater risk for suffering depressive symptoms than men (Hirschfeld & Cross, 1982; Steele, 1978; Weissman & Klerman, 1977). There is also strong evidence that rates of depressive symptoms are higher in lower SES samples than in middle or higher SES samples (Craig & Van Natta, 1979; Radloff & Rae, 1979; Steele, 1978). Research indicates that young, unmarried, low-SES women with children are more likely to self-report depressive symptoms (Bromet, Solomon, Dunn, & Nicklas 1982; Eaton & Kessler, 1981; Hall, 1990; Kaplan, Roberts, Camacho, & Coyne, 1987).

A number of studies have found a relationship between drug use and depressive symptoms (K. Burns, Melamed, W. Burns, Chasnoff, & Hatcher, 1985; Keeler, Taylor, & Miller, 1979; Mirin, Weiss, Michael, & Solloguls, 1986; Ross & Berzins, 1974; Weiss, Griffin, & Mirin, 1989; Weissman & Myers, 1980). Several researchers have reported that depression is a predictor of an increased likelihood of continued cocaine use (Neuspiel & Hamel, 1992; Ziedonis & Kosten, 1991). Williams and Roberts (1991) found that depression scores on the Beck Depression Inventory (BDI; Beck, Ward, Mendolson, Mock, & Erbaugh, 1961) are significantly higher for chemically dependent women who terminate drug treatment programs prematurely than for women who complete treatment.

It is not clear whether depression promotes drug use or drug use results in depression. There is some evidence that cocaine abusers undergoing treatment have an increased incidence of affective disorders (Gawin, 1986; Weiss, Mirin, Michael, & Sollogub, 1986). Griffin, Weiss, Mirin, and Lange (1989) found that depressive symptoms are more likely to occur in female cocaine users than male users, are more severe, and more often lead to a diagnosis of major depression.

The possibility of greater levels of depression in low-SES women using cocaine is of particular concern given the findings that children of depressed mothers are at risk for behavioral and emotional problems (Ghodsian, Zajicek, & Wolkind, 1984; Rutter, 1966; Zuckerman & Beardslee, 1987). There is evidence that depressed mothers demonstrate flat affect during interaction with their infants, provide less stimulation, and fail to modify their behavior according to the behavior of their infant (Cohn et al., 1986; Field, 1984; Field et al., 1985). Cohn and Tronick (1983) found that even brief experience with simulated maternal depression at 3 months old results in continued negative affect even when the mother returned to normal interaction. Egeland, Kalkoske, Gottesman, and Erickson (1990) found that children who did not exhibit behavioral stability in their withdrawn or acting-out behaviors from first to third grade had mothers with changes in depressive symptomology over that time. The number of self-reported depressive symptoms appears to directly affect the quality of care provided to children and to indirectly affect the quality and organization of the home environment.

Limited research has been published regarding the depressive symptoms of cocaine-using pregnant and postpartum women. We examined infant neurobehavior and maternal depressive symptoms both following delivery and at 1 month postpartum (Woods et al., 1993). We found that cocaine-using women reported significantly more depressive symptoms on the BDI (Beck et al., 1961) following delivery than did the matched control group. At 1 month postpartum, however, there was no longer a significant difference. Several possible reasons for this change were proposed. First, all of the cocaine-using women were under state-mandated investigation for child abuse at the time of the first depression assessment. Second, the cocaine-using women may have been suffering from withdrawal-induced depressive symptoms while they were in the hospital. Third, any initial concern and guilt over the effect of their cocaine use on their infants may have lessened after a month of caregiving.

Alessandri, Sullivan, Imaizumi, and Lewis (1993) recently studied the relationship between infant learning and emotional responsivity and maternal depressive symptoms and stress in women who had used cocaine during pregnancy. They found that at 4 to 8 months postpartum cocaine-using women did not report significantly more depressive symptoms on the BDI than did a control group drawn from the same prenatal population.

The Center for Epidemiologic Studies Depression (CES–D) Scale (Radloff, 1977) is a self-report depression measure. This 20-item scale assesses symptoms of depressed mood and psychophysiologic complaints using a 4-point Likert scale commonly ranging from "rarely or none of the time" (score = 0) to "most of the time" (score = 3). Total scale scores range from 0 to 60, with scores of 16 or greater commonly considered indicative of high depressive symptoms. This cutoff point corresponds to the 80th percentile of scores in community samples (Comstock & Helsing, 1976) and has been used extensively in other studies (Eaton & Kessler, 1981; Frerichs, Aneshensel, & Clark, 1981; Hall & Farel, 1988; Orr & James, 1984). The CES–D demonstrates high internal consistency and good test–retest reliability (Comstock & Helsing, 1976; Radloff, 1977; Weissman, Sholomskas, Pottenger, Prusoff, & Locke, 1977), and validity is supported by correlations with other self-report depression scales and with clinical ratings of depression (Myers & Weissman, 1980; Radloff, 1977; Weissman et al., 1977). Several studies have used the CES–D to evaluate depressive symptoms in pregnant women. Zuckerman, Amaro, Bauchner, and Cabral (1989) found that depressive symptoms are associated with increased life stress, decreased social support, poor weight gain, and the use of cigarettes, alcohol, and cocaine. When they controlled for income, all of the associations remained significant except for the use of cocaine. In another study Zuckerman and colleagues found that CES–D scores are associated with infant unconsolibility and excessive crying. This relationship remains even when controlling for a variety of potentially confounding factors, including cigarette, alcohol, marijuana, and cocaine use (Zuckerman, Bauchner, Parker, & Cabral, 1990).

In our longitudinal study mothers were asked to indicate how often they had experienced the various depressive symptoms during each of the trimesters of pregnancy on a 4-point scale labeled simply "most of the time," "some of the time," "rarely," or "never." At the time of delivery the mean CES–D score for the entire sample was 26.8 and the cocaine-using women had significantly more depressive symptoms ($M = 29.7$) than the nonusing women ($M = 23.2$), $F(1, 295) = 37.34, p < .0001$.

Locus of Control

Internal-external locus of control is a psychological variable that has been the subject of extensive study. *Internal* individuals believe that life events are dependent on their own behavior, whereas *external* individuals feel that life events are the result of fate, luck, or powers beyond their control (Rotter, 1966). The locus of control construct has been found to be a predictor of positive mental and physical health (Brown & Granick, 1983; Lefcourt, Martin, Fick, & Saleh, 1985). People who accept responsibility for most of the events that occur in their lives have been found to be healthier and more productive than individuals who believe that external factors control these events (Edwards & Waters, 1981; Johnson & Sarason, 1978).

The Levenson Locus of Control Scale (LOC) was used in our study to assess the extent to which each mother believed that she has control over her own life. The 24-item instrument is composed of three scales: internality, external powerful others, and external chance. Each scale has eight items scored on a 6-point Likert scale. Alpha coefficients and 1-week test–retest reliabilities range from .64 to .78 for all three scales. This measure is a useful predictor of adult communication patterns with difficult children (Bugental & Shennum, 1984). Stringer and La Greca (1985) found that perceptions of control by powerful others and by chance are related to the potential for abuse by mothers of children of both genders. In addition, a study of alcoholics found that patients with an external locus of control are more likely to relapse after remission (Castor & Parsons, 1977).

We found no significant difference between cocaine-using and nonusing women on internality scores. Our groups did differ, however, on their external powerful others scores, such that cocaine-using women ($M = 19.21$) indicated a greater belief in external powerful others than did nonusers ($M = 14.0$), $F(1, 280) = 13.8$, $p \leq .0002$. Cocaine-using women also had significantly higher scores regarding their belief in external chance ($M = 21.59$) than did nonusing women ($M = 20.09$), $F(1, 280) = 8.36$, $p < .0041$.

Self-Esteem

Self-esteem is generally considered to be the degree to which one values oneself. Two sources of self-esteem are our perceptions of our accomplishments and of how others perceive us (Rosenberg, 1965). It is reasonable to hypothesize that cocaine-using pregnant women might perceive others' opinions of them to be negative. Individuals with low self-esteem are more vulnerable to psychological problems than persons with high self-esteem (Ingham, Kreitman, Miller, Sashidharan, & Surtees, 1986; Meisenhelder, 1986; Robson, 1988). Kemp and Page (1987) found that women experiencing a high-risk pregnancy have significantly lower self-esteem scores on the Rosenberg Self-Esteem Scale (RSS) than do women experiencing a normal pregnancy. Beckman (1978) reported that female alcoholics have significantly lower self-esteem on the RSS than do male alcoholics or female controls. Magura, Siddiqi, Freeman, and Lipton (1991) found that low self-esteem predicts continued cocaine use in a sample of cocaine addicts in treatment.

There are currently no published data on self-esteem in cocaine-using mothers. Our study measured individual self-esteem through the use of the Rosenberg Self-Esteem Scale (Rosenberg, 1965). The RSS is a widely used self-report measure of the self-acceptance aspect of self-esteem (R. B. Burns, 1979). It appears to be a unidimensional measure of global self-esteem (O'Brien, 1985). The instrument consists of 10 items that are commonly scored using a 4- or 5-point Likert scale format from "strongly disagree" to "strongly agree" (Crandall, 1973). The scores for the five positively stated items are reversed when calculating the final score and higher scores indicate increased self-esteem. Silber and Tippett (1965) obtained a 2-week test–retest reliability coefficient of .85 and concurrent validity correlations ranging from .56 to .83. Our preliminary analysis on self-esteem at the time of delivery indicated that cocaine-using women reported lower self-esteem ($M = 29.09$) than did nonusing women ($M = 31.21$), $F(1, 291) = 22.02$, $p < .0001$.

Social Support

Support refers to the resources provided to individuals or families in response to their needs. The stress-reducing and health-maintaining benefits of social support are well documented (Cohen & Syme, 1985; Sarason & Sarason, 1985). Cobb (1976) argued that social support is information that leads an individual to believe that they are: (a) cared for and loved, (b) esteemed and valued, and (c) part of a network of communication and mutual obligation.

Researchers have shown the importance of social support by both the maintenance of drug abstinence during recovery when support is present and the facilitation of drug use when it is lacking (Boyd & Mieczkowski, 1990; Comfort, Shipley, White, & Griffith, 1990; Galanter, 1986; Guinan, 1990). Dunst, Vance, and Cooper (1986) found that social support, along with education level and SES, significantly predicts both delivery and postpartum outcomes. Dunst et al. also found that intervention to provide a support that has been indicated as needed by the family enhances positive parental perception of child functioning and indirectly influences a number of child behavior characteristics (Dunst, Trivette, & Cross, 1986).

Social support was measured in our study using the Family Support Scale (FSS). The FSS is an 18-item self-report measure that assesses the number of sources of support available to an individual and the degree to which the individual perceives them to be helpful. Ratings are made on a 5-point Likert scale ranging from "not at all helpful" to "extremely helpful." The FSS is widely used in research, is a reliable and valid instrument, and was found by Dunst et al. (1984) to be related to personal and familial well-being.

There was no significant difference in the number of sources of support reported by the cocaine-using women in our study ($M = 11.61$) and nonusing controls ($M = 11.47$). There was also no difference in how cocaine-using women in our study ($M = 37.03$) and the nonusing controls ($M = 34.08$) rated the helpfulness of their sources of support.

Life Stress

A life event is generally defined as any commonly experienced situation arising from personal, family, occupational, or financial events that requires change or adjustment in an individual's life pattern. Research indicates that exposure to numerous social stressors over a relatively short period of time increases an individual's susceptibility to disease or psychological distress (B. S. Dohrenwend & B. P. Dohrenwend, 1981).

The Life Experiences Survey (LES) is a 47-item questionnaire designed to assess the life events that have been experienced by an individual during the previous year. Subjects are also asked to indicate whether the events had a positive or negative impact and to rate the degree of impact. Life events included in the survey involve typically positive and negative experiences and experiences that could vary in their positivity or negativity for different individuals. Several types of scores can be calculated including a positive, a negative, and a total life events impact score. The LES includes three blank lines where the subject can list additional stressful events. Kale and Stenmark (1983) found that the LES significantly predicts emotional well-being and adjustment ($r^2 = .20$). Siegel, Johnson, and Sarason (1979) found that the LES is not unduly influenced by mood states such as depression. This is important because the assessment of life changes is retrospective in nature. It is possible that mood states such as depression could simply increase the probability that an individual would report more life changes or perceive them as more stressful.

Research using the LES has suggested that life stress during pregnancy may be related to greater anxiety and depression (Tilden, 1983). Also, mothers' life stress can significantly predict maternal attitudes and quality of mother–infant interaction in the first 4 months of life (Crnic, Greenberg, Robinson, & Ragozin, 1984).

In a longitudinal study of heroin addicts in methadone treatment, Rhoads (1983) found that female compared to male addicts are differentially susceptible to stressful life events, as measured by the LES. She also found that women tend to respond to those stressors with depression and cope through self-medication with heroin. Surprisingly, men and women in drug treatment experience a decrease in the number of positive life events. Rhoads hypothesized that many of the positive events in a drug abuser's life are associated with drug use.

A recent study compared life stress in 36 women who used cocaine during pregnancy to 36 matched controls when their infants were 4 to 8 months old (Alessandri et al., 1993). The groups were matched on maternal age ($\pm$ 3 years), maternal years of schooling, child gender, and number of children in the home. All mothers were African-American single parents with a high school education or less, and all were receiving Aid to Families with Dependent Children. The mothers were also matched for the amount and variability of their use of cigarettes, alcohol, and marijuana. There are no significant differences between the groups on the LES.

In our project the LES was modified so that life events were assessed during pregnancy rather than the customary preceding 12 months. The survey was administered following delivery and degree of impact ratings was on a 7-point Likert scale from "no effect" to "great effect." The reasons for selecting this instrument for our study included: its use of simple language and broad referent terms (spouse/partner), the assessment of the relative impact of each event, and adequate test–retest reliability. There was no significant difference in negative life event impact scores between our cocaine-using women ($M = 10.88$) and nonusing women ($M = 11.99$). Cocaine-using women reported significantly more positive life events ($M = 14.76$) than nonusing women ($M = 10.69$), $F(1, 260) = 11.74, p < .0007$. Cocaine-using women also had significantly higher total life event impact scores ($M = 26.76$) than nonusing women ($M = 21.57$), $F(1, 260) = 7.74, p \le .0058$.

In summary, preliminary analyses of several of our psychosocial measures indicated that the cocaine-using women in our study experienced greater impact from life events during their pregnancies—in particular greater positive life event impact. They also experienced more depressive symptoms and lower self-esteem and were more likely to believe in the influence of external chance and powerful others in their lives.

CONCLUSIONS

The investigation of cocaine use during pregnancy and its effects on infants and mothers is in its early stages. Currently our knowledge about infant effects is more complete than our knowledge about the impact on mothers and their parenting skills. It has become increasingly clear that researchers and the rest of society initially overreacted regarding the potential negative consequences of cocaine use during pregnancy (Chasnoff, 1993; Coles, 1993; Day & Richardson, 1993; Frank & Zuckerman, 1993; Hutchings, 1993; Koren, 1993; Neuspiel, 1993; Richardson & Day, 1994; Zuckerman & Frank, 1992). In many ways the mistakes that were made in the early conduct and dissemination of research in this area make it even more important that we continue the scientific pursuit of knowledge on this topic. A group of infants have been given the negative label "cocaine baby"; most parents, professionals, and citizens have been led to believe that these infants are abnormal and potentially brain damaged. Given this belief there is the realistic possibility that some of these children will develop problems simply because the adults with whom they interact will have negative expectations and will therefore interact with them differently (J. C. Condry & S. Condry, 1976; J. C. Condry & Ross, 1985; Rosenthal & Jacobson, 1968; Woods et al., 1994).

This potential for self-fulfilling prophecy may prevent us from determining the relationship between various risk factors and the children's problems. Poor developmental outcome could be a result of prenatal drug exposure, low adult expectations, or having a mother who has been or is currently drug addicted.

Projects with multidimensional models of analyses, like ours, will provide us with the opportunity to evaluate the differential effects of cocaine use on the physical, psychosocial, and environmental well-being of women and children. Most importantly we can compare their functioning and home environments to other low-SES, rural dyads, thereby clarifying the confounding influences of poverty and its related risks. It is likely that our control sample differs markedly from the general population of pregnant women in our country. The combined anecdotal experience of our trained interviewers indicates that our entire sample suffers from the disadvantages of poverty; including disorganized home environments, poor general health and nutrition, physical abuse from their partners, and poor psychosocial functioning compared to the general population. We expect to verify these strong impressions when complete data analyses are possible.

The limited early results from our longitudinal project have indicated that prenatal cocaine users are more likely than nonusers to experience depression and low self-esteem. Thus cocaine-using women may be at increased risk for poorer parenting. Research on women using other drugs of abuse indicates that the drug-abusing parent faces many adversities because of the interrelationships between drug use, physical abuse, psychological functioning difficulties, and chaotic lifestyles involving more stress and less adequate social support (Bauman & Dougherty, 1983; Blume, 1990; Finnegan, 1991; Finnegan et al., 1981; Goldstein, Bellucci, Spunt, & Miller, 1991; James & Coles, 1991; Murphy et al., 1991; Regan, Ehrlich, & Finnegan, 1987). It is vital that we determine what specific difficulties are faced by women using drugs if we hope to intervene on behalf of their children. If in fact we find that cocaine-exposed infants are at risk primarily due to self-fulfilling prophecy and maternal and environmental differences, then it is likely that traditional, family-centered early intervention can provide effective help (Anastasiow & Harel, 1993; Meisels & Shonkoff, 1990). If future research reveals that these children have in fact suffered biological damage from their prenatal drug exposure then we must work to determine if the damage can be reversed. That process understandably will involve early and intensive family-centered interventions.

ACKNOWLEDGMENTS

Portions of this study were supported by National Institute on Drug Abuse Grant DA05854 and by Clinical Research Center Grant RR00082.

REFERENCES

Alessandri, S. M., Sullivan, M. W., Imaizumi, S., & Lewis, M. (1993). Learning and emotional responsivity in cocaine-exposed infants. *Developmental Psychology, 29,* 989–997.

Anastasiow, N. J., & Harel, S. (1993). *At-risk infants: Interventions, families, and research.* Baltimore, MD: Brooks.

Bauman, P. S., & Dougherty, F. E. (1983). Drug-addicted mothers' parenting and their children's development. *International Journal of the Addictions, 18,* 291–302.

Beck, A. T., Ward, C. H., Mendolson, M., Mock, J., & Erbaugh, J. (1961). An inventory for measuring depression. *Archives of General Psychiatry, 4,* 561–571.

Beckman, L. J. (1978). Self-esteem in women alcoholics. *Journal of Studies on Alcohol, 39,* 491–498.

Behnke, M., Eyler, F. D., Conlon M., Woods, N. S., & Casanova, O. Q. (1994). Multiple risk factors do not identify cocaine use in rural obstetrical patients. *Neurotoxicology and Teratology, 16,* 479–484.

Bingol, N., Fuchs, M., Diaz, V., Stone, R. K., & Gromisoh, D. S. (1987). Teratogenicity of cocaine in humans. *Journal of Pediatrics, 110,* 93–96.

Blume, S. B. (1990). Chemical dependency in women: Important issues. *American Journal of Drug and Alcohol Abuse, 16,* 297–307.

Boyd, C. J., & Mieczkowski, T. (1990). Drug use, health, family and social support in "crack" cocaine users. *Addictive Behaviors, 15,* 481–485.

Brazelton, T. B. (1984). Neonatal behavioral assessment scale (2nd ed.). *Clinics in developmental medicine (Vol. 88).* Philadelphia: Lippincott.

Bromet, E., Solomon, Z., Dunn, L., & Nicklas, N. (1982). Affective disorder in mothers of young children. *British Journal of Psychiatry, 140,* 30–36.

Brown, B. R., & Granick, S. (1983). Cognitive and psychosocial differences between I and E Locus of Control aged persons. *Experimental Aging Research, 9,* 107–110.

Bugental, D. B., & Shennum, W. A. (1984). "Difficult" children as elicitors and targets of adult communication patterns: An attributional-behavioral transactional analysis. *Monographs of the Society for Research in Child Development, 49*(1).

Burns, K., Melamed, J., Burns, W., Chasnoff, I., & Hatcher, R. (1985). Chemical dependence and clinical depression in pregnancy. *Journal of Clinical Psychology, 41,* 851–854.

Burns, R. B. (1979). *The self-concept: Theory, measurement, development and behavior.* New York: Longman.

Cartwright, P. S., Schorge, J. O., & McLaughlin, F. J. (1991). Epidemiologic characteristics of drug use during pregnancy: Experience in a Nashville hospital. *Southern Medical Journal, 84,* 867–870.

Castor, D., & Parsons, O. (1977). Locus of control in alcoholics and treatment outcome. *Journal of Studies on Alcohol, 38,* 2087–2095.

Chasnoff, I. J. (1989). Cocaine, pregnancy, and the neonate. *Women and Health, 15,* 23–35.

Chasnoff, I. J. (1993). Missing pieces of the puzzle. *Neurotoxicology and Teratology, 15,* 287–288.

Chasnoff, I. J., Burns, W. J., Schnoll, S. H., & Burns, K. A. (1985). Cocaine use in pregnancy. *New England Journal of Medicine, 313,* 666–669.

Chasnoff, I. J., Griffith, D. R., MacGregor, S., Dirkes, K., & Burns, K. A. (1989). Temporal patterns of cocaine use in pregnancy. *Journal of the American Medical Association, 261,* 1741–1744.

Chasnoff, I. J., Keith, L. G., & Schnoll, S. H. (1986). Perinatal aspects of maternal addiction. *Current Problems in Obstetrics, Gynecology, and Fertility, 9,* 401–440.

Chasnoff, I. J., Landress, H. J., & Barrett, M. E. (1990). The prevalence of illicit-drug or alcohol use during pregnancy and discrepancies in mandatory reporting in Pinellas County, Florida. *New England Journal of Medicine, 322,* 1202–1206.

Cherukuri, R., Minkoff, H., Feldman, J., Parekh, A., & Glass, L. (1988). A cohort study of alkaloidal cocaine ("crack") in pregnancy. *Obstetrics and Gynecology, 72,* 147–151.

Cobb, S. (1976). Social support as a moderator of life stress. *Psychosomatic Medicine, 38,* 300–314.

Cohen, S., & Syme, S. L. (1985). *Social support and health.* Orlando: Academic Press.

Cohn, J. F., Matis, R., Tronick, E. Z., Connell, D., & Lyons-Ruth, K. (1986). Face-to-face interactions of depressed mothers and their infants. In E. Z. Tronick & T. Field (Eds.), *New directions for child development: Vol. 34. Maternal depression and infant disturbance.* San Francisco: Jossey-Bass.

Cohn, J. F., & Tronick, E. Z. (1983). Three-month-old infants' reactions to simulated maternal depression. *Child Development, 54,* 185–193.

Coles, C. D. (1993). Saying "goodbye" to the "crack baby." *Neurotoxicology and Teratology, 15,* 290–292.

Coles, C. D., Platzman, K. A., Smith, I., James, M. E., & Falek, A. (1992). Effects of cocaine and alcohol use in pregnancy on neonatal growth and neurobehavioral status. *Neurotoxicology and Teratology, 14,* 23–33.

Comfort, M., Shipley, T. E., White, K., & Griffith, E. M. (1990). *Alcoholism Treatment Quarterly, 7,* 129–147.

Comstock, G., & Helsing, K. (1976). Symptoms of depression in two communities. *Psychological Medicine, 6,* 551–563.

Condry, J. C., & Condry, S. (1976). Sex differences: A study in the eye of the beholder. *Child Development, 47,* 812–819.

Condry, J. C., & Ross, D. F. (1985). Sex and aggression: The influence of gender label on the perception of aggression in children. *Child Development, 56,* 225–233.

Craig, T. J., & Van Natta, P. A. (1979). Influence of demographic characteristics on two measures of depressive symptoms. The relation of prevalence and persistence of symptoms with sex, age, education, and marital status. *Archives of General Psychiatry, 36,* 149–154.

Crandall, R. (1973). The measurement of self-esteem and related constructs. In J. Robinson & P. Shaver (Eds.), *Measures of social psychological attitudes* (pp. 45–167). Ann Arbor, MI: Survey Research Center for Institutional for Social Research.

Crnic, K. A., Greenberg, M. T., Robinson, N. M., & Ragozin, A. A. (1984). Maternal stress and social support: Effects on the mother–infant relationship from birth to eighteen months. *American Journal of Orthopsychiatry, 54,* 224–235.

Day, N. L., & Richardson, G. A. (1993). Cocaine use and crack babies: Science, the media, and the miscommunication. *Neurotoxicology and Teratology, 15,* 293–294.

Day, N. L., Wagener, D. K., & Taylor, P. M. (1985). Measurement of substance abuse during pregnancy: Methodologic issues. In T. M. Pinkert (Ed.), *Current research on the consequences of maternal drug abuse* (Research Monograph No. 59) (pp. 36–47). Rockville, MD: National Institute on Drug Abuse.

Dohrenwend, B. S., & Dohrenwend, B. P. (1981). *Stressful life events and their contexts.* New York: Prodist.

Dombrowski, M. P., Wolfe, H. M., Welch, R. A., & Evans, M. I. (1991). Cocaine abuse is associated with abruptio placentae and decreased birth weight, but not shorter labor. *Obstetrics and Gynecology, 77,* 139–141.

Dunst, C. J., Jenkins, V., & Trivette, C. M. (1984). The family support scale: Reliability and validity. *Journal of Individual, Family, and Community Wellness, 1,* 45–52.

Dunst, C. J., Trivette, C. M., & Cross, A. (1986). Mediating influences of social support: Personal, family, and child outcomes. *American Journal of Mental Deficiency, 90,* 403–417.

Dunst, C. J., Vance, S. D., & Cooper, S. (1986). A social systems perspective of adolescent pregnancy: Determinants of parent and parent–child behavior. *Infant Mental Health Journal, 7,* 34–48.

Eaton, W., & Kessler, L. (1981). Rates of symptoms of depression in a national sample. *American Journal of Epidemiology, 114,* 528–538.

Edwards, J. E., & Waters, L. K. (1981). Relationship of locus of control to academic ability, academic performance, and performance-related attributions. *Educational and Psychological Measurement, 41,* 529–531.

Egeland, B., Kalkoske, M., Gottesman, N., & Erickson, M. F. (1990). Preschool behavior problems: Stability and factors accounting for change. *Journal of Child Psychology and Psychiatry, 31,* 891–909.

Eisen, L. N., Field, T. M., Bandstra, E. S., Roberts, J. P., Morrow, C., Larson, S. K., & Steele, B. M. (1991). Perinatal cocaine effects on neonatal stress behavior and performance on the Brazelton Scale. *Pediatrics, 88*, 477–480.

Eyler, F. D., Behnke, M., Conlon, M., Woods, N. S., & Frentzen, B. (1994). Prenatal cocaine use: A comparison of neonates matched on maternal risk factors. *Neurotoxicology and Teratology, 16*, 81–87.

Farrar, H. C., & Kearns, G. L. (1989). Cocaine: Clinical pharmacology and toxicology. *Journal of Pediatrics, 115*, 665–675.

Field, T. (1984). Early interactions between infants and their postpartum mothers. *Infant Behavior and Development, 7*, 527–532.

Field, T., Healy, B., Goldstein, S., Perry, S., Bendell, D., Schanberg, S., Zimmerman, E. A., & Kuhn, C. (1988). Infants of depressed mothers show "depressed" behavior even with nondepressed adults. *Child Development, 59*, 1569–1579.

Field, T., Sandberg, D., Garcia, R., Vega-Lahr, N., Goldstein, S., & Guy, L. (1985). Prenatal problems, postpartum depression, and early mother–infant interactions. *Developmental Psychology, 12*, 1152–1156.

Finnegan, L. P. (1991). Perinatal substance abuse: Comments and perspectives. *Seminars in Perinatology, 15*, 331–339.

Finnegan, L., Oehlberg, S. M., Regan, D. O., & Rudraveff, M. E. (1981). Evaluation of parenting, depression, and violence profiles in methadone-maintained women. *Child Abuse and Neglect, 5*, 267–273.

Frank, D. A., & Zuckerman, B. S. (1993). Children exposed to cocaine prenatally: Pieces of the puzzle. *Neurotoxicology and Teratology, 15*, 298–300.

Frank, D. A., Zuckerman, B. S., Amaro, H., Aboagye, K., Cabral, H., Fried, L., Hingson, R., Kayne, H., Levenson, S. M., Parker, S., Reece, H., & Vinci, R. (1988). Cocaine use during pregnancy: Prevalence and correlates. *Pediatrics, 82*, 888–895.

Frerichs, R. R., Aneshensel, C. S., & Clark, V. A. (1981). Prevalence of depression in Los Angeles County. *American Journal of Epidemiology, 113*, 691–699.

Galanter, M. (1986). Social network therapy for cocaine dependence. *Advances in Alcohol and Substance Abuse, 6*, 159–175.

Gawin, F. H. (1986). New uses of antidepressants in cocaine abuse. *Psychosomatics, 27*, 27–29.

George, S. K., Price, J., Hauth, J. C., Barnette, D. M., & Preston, P. (1991). Drug abuse screening of childbearing women in Alabama public health clinics. *American Journal of Obstetrics and Gynecology, 165*, 924–927.

Ghodsian, M., Zajicek, E., & Wolkind, S. (1984). A longitudinal study of maternal depression on child behavior problems. *Journal of Child Psychology and Psychiatry, 25*, 91–109.

Gilbaud-Wallston, J., & Wandersman, L. P. (1978, November). *Development and utility of the Parenting Sense of Competence Scale.* Paper presented at the meeting of the American Psychological Association, Toronto, Canada.

Gillogley, K. M., Evans, A. T., Hansen, R. L., Samuels, S. J., & Batra, K. K. (1990). The perinatal impact of cocaine, amphetamine, and opiate use detected by universal intrapartum screening. *American Journal of Obstetrics and Gynecology, 163*, 1535–1542.

Golding, J., & Butler, N. R. (1984). The socioeconomic factor. In F. Falkner (Ed.), *Prevention of perinatal mortality and morbidity* (pp. 31–46). Basel: Karger.

Goldstein, P. J., Bellucci, P. A., Spunt, B. J., & Miller, T. (1991). Volume of cocaine use and violence: A comparison between men and women. *Journal of Drug Issues, 21*, 345–367.

Griffin, M. L., Weiss, R. D., Mirin, S. M., & Lange, U. (1989). *Archives of General Psychiatry, 46*, 122–126.

Guinan, J. F. (1990). Extending the system for the treatment of chemical dependencies. *Journal of Strategic and Systemic Therapies, 9*, 11–20.

Hadeed, A. J., & Siegel, S. R. (1989). Maternal cocaine use during pregnancy: Effect on the newborn infant. *Pediatrics, 84*, 205–210.

Hall, L. A. (1990). Prevalence and correlates of depressive symptoms in mothers of young children. *Public Health Nursing, 7*, 71–79.

Hall, L. A., & Farel, A. M. (1988). Maternal stresses and depressive symptoms: Correlates of behavior problems in young children. *Nursing Research, 37*, 156–161.

Handler, A., Kistin, N., Davis, F., & Ferré, C. (1991). Cocaine use during pregnancy: Perinatal outcomes. *American Journal of Epidemiology, 133*, 818–825.

Hans, S. L. (1989). Developmental consequences of prenatal exposure to methadone. *Annals of the New York Academy of Science, 562*, 195–207.

Hirschfeld, R. M. A., & Cross, C. K. (1982). Epidemiology of affective disorders. *Archives of General Psychiatry, 39*, 35–46.

Hollingshead, A. B. (1975). *Four Factor Index of Social Status.* Unpublished manuscript.

Hollinshead, W. H., Griffin, J. F., Scott, H. D., Burke, M. E., Coustan, D. R., & Vest, T. A. (1990). Statewide prevalence of illicit drug use by pregnant women—Rhode Island. *Morbidity and Mortality Weekly Report, 39*, 225–227.

Hume, R. F., O'Donnell, K. J., Stanger, C. L., Killam, A. P., & Gingras, J. L. (1989). In utero cocaine exposure: Observations of fetal behavioral state may predict neonatal outcome. *American Journal of Obstetrics and Gynecology, 161*, 685–690.

Hutchings, D. E. (1993). The puzzle of cocaine's effects following maternal use during pregnancy: Are there reconcilable differences? *Neurotoxicology and Teratology, 15*, 281–286.

Ingham, J. G., Kreitman, N. B., Miller, P. M., Sashidharan, S. P., & Surtees, P. G. (1986). Self-esteem, vulnerability, and psychiatric disorder in the community. *British Journal of Psychiatry, 148*, 375–395.

James, M. E., & Coles, C. D. (1991). Cocaine abuse during pregnancy: Psychiatric considerations. *General Hospital Psychiatry, 13*, 399–409.

Johnson, J. H., & Sarason, I. G. (1978). Life stress, depression, and anxiety: Internal-external control as a moderator variable. *Journal of Psychosomatic Research, 22*, 205–208.

Kale, W. L., & Stenmark, D. E. (1983). A comparison of four life event scales. *American Journal of Community Psychology, 11*, 441–458.

Kaplan, G., Roberts, R., Camacho, T., & Coyne, J. (1987). Psychosocial predictors of depression. *American Journal of Epidemiology, 125*, 206–220.

Keeler, M. H., Taylor, C. I., & Miller, W. C. (1979). Are all recently detoxified alcoholics depressed? *American Journal of Psychiatry, 136*, 586–588.

Keith, L. G., MacGregor, S., Friedell, S., Rosner, M., Chasnoff, I. J., & Sciarra, J. J. (1989). Substance abuse in pregnant women: Recent experience at the Perinatal Center for Chemical Dependence of Northwestern Memorial Hospital. *Obstetrics and Gynecology, 73*, 715–720.

Kemp, V. H., & Page, C. (1987). Maternal self-esteem and prenatal attachment in high-risk pregnancy. *Maternal–Child Nursing Journal, 16*, 195–206.

Kessel, S. S., Kleinman, J. C., Koontz, A. M., Hogue, C. J. R., & Berendes, H. W. (1988). Racial differences in pregnancy outcomes. *Clinics in Perinatology, 15*, 745–754.

Koren, G. (1993). Cocaine and the human fetus: The concept of teratophilia. *Neurotoxicology and Teratology, 15*, 301–304.

Lefcourt, H. M., Martin, R. A., Fick, C. M., & Saleh, W. E. (1985). Locus of control for affiliation and behavior in social interactions. *Journal of Personality and Social Psychology, 48*, 755–759.

Levenson, H. (1974). Activism and the powerful others: Distinctions within the concept of internal-external control. *Journal of Personality Assessment, 38*, 377–383.

Little, B. B., & Snell, L. M. (1991). Brain growth among fetuses exposed to cocaine in utero: Asymmetrical growth retardation. *Obstetrics and Gynecology, 77*, 361–364.

Little, B. B., Snell, L. M., Klein, V. R., & Gilstrap, L. C. (1989). Cocaine abuse during pregnancy: Maternal and fetal implications. *Obstetrics and Gynecology, 73*, 157–160.

Little, B. B., Snell, L. M., Palmore, M. K., & Gilstrap, L. C. (1988). Cocaine use in pregnant women in a large public hospital. *American Journal of Perinatology, 5*, 206–207.

MacGregor, S., Keith, L. G., Bachicha, J. A., & Chasnoff, I. J. (1989). Cocaine abuse during pregnancy: Correlation between prenatal care and perinatal outcome. *Obstetrics and Gynecology, 74*, 882–885.

MacGregor, S. N., Keith, L. G., Chasnoff, I. J., Rosner, M. A., Chisum, G. M., Shaw, P., & Minogue, J. P. (1987). Cocaine use during pregnancy: Adverse perinatal outcome. *American Journal of Obstetrics and Gynecology, 157*, 686–690.

Magura, S., Siddiqi, Q., Freeman, R. C., & Lipton, D. S. (1991). Changes in cocaine use after entry to methadone treatment. *Journal of Addictive Diseases, 10*, 31–45.

Matera, C., Warren, W. B., Moomjy, M., Fink, D. J., & Fox, H. E. (1990). Prevalence of use of cocaine and other substances in an obstetric population. *American Journal of Obstetrics and Gynecology, 163*, 797–801.

McCalla, S., Minkoff, H. L., Feldman, J., Delke, I., Salwin, M., Valencia, G., & Glass, L. (1991). The biologic and social consequences of perinatal cocaine use in an inner-city population: Results of an anonymous cross-sectional study. *American Journal of Obstetrics and Gynecology, 164*, 625–630.

Meisels, S. J., & Shonkoff, J. P. (1990). *Handbook of early childhood intervention.* New York: Cambridge University Press.

Meisenhelder, J. B. (1986). Self-esteem in women: The influence of employment and perception of husband's appraisals. *Image, 18*, 8–14.

Minkoff, H. L., McCalla, S., Delke, I., Stevens, R., Salwen, M., & Feldman, J. (1990). The relationship of cocaine use to syphilis and human immunodeficiency virus infections among inner city parturient women. *American Journal of Obstetrics and Gynecology, 163*, 521–526.

Mirin, S. M., Weiss, R. D., Michael, J. L., & Solloguls, A. C. (1986). Psychopathology in chronic cocaine abusers. *American Journal of Drug and Alcohol Abuse, 12*, 17–29.

Mule, S. J., & Casella, G. A. (1988). Confirmation of marijuana, cocaine, morphine, codeine, amphetamine, methamphetamine, phencyclidine by GC/MS in urine following immunoassay screening. *Journal of Analytical Toxicology, 12*, 102–107.

Murphy, J. M., Jellinek, M., Quinn, D., Smith, G., Poitrast, F. G., & Goshko, M. (1991). Substance abuse and serious child maltreatment: Prevalence, risk, and outcome in a court sample. *Child Abuse and Neglect, 15*, 197–211.

Myers, J. K., & Weissman, M. M. (1980). Use of a self-report symptom scale to detect depression in a community sample. *American Journal of Psychiatry, 137*, 1081–1084.

Nanda, D., Feldman, J., Delke, I, Chintalapally, S., & Minkoff, H. (1990). Syphilis among parturients at an inner city hospital: Association with cocaine use and implications for congenital syphilis rates. *New York State Journal of Medicine, 90*, 488–490.

National Institute of Medicine. (1985). *Preventing low birthweight.* Washington, DC: National Academy Press.

Neerhof, M. G., MacGregor, S. N., Retzky, S. S., & Sullivan, T. P. (1989). Cocaine abuse during pregnancy: Peripartum prevalence and perinatal outcome. *American Journal of Obstetrics and Gynecology, 161*, 633–638.

Neuspiel, D. R. (1993). Cocaine and the fetus: Mythology of severe risk. *Neurotoxicology and Teratology, 15*, 305–306.

Neuspiel, D. R., & Hamel, S. C. (1991). Cocaine and infant behavior. *Developmental and Behavioral Pediatrics, 12*, 55–64.

Neuspiel, D. R., & Hamel, S. C. (1992). Cocaine use and post partum psychiatric symptoms. *Psychological Reports, 70*, 51–56.

Neuspiel, D. R., Hamel, S. C., Hochberg, E., Greene, J., & Campbell, D. (1991). Maternal cocaine use and infant behavior. *Neurotoxicology and Teratology, 13*, 229–233.

O'Brien, E. J. (1985). Global self-esteem scales: Unidimensional or multidimensional? *Psychological Reports, 57*, 383–389.

Olson, D. H., Portner, J., & Lavee, Y. (1985). *FACES III.* St. Paul, MN: Family Social Science, University of Minnesota.

O'Malley, P. M., Bachman, J. G., & Johnston, L. D. (1988). Period, age, and cohort effects on substance use among young Americans: A decade of change, 1976–86. *American Journal of Public Health, 78*, 1315–1321.

Orr, S., & James, S. (1984). Maternal depression in an urban pediatric practice: Implications for health care delivery. *American Journal of Public Health, 74,* 363–364.

Ostrea, E. M., Brady, M., Gause, S., Raymundo, A. L., & Stevens, M. (1992). Drug screening of newborns by meconium analysis: A large-scale, prospective, epidemiologic study. *Pediatrics, 89,* 107–113.

Parker, S., Greer, S., & Zuckerman, B. (1988). Double jeopardy: The impact of poverty on early child development in children at risk: Current social and medical challenges. *Pediatric Clinics of North America, 35,* 1227–1240.

Radloff, L. (1977). The CES-D scale: A self-report depression scale for research in the general population. *Applied Psychological Measurement, 1,* 385–401.

Radloff, L. S., & Rae, D. S. (1979). Susceptibility and precipitating factors in depression: Sex differences and similarities. *Journal of Abnormal Psychology, 88,* 174–181.

Regan, D. O., Ehrlich, S. M., & Finnegan, L. P. (1987). Infants of drug addicts: At risk for child abuse, neglect, and placement in foster care. *Neurotoxicology and Teratology, 9,* 315–319.

Rhoads, D. L. (1983). A longitudinal study of life stress and social support among drug abusers. *International Journal of the Addictions, 18,* 195–222.

Richardson, G. A., & Day, N. L. (1991). Maternal and neonatal effects of moderate cocaine use during pregnancy. *Neurotoxicology and Teratology, 13,* 455–460.

Richardson, G. A., & Day, N. L. (1994). Detrimental effects of prenatal cocaine exposure: Illusion or reality? *Journal of the American Academy of Child and Adolescent Psychiatry, 33,* 28–34.

Robson, P. J. (1988). Self-esteem: A psychiatric view. *British Journal of Psychiatry, 153,* 6–15.

Rolfs, R. T., Goldberg, M., & Sharrar, R. G. (1990). Risk factors for syphilis: Cocaine use and prostitution. *American Journal of Public Health, 80,* 853–857.

Rosenberg, M. (1965). *Society and the adolescent self-image.* Princeton, NJ: Princeton University Press.

Rosenthal, R., & Jacobson, L. (1968). *Pygmalion in the classroom.* New York: Holt, Rinehart & Winston.

Ross, F., & Berzins, J. (1974). Personality characteristics of female addicts on the MMPI. *Psychological Reports, 35,* 779–784.

Rotter, J. B. (1966). Generalized expectancies for internal versus external control of reinforcement. *Psychological Monographs, 80*(609).

Rutter, M. (1966). The developmental psychopathology of depression: Issues and perspectives. In M. Rutter, C. E. Izard, & P. B. Read (Eds.), *Depression in young people* (pp. 3–30). New York: Guilford.

Sameroff, A. J., & Chandler, M. J. (1975). Reproductive risk and the continuum of caretaking casualty. In F. D. Horowitz (Ed.), *Review of child development research* (pp. 187–244). Chicago: University of Chicago Press.

Sameroff, A. J., & Feil, L. A. (1984). Parental concepts of development. In I. Sigel (Ed.), *Parental belief systems: The psychological consequences for children* (pp. 83–104). Hillsdale, NJ: Lawrence Erlbaum Associates.

Sarason, I., Johnson, H., & Siegal, M. (1978). Assessing the impact of life-changes: Development of the life experiences survey. *Journal of Consulting and Clinical Psychology, 46,* 932–946.

Sarason, I. G., & Sarason, B. R. (1985). *Social support: Theory, research and applications.* Dordrecht, The Netherlands: Nijhoff.

Schutzman, D. L., Frankenfield-Chernicoff, M., Clatterbaugh, H. E., & Singer, J. (1991). Incidence of intrauterine cocaine exposure in a suburban setting. *Pediatrics, 88,* 825–827.

Shiono, P. H., & Klebanoff, M. A. (1993). A review of risk scoring for preterm birth. *Clinics in Perinatology, 20,* 107–125.

Siegel, J. M., Johnson, J. H., & Sarason, I. G. (1979). Mood states and the reporting of life changes. *Journal of Psychosomatic Research, 23,* 103–108.

Silber, E., & Tippett, J. (1965). Self-esteem: Clinical assessment and measurement validation. *Psychological Reports, 16,* 1017–1071.

Sloan, L. B., Gay, J. W., Snyder, S. W., & Bales, W. R. (1992). Substance abuse during pregnancy in a rural population. *Obstetrics and Gynecology, 79,* 245–248.

Steele, R. E. (1978). Relationship of race, sex, social class, and social mobility to depression in normal adults. *Journal of Social Psychology, 104,* 37–47.

Streissguth, A. P., Grant, T. M., Barr, H. M., Brown, Z. A., Martin, J. C., Mayock, D. E., Ramey, S. L., & Moore, L. (1991). Cocaine and the use of alcohol and other drugs during pregnancy. *American Journal of Obstetrics and Gynecology, 164,* 1239–1243.

Stringer, S. A., & La Greca, A. M. (1985). Correlates of child abuse potential. *Journal of Abnormal Child Psychology, 13,* 217–226.

Tilden, V. P. (1983). The relation of life stress and social support to emotional disequilibrium during pregnancy. *Research in Nursing and Health, 6,* 167–174.

Vega, W. A., Kolody, B., Hwang, J., & Noble, A. (1993). Prevalence and magnitude of perinatal substance exposures in California. *New England Journal of Medicine, 329,* 850–854.

Weathers, W. T., Crane, M. M., Sauvain, K. J., & Blackhurst, D. W. (1993). Cocaine use in women from a defined population: Prevalence at delivery and effects on growth in infants. *Pediatrics, 91,* 350–354.

Webber, M. P., Lambert, G., Bateman, D. A., & Hauser, W. A. (1993). Maternal risk factors for congenital syphilis: A case-control study. *American Journal of Epidemiology, 137,* 415–422.

Weiss, R. D., Griffin, M. L., & Mirin, M. (1989). Diagnosing major depression in cocaine abusers: The use of depression rating scales. *Psychiatry Research, 28,* 335–343.

Weiss, R. D., Mirin, S. M., Michael, J. L., & Sollogub, A. C. (1986). Psychopathology in chronic cocaine abusers. *American Journal of Alcohol and Drug Abuse, 12,* 17–29.

Weissman, M., & Klerman, G. (1977). Sex differences and epidemiology of depression. *Archives of General Psychiatry, 34,* 98–111.

Weissman, M. M., & Myers, J. K. (1980). Clinical depression in alcoholics. *American Journal of Psychiatry, 137,* 372–373.

Weissman, M. M., Sholomskas, D., Pottenger, M., Prusoff, B. A., & Locke, B. Z. (1977). Assessing depressive symptoms in five psychiatric populations: A validation study. *American Journal of Epidemiology, 106,* 203–214.

Williams, M. T., & Roberts, C. S. (1991). Predicting length of stay in long-term treatment for chemically dependent females. *International Journal of the Addictions, 26,* 605–613.

Woods, N. S., Eyler, F. D., Behnke, M., & Conlon, M. (1993). Cocaine use during pregnancy: Maternal depressive symptoms and infant neurobehavior over the first month. *Infant Behavior and Development, 16,* 83–98.

Woods, N. S., Eyler, F. D., Conlon, M., Wobie, K., Behnke, M., Anderson, C., & Maag, L. (1994, June). *Pygmalion in the cradle: Observer bias against cocaine-exposed infants.* Paper presented at the Ninth International Conference on Infant Studies, Paris.

Ziedonis, D. M., & Kosten, T. R. (1991). Depression as a prognostic factor for pharmacological treatment of cocaine dependence. *Psychopharmacology Bulletin, 27,* 337–343.

Zuckerman, B., Amaro, H., Bauchner, H., & Cabral, H. (1989). Depressive symptoms during pregnancy: Relationship to health behaviors. *American Journal of Obstetrics and Gynecology, 160,* 1107–1111.

Zuckerman, B., Bauchner, H., Parker, S., & Cabral, H. (1990). Maternal depressive symptoms during pregnancy, and newborn irritability. *Developmental and Behavioral Pediatrics, 11,* 190–194.

Zuckerman, B. S., & Beardslee, W. R. (1987). Maternal depression: A concern for pediatricians. *Pediatrics, 79,* 110–117.

Zuckerman, B., & Bresnahan, K. (1991). Developmental and behavioral consequences of prenatal drug and alcohol exposure. *Pediatric Clinics of North America, 38,* 1387–1406.

Zuckerman, B., & Frank, D. A. (1992). "Crack kids": Not broken. *Pediatrics, 89,* 337–339.

Zuckerman, B., Frank, D. A., Hingson, R., Amaro, H., Levenson, S. M., Kayne, H., Parker, S., Vinci, R., Aboagye, K., Fried, L. E., Cabral, H., Timperi, R., & Bauchner, H. (1989). Effects of maternal marijuana and cocaine use on fetal growth. *New England Journal of Medicine, 320,* 762–768.

IV

INTERVENTION

The need to intervene in the lives of families with children who have been exposed to cocaine is obvious. There have been many systematic attempts to address these problems. Although the results of such intervention remain to be determined, there is no question as to the importance of intervention itself. The two chapters in this section highlight the types of approaches that can be taken. Brinker and his colleagues attempt to address the intervention from an ecological point of view, in which the family and child are treated. An ecological point of view stresses the multiply determined nature of the problem. It is a broad perspective that treats the cocaine-exposed child and family to a set of interventions that seeks to not only improve the cognitive and emotional well-being of the child but to work with the family, teaching them new social skills.

A somewhat contrasting model is the work of Field and her group. Field proposes a highly specific intervention procedure, one where the child is the target of the intervention. These two points of view and models serve to contrast what are perhaps two of the important ways of treating children and families. The first argues for a broad approach and is predicated on the principle that cocaine exposure requires a broad intervention approach, including the family as well as the child. It is an intervention strategy that can hold for any problem area and as such represents what can be called the *broad* model of intervention. Its negative feature resides in its lack of specificity vis-à-vis a particular disorder, in this case cocaine exposure. Although it is clear that cocaine exposure is brought about by a diverse set of factors and that a large number of problems need to be met in an intervention strategy, one could substitute any problem for the cocaine exposure and the same intervention would be used. A contrasting approach is best seen in medicine, where a particular infection is treated with particular antibiotics in order to focus treatment that is specifically related to a disorder. One hopes that when we know enough about the causes of development, such specific treatments will become available.

Field's intervention for cocaine-exposed children is specific, namely massage. Such a treatment strategy presents us with the type of alternative model we seek. Although massaging infants appears to be successful in treating cocaine-exposed children, more data are necessary. This approach, looking at a specific intervention strategy, does contrast to the more general approach taken by the Brinker Group.

Of course, these approaches bring to mind the problem of who should be treated for the difficulty. Obviously the cocaine-exposed child may be at risk for multiple disorders, including attentional difficulties, impulse control, and so on. However, as this volume attempts to make clear, a large part of the developmental failures may be due to the environmental factors associated with families in which cocaine is used. If this is the case, intervention at the level of the family is critical, not only for the prevention of further cocaine exposure, such as in passive receiving of cocaine in a family continuing to use it, but in terms of making sure the family interacts with the cocaine-exposed infant in a constructive and facilitating fashion, a fashion in which the child's capacities can be strengthened.

Intervention research is relatively undeveloped. This is because we have not yet been able to identify specific intervention strategies for specific difficulties. However, our model appears to suggest that poor outcomes of children exposed to cocaine are due primarily to the environments in which they live. If this proves to be the case, our research strategies in terms of intervention should be focused on familial variables. If, however, our research confirms specific deficits located in the child as a function of the exposure, then our interventions obviously need to be directed toward the child. Without sufficient information about the cause of developmental difficulties one can only proceed under the assumption that intervention programs need to address both the child and the family. We have chosen to focus on intervention programs targeting the child. We recognize that a large and concerted effort is being expended toward drug treatment intervention in the lives of cocaine-using pregnant women.[1] These two chapters, then, reflect only part of the overall effort in intervention research.

---

[1]The Perinatal 20 Treatment Research Demonstration Program of the National Institute on Drug Abuse is evaluating 20 different approaches to drug treatment interventions. Strategies range from home-based services to residential treatment for women in different cities in a variety of living situations. This project perhaps represents the most fruitful approach, as the best intervention for children is prevention of drug exposure and provision of a drug-free home.

17

▼▼▼▼▼▼▼

Effective Early Intervention for Children Prenatally Exposed to Cocaine in an Inner-City Context

Abigail Baxter
Linda S. Butler
Richard P. Brinker
Wynetta A. Frazier
Delores M. Wedgeworth
University of Illinois at Chicago

Since the mid-1980s, cocaine use has been a focal point in political and legal arenas as its consumption has escalated across all socioeconomic classes, ethnicities, races, and ages (Chasnoff, 1989; Gold, 1987). Cocaine is reported to be the most prevalent illicit drug used by women of childbearing age, with between 8% and 30% of mothers using it during their pregnancies (Bandstra et al., 1989; Brodsky, Hurt, & Webb, 1992; Chasnoff, 1989; Clayton, 1986; Frank et al., 1988; Little, Snell, Palmore, & Gilstrap, 1988; Pollin, 1985; Vega, Kolody, Hwang, & Noble, 1993). The actual percentages of use may be even higher because the lack of legal mandates and funds to systematically perform drug screening as part of routine obstetric care and upon delivery (Moore, 1992) and women's reluctance to report prenatal substance use (Segal, 1991) make obtaining actual prevalence rates extremely difficult. These obstacles may become more difficult as drug prosecution and child abuse laws become more stringent, resulting in drug-using mothers opting for nonhospital deliveries. Maternal fear of referral to child protective services for abuse or neglect also deters many women, especially those of low socioeconomic status (SES), from reporting their drug use. Despite the diversity in prevalence figures due to differences in geographic areas, methods of collecting data, and SES levels, the ramifications of cocaine use by women of childbearing age warrant attention. Equally important are the effects of prenatal cocaine exposure on the exposed child's subsequent development.

INITIAL MEDICAL OUTCOME RESEARCH
AND MEDIA ATTENTION

In 1983 the first report of an association between prenatal cocaine use and adverse perinatal effects appeared in the medical literature (Acker, Sachs, Tracey, & Wise, 1983). Two years later the first empirical study revealing neonatal and perinatal anomalies in infants prenatally exposed to cocaine was published (Chasnoff, W. J. Burns, Schnoll, & K. A. Burns, 1985). In subsequent years published studies were mostly anecdotal descriptions of clinical findings by pediatric physicians and researchers, or had small sample sizes and questionable methodologies (Bingol et al., 1986; Chasnoff, Lewis, Griffith, & Willey, 1989; Cohen, Anday, & Leitner, 1989; Dixon, Coen, & Crutchfield, 1987; Geggel, McInerny, & Estes, 1989; Isenberg, Spierer, & Inkelis, 1987; Riley & Porat, 1987). All these studies shared the common premise that an unhealthy and dangerous adult drug could cause nothing but biological and developmental harm to the neonate. The media have taken a similar position and presented "cocaine babies" in a very negative light (Besharov, 1989; Daley, 1991; Hopkins, 1990; Howze & Howze, 1991; Toufexis, 1991; Viadero, 1989; Waller, 1992–1993). The majority of media information has been exaggerated and presumptuous, and projects an inaccurate vision of the group of cocaine-exposed children as a "biounderclass" (Rist, 1991, p. 5). Recently, however, fewer negative stories have emerged in the media (Gerber, 1990; Viadero, 1992) and scientific research has become more methodologically refined.

RECENT MEDICAL, DEVELOPMENTAL,
AND BEHAVIORAL RESEARCH

In the late 1980s, much of the empirical research on prenatal cocaine exposure, using larger samples, continued to report negative medical consequences (Kaye, Elkind, Goldberg, & Tytun, 1989; Zuckerman et al., 1989). Although several biomedical outcomes, including preterm labor (Acker et al., 1983; Keith et al., 1989; MacGregor et al., 1987; Young, Vosper, & Phillips, 1992) and intrauterine growth retardation (Bingol, Fuchs, Diaz, Stone, & Gromisch, 1987; Hadeed & Siegel, 1989; Ryan, Ehrlich, & Finnegan, 1987; Young et al., 1992) were sometimes present in the neonatal period, conclusive medical sequelae of children prenatally exposed to cocaine in utero were indeterminable. Nevertheless, medical research continued to describe biomedical characteristics in some children (Kelley, Walsh, & Thompson, 1991). Overall, this research indicates that, unlike prenatal alcohol exposure resulting in fetal alcohol syndrome, prenatal exposure to cocaine does not lead to a specified cluster of anomalies or sequelae (Abel, 1984; Clarren & Smith, 1978; Day et al., 1989; Jones, Smith, Ulleland, & Streissguth, 1973).

Beyond medical sequelae, what *is* known about children prenatally exposed to cocaine is anecdotal and remains to be demonstrated empirically. There are relatively fewer studies detailing the effects of prenatal cocaine exposure in infancy and childhood. Follow-up with older children is complicated by high rates of family mobility, financial instability, disenfranchisement from social and medical services, and often continued maternal drug abuse (Hansen & Ulrey, 1993). Some studies have reported atypical emotional expression (Alessandri, Sullivan, Imaizumi, & Lewis, 1993; Lester et al., 1991), motor disabilities (Schneider, Griffith, & Chasnoff, 1989), qualitative differences in play (Rodning, Beckwith, & Howard, 1989, 1991), and different patterns of learning (Alessandri et al., 1993). Other studies have reported average performance on the Bayley Scales of Infant Development (Chasnoff, Griffith, Freier, & Murray, 1992); however studies of visual recognition memory (Struthers & Hansen, 1992) and contingency learning (Alessandri et al., 1993) suggest differences between cocaine-exposed and nonexposed children. These studies are too recent and too few to lead to any conclusive results about the effects of prenatal cocaine exposure on intellectual and social development.

Thus, a single medical, behavioral, or developmental effect or group of effects common to all infants and children prenatally exposed to cocaine has yet to be determined. Because the literature on the consequences of prenatal cocaine exposure is itself in its infancy, especially in terms of knowledge about developmental outcome for these children, there is no evidence to suggest the necessity of the label of *fetal cocaine syndrome* (Hansen & Ulrey, 1993; Schutter & Brinker, 1992). As Myers, Olson, and Kaltenbach (1992) asserted, "the simple truth at this point is that we do not yet know what the effects are" (p. 1).

CONFOUNDS TO ACQUIRING KNOWLEDGE ABOUT PRENATAL COCAINE EXPOSURE

The investigation of the effects of prenatal cocaine exposure is a relatively new field and it is plagued with inadequate research designs and multiple confounds. It is often impossible to quantify the amount and frequency of maternal cocaine use. Toxicologies can only detect cocaine use within the past 3 days and often maternal report is the only indicator of drug use available to researchers (Hansen & Ulrey, 1993). Many women and exposed children are not identified because toxicology screening is not a standardized, national procedure (Marshall, 1991; Moore, 1992). Most investigations of the effects of prenatal cocaine exposure have been conducted on poor minority women and their children, perhaps because they are more likely to be identified. Hence, research has used biased samples and may not accurately represent the extent of the problem.

In addition to prenatal cocaine use, studies are confounded by other factors in these families' lives that put these children at risk for developmental difficulties. Factors such as extreme poverty, exclusion from society's mainstream, and continued cocaine use may also lead to developmental delay. These other variables also interfere with maintaining consistent contact with families, resulting in difficulty implementing longitudinal designs (Hansen & Ulrey, 1993). The inability to follow specific families for relatively long periods of time precludes the actual investigation of the long-term effects of cocaine on the child and the family. Thus, we are forced to use cross-sectional research designs that do not capture individual developmental trajectories.

Additionally, maternal lifestyles present difficulties in separating direct effects of cocaine from indirect effects of other variables such as poverty, poor nutrition, and poor prenatal care. Biologically, the physical condition of the pregnant cocaine-using woman contributes to the deteriorating health of the cocaine-exposed fetus. Pregnant women who use substances exhibit a higher rate of infectious diseases than drug-free women (Chasnoff, 1987; Chasnoff & Chisum, 1987; Frank et al., 1988). Vitamin deficiencies are especially prevalent in cocaine users due to cocaine's anorexic action (Ryan et al., 1987). Women who use cocaine often have decreased interest in bodily needs and irregular menstrual cycles that delay awareness of pregnancy and increase fetal risk due to excessive and strenuous activity (Chasnoff, 1987). Several studies report that 60% to 70% of cocaine-abusing pregnant women received no prenatal care (Cherukuri, Minkoff, Feldman, Parekh, & Glass, 1988; Dixon & Bejar, 1989; Oro & Dixon, 1987). Clearly, these concomitants of cocaine use contribute to reduced maternal and fetal health, and present potential complications in labor, delivery, and neonatal health.

EARLY INTERVENTION FOR CHILDREN
PRENATALLY EXPOSED TO COCAINE

In some states, children with histories of prenatal cocaine exposure may be excluded from receiving early intervention (EI). Although prenatal cocaine exposure does not automatically lead to developmental delay, exposed infants are often considered to be at risk for delay and thus in need of EI as a form of primary prevention. However, some states do not mandate EI services for at-risk children. Thus, it may only be cocaine-exposed children with identifiable disabilities who become enrolled in EI programs. Unfortunately this invites inaccurate attribution of the disability to the prenatal cocaine exposure, and excludes from eligibility cocaine-exposed children who may, in fact, benefit from EI.

An Ecological Framework for Early Intervention

Effective EI views the child and his or her social environment from an ecological perspective. Incorporating a child's own constitution and influential surroundings into a model for EI requires a framework that appreciates an entire range of contextual variables. An ecological framework allows attention to be shifted away from linear cause-and-effect relationships toward consideration of the child in a holistic manner. This perspective is different from intervention strategies used in the 1960s that focused primarily on prevention of cognitive deficits (Simeonsson, Cooper, & Scheiner, 1982) and treatment of the individual child (Zeanah & McDonough, 1989).

An ecological viewpoint holds two assumptions (Stokols, 1992). The first is that in any situation or setting, multiple physical and social effects jointly and developmentally influence outcomes. The development of children is determined by interactive, reciprocal, immediate, relational, societal, intrinsic, and extrinsic factors, all exerting force in varying degrees (Evans, 1992). The second assumption heralds the strength of personal attributes, including psychological dispositions and behavioral patterns. Although individual cases can be cited in which personal attributes overcame environmental forces, the multifarious interaction between both forces is elusive. The ecological viewpoint advocates for consideration of, investigation of, and intervention on the interplay between constitutional and environmental factors that influence child health and developmental outcomes. Such a broad perspective is necessary to avoid mistakenly identifying precursors of pathology based on the consideration of less than adequate ecological variables (Cicchetti & Manly, 1990; Rutter, 1982). This is especially true for children prenatally exposed to cocaine. Intervention strategies must recognize that prenatal drug exposure may compromise the individual, but environmental factors may also exert remediating forces (Hansen & Ulrey, 1993). Alternatively, environmental factors, and not cocaine exposure, may negatively impact development.

Systems Theory.   Systems theory offers a foundation for building ecologically based EI. Bronfenbrenner (1977) proposed a detailed model of systemic influences that incorporates the multiple strata of interacting forces comprising an individual's ecologies. These layers—termed *microsystem, mesosystem, exosystem,* and *macrosystem*—influence developmental processes and can be perceived as moving from most proximal to most distal in terms of vicinity to an individual. The microsystem involves an individual's relationships to significant and immediate people and activities. Caregiver–child relationships are an important microsystem for children. The mesosystem includes the relationships between these microsystemic people and settings. For children, significant mesosystem elements include mother–father or aunt–grandmother relationships. The exosystem is composed of environmental aspects that indirectly modify the context of an individual's ecology. A neighborhood, its culture, and its opportunities and limitations are exosystemic variables. The macrosystem includes the social, political, and economic structures that impact an individual's world, such as social service provisions and legal boundaries. The child and family are part of a larger macrosystem that includes societal influences, SES factors, and current living conditions.

Systems theory maintains that the microsystem, mesosystem, exosystem, and macrosystem are all interconnected in their organizational influence on a person's world (Bronfenbrenner, 1977). To intervene at just one level of the system offers a limited view of the individual. According to systems theory, functioning is only observable and understood when both the individual and the life situation are studied. Sameroff and Fiese (1990) reviewed research and concluded that the *number* of risk factors better determines outcome than the specific factors present. Sameroff (1975) contended that "in many cases, family and cultural factors may be more important than factors in the child" (p. 192) in preventing developmental disabilities.

Because research suggests that there is little evidence of cognitive impairment due to prenatal cocaine exposure alone, examination of other domains of child competence and behavior beyond those defined by IQ or developmental quotient scores is clearly indicated (Shonkoff, Hauser-Cram, Krauss, & Upshur, 1992). The multifaceted developmental outcomes of children are multiply determined by variables including maternal childrearing attitudes, beliefs and coping skills, psychological characteristics (Sameroff & Seifer, 1983), and stimulation within the home environment (Silber, 1989; Solnit, 1984). Developmental disabilities in the majority of children are due to psychological and social factors. Only the most seriously biologically insulted children will be unresponsive to social and environmental persuasion (Sameroff, 1986). Hence, EI focusing on multiple areas of development increases the identification of important risk factors and offers a more accurate portrait and prediction of development.

Transactional Model of Development. Sameroff and Chandler's (1975) transactional model of development posits mutual contributions of both environmental and constitutional variables. The model also maintains that "the complex mutual influences that operate between the child and his environment . . . together serve to dissipate or amplify the effects of earlier developmental insults" (p. 189). As with considering systemic levels' influence on development, the consideration of both reproductive and caretaking factors offers more successful developmental predictions. The transactional model addresses the complexities among constitutional and environmental forces, emphasizing dyadic interactions between caregiver and child. The model stresses the dynamic nature of both factors, elaborating on a two-dimensional interactional model that regards constitution and environment in a static manner. Thus, the transactional model addresses the continual interplay, mutual influence, and interdependency of caregiver and child, and validates the ecological framework.

Hence, effective EI for children prenatally exposed to cocaine calls for a framework that reaches beyond the child. Addressing ecological risk factors at multiple systemic levels of child proximity ensures more comprehensive and effective EI. This entails exploring and addressing multiple child domains as well as underdeveloped or malfunctioning systemic influences including parents, family members, and sociocultural conditions.

Effective Early Intervention Strategies

The Three Rs. A working synthesis for EI incorporating systems and transactional perspectives is the "three Rs": *remediation, redefinition,* and *re-education* (Sameroff & Fiese, 1990). Remediation is changing the child through medical, therapeutic or educational interventions. Regardless of the etiology of the behavioral symptoms (e.g., maternal drug use, poor parenting environment), remediation is used to change the child's behavior. It is presumed that by changing the child's behavior there will also be systemic changes. Remediation is utilized when there is an identifiable problem in the child that can be changed. For example, remediation may be used to teach a child to vocalize rather than use gestures when he or she wants to indicate something to a caregiver.

Redefinition involves altering the caregiver's interpretation of the child and/or his or her behavior. Redefinition is used in instances in which a child may or may not have an identifiable problem but the caregiver's relationship with the child is limiting his or her development (Sameroff & Fiese, 1990). Redefinition may help the caregiver of a child with very little affective expression view these behaviors as manifestations of biological or temperamental differences rather than rejection of the caregiver.

Re-education occurs when caregivers are taught a different or new way of reacting to a child's behavior. Re-education is only used when there are no changes that can be brought about in the child and caregivers have been identified as needing certain skills or knowledge that are necessary for optimal parenting. The caregiver of a child who is very active and described as "bad" may learn to "catch the child being good" as a strategy for decreasing the rate of negative behaviors and increasing the rate of positive behaviors seen in the child. These three methods of intervention may occur at all levels of the family system through the mechanism of the Individualized Family Service Plan (IFSP).

The Individualized Family Service Plan. Federal law (Public Law 99-457) mandates that the IFSP serve as the treatment plan for EI. The IFSP is the backbone of EI services and is used to implement comprehensive EI. It details strengths that the child and family possess, as well as needs and concerns for both the family and the individual child. A child has a much better chance of thriving in a family that is thriving (Davidson, 1991). As there is not a "typical" child exposed to cocaine, there is not a "typical" curriculum for children with histories of prenatal cocaine exposure. EI services should be based on "existing knowledge of effective developmental and educational strategies used in other high-risk groups of children and their families" (Hansen & Ulrey, 1993, p. 123). For example, if a child has cerebral palsy, whether or not his or her mother used cocaine during the pregnancy, there are EI strategies to use with that child to make the cerebral palsy less limiting.

As with any other child with developmental delays or at risk for developmental delay, EI for the prenatally cocaine-exposed child is individually based with extensive family involvement in the development of the IFSP. Needs and concerns are articulated by the family rather than originating from the professionals' analyses of the child and the family. Caregivers and professionals are required to work as partners to develop and implement the IFSP. An assessment of the child's health status is completed, along with measures assessing his or her level of development in each of the following developmental domains: fine motor, gross motor, cognitive, speech/language, social, and activities of daily living. Based on the specific constellation of strengths, needs, and concerns in each of the child domains, as well as families' needs and goals as they relate to optimal child development, the IFSP is developed and serves as the child's and the family's EI treatment plan.

Development of an IFSP with children and families with a history of maternal cocaine use may not be a simple procedure. Remediation can be used when determining child goals for the IFSP, but may be more difficult to implement for the child with a history of prenatal cocaine exposure. It may be necessary for the child to have a complete physical examination and diagnostic work-up. The child may require vaccinations due to inconsistent medical care in the past. Engaging the caregiver to participate in developing the child goals may prove difficult, as many caregivers ordered by the courts to attend EI programs because of drug use often do not see the need for EI services. Caregivers often state that their child is developing appropriately and does not need EI. This puts the EI professional in the position of having to engage the caregiver in a process that he or she does not value.

In conducting remediation with a child one must view the child in terms of his or her particular developmental needs and the strengths and resources available in his or her social ecology. Children's individual learning styles are also important to consider. Rather than insisting that the child learn in the manner prescribed by the EI professional or even the caregiver, remediation is attempted based on the child's way of approaching new tasks. Observation of the child provides information about his or her learning style, preferences, and strengths.

Redefinition can be utilized to validate, expand, or otherwise change caregivers' perceptions of their children. Instead of concentrating on children's specific strengths or needs, redefinition involves asking caregivers to identify broader, developmental goals for their children. An understanding of child development may prove beneficial to caregivers as an effective EI redefinition strategy, as many families do not believe they can have any control over or impact on their children's development (Bickerstaff, 1980). Additionally, families may not understand that parenting behaviors and intervention efforts can alleviate future developmental problems (Badger, 1985; Bickerstaff, 1980; Bromwich, 1990; Ogbu, 1987). EI providers can facilitate redefinition by building and engaging caregivers in a relationship of open exchange of concerns and goals about the target child. This may take the form of jointly observing the child's behavior and discussing alternative interpretations.

Redefinition through intervention at a child–caregiver dyadic level is also important. Although infant competency (a potent target of remediation) influences parental bonding, enhancing dyadic transactions may also require direct attention (Stump, 1992). Interventions that target caregiver–child interactions have an increased potential for long-term effects compared to interventions that merely teach infants skills (Bromwich, 1990). One way to enhance dyadic relationships is to effectively facilitate caregivers' interactions with the child. For example, interventionists may want to help caregivers detect children's attentional bids, interpret gestures, and follow the child's lead.

In developing a successful IFSP for children prenatally exposed to cocaine, the greatest attention may be focused on re-education strategies for the caregiver and entire family. To promote a healthy climate for child development and growth, continuing caregiver drug use must be addressed. For the drug-using caregiver, re-education extends beyond learning new ways of reacting to a child, to altering one's own proactive behaviors. An increase in the incidence of child abuse and neglect can be traced in part to an escalation in drug use (Children's Defense Fund, 1990; Fanshel, 1975). Hence addressing and servicing the substance-using caregiver as part of EI may contribute to the alleviation of child abuse and neglect. EI techniques, then, may target the caregiver's drug use and include group therapy, relapse prevention, individual therapy, and 12-step meetings. However, because EI programs are often not equipped to provide substance abuse treatment, at minimum, EI must refer drug-using caregivers to substance abuse programs. That is, EI must at least ensure a linkage of drug-using caregivers to outside case management agencies that can help drug-using women access services that provide postnatal care, transportation, child care, job training, and substance abuse treatment (Segal, 1991).

However, accessing drug treatment services is very difficult for poor, inner-city women with children. Many drug treatment programs have extremely long waiting lists, and more deny admission to mothers and pregnant women ("Punishing women," 1993). Even when mothers or pregnant women *do* admit themselves for drug treatment, federal laws limiting the number of Medicaid beds allocated for this type of care severely restrict the number of women who can be effectively treated. In addition, inpatient hospitalization is often not a viable alternative for women with children because public assistance often requires that women pay over 75% of their welfare check for treatment. This stipulation does not allow mothers to financially support their families while they are receiving inpatient drug treatment. Even if women are able to complete a drug treatment program, returning to an environment of continuing poverty, personal demoralization, physical illness, and social instability (Fanshel, 1975; Lawson & Wilson, 1980; Nichtern, 1973) makes sobriety difficult. Despite the best intentions to remain drug free, the nature of addiction along with the lack of adequate support systems and ineffective coping skills will inevitably result in relapse (Howard & Kropenske, 1990).

Re-education may also be used with caregivers' parenting skills. Although parenting proficiency has not been definitively determined to be poorer for the drug-using caregiver (Bauman, 1978; Lief, 1976), some studies have reported that drug-using caregivers provide inadequate parenting (Bauman & Dougherty, 1983; Carr, 1975; Coles & Platzman, 1992; Coppolillo, 1975; Escamilla-Mondanaro, 1975; Lief, 1985; Nichtern, 1973; Smith, 1992) and have children who are at a higher risk for neglect, abuse, and abandonment (Children's Defense Fund, 1990; Fanshel, 1975; Lawson & Wilson, 1980). In fact, positive parenting models are not common with drug-using women. Many were reared in physically, sexually, and emotionally abusive homes by drug-using caregivers (Mayer & Black, 1977; Steele, 1987), contributing to an intergenerational cycle of inadequate parenting. These mixed findings on parenting skills illuminate the complexity involved in determining parenting behavior and child developmental outcome and the need to consider each family system individually. Caregiver psychopathology (e.g., drug use, stress, depression), expectations and beliefs about their child and child development, perceptions about the severity and life impact of their child's condition, and community support are important factors in the facilitation of child development (Silber, 1989). Additionally, child vulnerabilities may activate potential resources, or exacerbate dysfunctional coping within caregivers (Solnit, 1984). Thus, interventions with caregivers may need to focus on parenting skills, as well as practical life skills (e.g., budgeting, cooking, health education, public assistance, parenting), and psychological issues (e.g., resolving guilt about prenatal drug use). However, EI providers often must focus efforts on maintaining contact and engaging drug-using caregivers and their children in EI due to inconsistent attendance. Nevertheless, EI aimed at improving family functioning is effective (Heinicke, Beckwith, & Thompson, 1988) and can be used to break the intergenerational cycle of inadequate parenting.

Comprehensive EI rooted in an ecological foundation, recognizing multiple child developmental and behavioral domains, and family strengths and needs, provides sensitive and responsive services to children and families. The factors influencing the developmental outcomes of children prenatally exposed to cocaine are complex, multifaceted, and multifarious. Only by considering the at-risk child in a holistic manner can concrete interventions be generated to enhance such children's development.

Benefits of Ecological EI

Ecologically based EI that considers each child individually will lead to the extinction of the average child and family situation that has become characteristic of the majority of research on the treatment of children with disabilities (Shonkoff et al., 1992). Because the causal mechanisms of developmental disabilities are not wholly understood, it is inappropriate to extend population inferences to individuals in a population. Just as applying an "average" prototype to children with similar disabilities threatens their individuality, implementing a "standard" intervention ignores individual strengths and weaknesses. Prenatally cocaine-exposed children vary greatly and so should the interventions used with them.

From the standpoint of special education, an issue is whether children prenatally exposed to cocaine are or should be considered developmentally delayed or in need of EI. Only by examining these children's individual needs in their personal contexts can special educators effectively determine useful protocols of special education interventions or, more likely, advocate for a more varied, customized, and less categorized plan to assist prenatally cocaine-exposed children in need. If prenatally cocaine-exposed children receive EI services, such services must be valid and useful. Hence areas of concern and need, in terms of various child domains and ecosystemic variables, are required to best develop and tailor effective EI. Systemic intervention for prenatally cocaine-exposed children and their families is our best hope for facilitating optimal child development and healthy family functioning. In fact, programs that simultaneously target intervention efforts at many levels of the child's social ecology may be more successful than those treating each level independently (Schutter & Brinker, 1992).

Common Issues for Inner-City EI

Facilitating Attendance. Children prenatally exposed to cocaine who also live in poverty present additional challenges to EI service delivery and research. Consistent attendance at EI sessions is associated with intervention effectiveness (Heinicke et al., 1988), but the difficulties of these families' everyday lives pose barriers to their participation in research and also impede service delivery. Inconsistent attendance is common for families who often have other appointments (e.g., clinics, supplemental food programs) at the same time as the EI session, and transportation may be difficult to access without financial assistance. In addition, many families may not be invested in receiving EI, as McLloyd (1990) found that research is a very low priority for severely disadvantaged families. Caregivers may feel disenfranchised from the EI process due to previous unsuccessful interactions with agencies. Families often mistrust researchers' motives because no change or help is perceived to have resulted from involvement in previous studies. Thus, caregivers may not believe that a partnership can develop with the EI provider, especially if the EI program is unfamiliar or does not have a positive reputation in the community.

In many states, when an infant is found to be drug exposed by a toxicology screening conducted at birth, the family becomes involved with the judicial and child protection systems. In many cases, EI is required for the family and involvement in an EI program is one of the conditions for family preservation. Thus, these families have not sought EI out of concern for their child's development; they are simply attempting to retain custody of the child through compliance with court orders. Thus, EI programs may have to develop more flexible procedures to engage and maintain involvement of poor, inner-city families in EI. This may be especially true for families with histories of substance abuse. Home-based services, intensified follow-up, and transportation services may be necessary to facilitate families' participation in EI programs.

This lack of participation, however, may not be solely a compliance issue. Dunst (1987) viewed family needs as organized into a categorical hierarchy. Individuals strive to fill needs at the top of their hierarchy before meeting lesser needs (Hull, 1943; Lewin, 1931; Maslow, 1954; Murray, 1938). Survival needs (e.g., shelter, food) must be met before less basic needs are addressed (Dunst, 1987). *Environmental press*—that environmental conditions play a role in shaping and guiding individual's behavior—(Garbarino, 1982) generates the hierarchy of needs that are most important to a family at a particular time. Certainly in an inner-city setting, the interplay among family resources, economic issues, and individual priorities require that basic family needs be met before families invest time and energy in EI services. The Beethoven Project, an inner-city early childhood development and family support program, found that in order to build relationships with families in poverty, attention must be paid to immediate family needs before research-related services can be provided (*Beethoven's Fifth*, 1993). However, even when tangible incentives are given to maintain participation in programs and research, families often drop out (Brinker, Frazier, & Baxter, 1992; Lasky et al., 1987). Brinker et al. (1992) concluded that efforts to reach out to low-SES and minority families must extend beyond the family–child system to the community and social systems in the families' ecologies. Unfortunately, while EI can offer families developmental information about their children, such information is not a primary need for families without housing and food.

Not surprisingly then, inconsistent attendance also leads to difficulties in implementing IFSPs, requiring EI programs to be more creative in IFSP development. Long absences may lead to the need for continual reassessment of the child's skills before an IFSP can be generated. EI professionals may need to go to families' homes to develop IFSPs and to get them signed.

Children may also find periodic attendance at the program to be problematic. For example, stranger anxiety may be a continually disruptive dynamic because the child does not have enough encounters with the EI providers to experience them as anyone but strangers. In addition, programs may need to adjust services to better engage families in EI services. Home-based services (either individual or small group) may be more successful in reaching out to these families than large center-based programs. Assisting with transportation costs may also improve families' attendance at EI programs.

The Importance of Social Support. In working with inner-city families with cocaine-exposed children, social support services are often a major part of the IFSP. Families are often in need of safe and adequate housing, food, job training, and medical care. This support may be limited to informal social support such as the assistance of the extended family or may also include formal social support such as intensified case management available through initiatives aimed at reducing infant mortality.

Informal social support for inner-city African-American families is usually centered around grandparents and other elders. Most members of the extended family seek the approval of grandparents for interventions that have been recommended. When a drug-exposed infant and his or her family are referred to EI grandparents often come to the forefront by attending the EI program in addition to or instead of the parent. Strongly religious families often believe that prayer will help a substance user to stop using drugs. Many grandparents urge their adult children to "turn their lives over to Christ" for help in treating their addiction. Such a perspective may be at odds with the IFSP goals of seeking professional assistance in battling the addiction. Alternatively, as there are often not enough treatment beds available for women with children, the family and the church may have to serve as addiction counselors.

Formal social support is currently provided for some families by a new wave of initiatives that have been launched by both state and federal governments to help prevent infant mortality and reach currently underserved populations. Federal initiatives include Healthy Start and Early Prevention, Screening, Diagnosis and Treatment. Illinois also has several programs targeted at these populations: Healthy Moms/Healthy Kids, the Illinois Technical Assistance Project Parent Resource Centers and the Help Me Grow Campaign. Similar programs exist in other states. These initiatives provide case management services and intensified case coordination. They employ family support strategies to include multiple members of the child's family. For example, the initiatives provide individual and group counseling, emergency food, warm clothing, transitional housing, enrollment in supplemental food programs, and child care. However, some of these resources are only available if the family resides in a community with a high rate of infant mortality. Furthermore, these state and federal initiatives do not make provisions for drug treatment. Drug Free Families With a Future (DFFWF), a program in Illinois that served drug-using women of childbearing age, has been phased out and replaced by another program called Healthy Moms/Healthy Kids. Unlike DFFWF, this new program does not emphasize addiction, even though the rate of drug use by pregnant women continues to increase.

Foster Care Families.   Many children in low-SES families attending EI in the inner city are cared for by someone other than their natural parents, often a grandmother. Relative foster care is especially prevalent among children prenatally exposed to cocaine. During the first 3 years of life, when EI is provided for children, the legal transitions of child guardianship and custody can change multiple times. For EI providers, this presents an additional area of focus, in terms of obtaining proper signatures for EI attendance and coordinating cases and treatment issues with case management and social service agencies.

EI professionals must be sensitive to the special needs of foster caregivers and children in foster care. Before being placed in foster care, a child's quality of life is usually less than optimal. Neglect or abuse led to involvement of the child welfare agency. After being removed from the parent, the child must form a new attachment with one or more new caregivers. This disruption of continuity in the attachment relationship impacts upon developmental achievements (Goldstein, Freud, & Solnit, 1979). The foster grandparent may not be physically able to care for the child as well as a younger caregiver, or the foster parent may have multiple foster and/or biological children to care for, decreasing the time that can be spent with each child. This may further impact the child's attachment relationships.

Foster caregivers also face additional burdens. Many foster grandmothers are relatively young and may not be content with having to care for their grandchildren. Instead they may have planned to continue their education, seek employment, or avail themselves of opportunities that did not exist when they were younger (Costin, Bell, & Downs, 1991). Financial compensation for foster care also may reduce the family's other forms of income at the same time that the child welfare agency is suggesting changes to make the home an acceptable placement.

EI providers must be sensitive to both children's and foster parents' issues. These families must be viewed as families in transition. They may need a great deal of social support from EI programs even though they are involved with the child welfare system.

CONCLUSION

Although prenatal cocaine exposure does not universally lead to developmental delay, children prenatally exposed to cocaine can be considered to be at risk for developmental delay. The *at risk* classification is the result of the cocaine exposure and the child's social environment. Individually based EI from an ecological perspective may be most effective in working with these children and their families. A transactional and family systems perspective allows the EI provider to better understand the family and its needs and more effectively plan interventions for both the child and the family.

ACKNOWLEDGMENTS

The contributions of the first two authors were equal. Richard P. Brinker passed away before this chapter was complete but contributed many ideas to this work. He will be missed by his colleagues and the families he was committed to serving. The authors thank Adam Kennedy for his thoughtful comments on this chapter.

REFERENCES

Abel, E. L. (1984). *Fetal alcohol syndrome/fetal alcohol effects*. New York: Plenum.

Acker, D., Sachs, B. P., Tracey, K. J., & Wise, W. E. (1983). Abruptio placentae associated with cocaine use. *American Journal of Obstetrics and Gynecology, 2,* 220–221.

Alessandri, S. M., Sullivan, M. W., Imaizumi, S., & Lewis, M. (1993). Learning and emotional responsivity in cocaine-exposed infants. *Developmental Psychology, 29,* 989–997.

Badger, E. (1985). *Intervention with low income children and families*. Paper presented at the NICHD Conference on Behavioral Intervention with High Risk Infants, Bethesda, MD.

Bandstra, E. S., Steele, B. W., Burkett, G. T., Palow, D. C., Levandoski, N., & Rodriguez, V. (1989). Prevalence of perinatal cocaine exposure in an urban multi-ethnic population. *Pediatric Research, 25,* 247A.

Bauman, P. S. (1978). *Childrearing attitudes of drug abusing mothers*. Unpublished master's thesis, California School of Professional Psychology, San Francisco, CA.

Bauman, P. S., Dougherty, F. E. (1983). Drug-addicted mothers' parenting and their children's development. *International Journal of the Addictions, 18*(3), 291–302.

Beethoven's fifth: The first five years of the Center for Successful Child Development. (1993, May). Executive Summary. Chicago: Ounce of Prevention Fund.

Besharov, D. J. (1989, Fall). The children of crack: Will we protect them? *Public Welfare*, pp. 6–11, 42–43.

Bickerstaff, J. (1980). Serving parents and families of young Black children with special needs. In E. Jackson (Ed.), *The young Black exceptional child: Providing programs and services*. Chapel Hill, NC: Technical Assistance and Development System.

Bingol, N., Fuchs, M., Diaz, V., Stone, R. K., & Gromisch, D. S. (1987). Teratogenicity of cocaine in humans. *Journal of Pediatrics, 110,* 93–96.

Bingol, N., Fuchs, M., Holipas, N., Henriquez, R., Pagan, M., & Diaz, V. (1986). Prune belly syndrome associated with maternal cocaine abuse [Abstract]. *American Journal of Human Genetics, 39,* A49.

Brinker, R. P., Frazier, W. A., & Baxter, A. (1992). Maintaining the involvement of inner city families in EI through a program of incentives: Looking beyond family systems to societal systems. *OSERS Newsline, 4*(3), 8–17.

Brodsky, N. L., Hurt, H., & Webb, D. (1992). *One thousand babies: Report on the findings from two studies*. Philadelphia: Philadelphia Perinatal Society and the Philadelphia Department of Public Health, Office of Maternal and Child Health.

Bromwich, R. M. (1990). The interactional approach to EI. *Infant Mental Health Journal, 1,* 66–79.

Bronfenbrenner, U. (1977). Toward an experimental ecology of human development. *American Psychologist, 32,* 513–531.

Carr, J. N. (1975). Drug patterns among drug-addicted mothers: Incidence, variance in use, and effects on children. *Pediatrician Annuals, 4,* 408–417.

Chasnoff, I. J. (1987). Perinatal effects of cocaine. *Contemporary Obstetrics and Gynecology, 29,* 163–179.

Chasnoff, I. J. (1989). Drug use and women: Establishing a standard of care. *Annals of the New York Academy of Sciences, 562,* 208–210.

Chasnoff, I. J., Burns, W. J., Schnoll, S. H., & Burns, K. A. (1985). Cocaine use in pregnancy. *New England Journal of Medicine, 313*(11), 666–669.

Chasnoff, I. J., & Chisum, G. (1987). Genitourinary tract dysmorphology and maternal cocaine use [Abstract]. *Pediatric Research, 2,* 22A.

Chasnoff, I. J., Griffith, D. R., Freier, C., & Murray, J. (1992). Cocaine/polydrug use in pregnancy: Two-year follow-up. *Pediatrics, 89,* 284–289.

Chasnoff, I. J., Lewis, D. E., Griffith, D. R., & Willey, S. (1989). Cocaine and pregnancy: Clinical and toxicological implications for the neonate. *Clinical Chemistry, 35,* 1276–1278.

Cherukuri, R., Minkoff, H., Feldman, J., Parekh, A., & Glass, L. (1988). A cohort study of alkaloidal cocaine ("crack") in pregnancy. *Obstetrics and Gynecology, 72,* 147–151.

Children's Defense Fund (1990). *SOS America.* Washington, DC: Author.

Cicchetti, D., & Manly, J. T. (1990). A personal perspective on conducting research with maltreating families: Problems and solutions. In G. H. Brody & I. E. Sigel (Eds.), *Methods of family research* (Vol. 2, pp. 87–133). Hillsdale, NJ: Lawrence Erlbaum Associates.

Clarren, S. K., & Smith, D. W. (1978). The fetal alcohol syndrome. *New England Journal of Medicine, 298,* 1063–1067.

Clayton, R. R. (1986). Cocaine use in the U.S.: In a blizzard or just being snowed. *NIDA Research Monographs, 65,* 8–34.

Cohen, M. E., Anday, E. K., & Leitner, D. S. (1989). Effects of in-utero cocaine exposure on sensorineural reactivity. *Annals of the New York Academy of Sciences, 562,* 344–346.

Coles, C. D., & Platzman, K. A. (1992). Fetal alcohol effects in preschool children: Research, prevention and intervention. *OSAP Prevention Monograph 11: Identifying the needs of drug-affected children: Public policy issues* (pp. 59–86). Rockville, MD: U.S. Dept. of Health and Human Services, Alcohol, Drug Abuse, and Mental Health Administration, Office of Substance Abuse Prevention.

Coppolillo, H. P. (1975). Drug impediments to mothering behavior. *Addictive Disorders, 2*(1), 201–208.

Costin, L. B., Bell, C. A., & Downs, S. W. (1991). *Child welfare policies and practice.* New York: Longman.

Daley, S. (1991, February 7). Born on crack, and coping with kindergarten. *New York Times,* pp. A1, A13.

Davidson, C. E. (1991). Attachment issues and the cocaine exposed dyad. *Child and Adolescent Social Work, 8*(4), 269–284.

Day, N. L., Jasperse, D., Richardson, G., Robies, N., Sambamoorthi, U., Taylor, P., Scher, M., Stoffer, D., & Cornelius, M. (1989). Prenatal exposure to alcohol: Effect on infant growth and morphologic characteristics. *Pediatrics, 84*(3) 536–541.

Dixon, S. D., & Bejar, R. (1989). Echoencephalographic findings in neonates associated with maternal cocaine and methamphetamine use: Incidence and clinical correlates. *Journal of Pediatrics, 115,* 770–778.

Dixon, S. D., Coen, R. W., & Crutchfield, S. (1987). Visual dysfunction in cocaine-exposed infants. *Pediatric Research, 21,* 359A.

Dunst, C. J. (1987, December). *What is effective helping?* Plenary session paper presented to the Fifth Bienneial Training Institute for the National Center for Clinical Infant Programs, Washington, DC.

Escamilla-Mondanaro, J. (1975). Mothers on methadone—Echoes of failure. *Proceedings of the National Drug Abuse Convention,* 41–49.

Evans, R. I. (1992). Commentary on an emerging research field. *Journal of Applied Developmental Psychology, 13,* 151–152.

Fanshel, D. (1975). Parental failure and consequences for children: The drug-abusing mothers whose children are in foster care. *American Journal of Public Health and National Health, 65,* 604–612.

Frank, D. A., Zuckerman, B. S., Amaro, H., Aboagye, K., Bauchner, H., Cabral, H., Fried, L., Hingson, R., Kayne, H., Levenson, S. M., Parker, S., Reece, H., & Vinci, R. (1988). Cocaine use during pregnancy: Prevalence and correlates. *Pediatrics, 82,* 888–895.

Garbarino, J. (1982). *Children and families in the social environment.* Hawthorne, NY: Aldine.

Geggel, R. L., McInerny, J., & Estes, N. A. M. (1989). Transient neonatal ventricular tachycardia associated with maternal cocaine use. *American Journal of Cardiology, 63,* 383–384.

Gerber, M. M. (1990, November 11). Cocaine children: Crack babies don't deserve to be stigmatized by media. *Santa Barbara News-Press,* p. 1.

Gold, M. S. (1987). Crack abuse: Its implications and outcomes. *Resident and Staff Physicians, 33,* 45–53.

Goldstein, J., Freud, A., & Solnit, A. J. (1979). *Beyond the best interests of the child.* New York: The Free Press.

Hadeed, A. J., & Siegel, S. R. (1989). Maternal cocaine use during pregnancy: Effect on the newborn infant. *Pediatrics, 84,* 205–210.

Hansen, R. L., & Ulrey, G. L. (1993). Knowns and unknowns in the outcomes of drug-dependent women. In N. J. Anastasiow & S. Harel (Eds.), *At-risk infants: Interventions, families, and research* (pp. 115–126). Baltimore: Brookes.

Heinicke, C. M., Beckwith, L., & Thompson, A. (1988). Early intervention in the family system: A framework and review. *Infant Mental Health Journal, 9,* 111–141.

Hopkins, E. (1990, October 18). Childhood's end. *Rolling Stone,* pp. 66–72, 108, 110.

Howard, J., & Kropenske, V. (1990). A preventive intervention model for chemically dependent parents. In S. E. Goldstein, J. Yager, C. M. Heinicke, & R. S. Pynoos (Eds.), *Preventing mental health disturbances in childhood* (pp. 71–84). Washington, DC: American Psychiatric Press.

Howze, K., & Howze, W. M. (1991, April). *Cocaine's kids: Is exceptional education ready?* Paper presented at the Annual Convention of the Council For Exceptional Children, Atlanta, GA.

Hull, C. L. (1943). *Principles of behavior.* New York: Appleton-Century-Crofts.

Isenberg, S. J., Spierer, A., & Inkelis, S. H. (1987). Ocular signs of cocaine intoxication in neonates. *American Journal of Opthamology, 102,* 211–214.

Jones, K. L., Smith, D. W., Ulleland, C. N., & Streissguth, A. P. (1973). Pattern of malformation in offspring of chronic alcoholic mothers. *Lancet, 1,* 676–680.

Kaye, K., Elkind, L., Goldberg, D., & Tytun, A. (1989). Birth outcomes for infants of drug abusing mothers. *New York State Journal of Medicine, 89,* 256–261.

Keith, L. G., MacGregor, S., Friedell, S., Rosner, M., Chasnoff, I. J., & Sciarra, J. J. (1989). Substance abuse in pregnant women: Recent experience at the perinatal center for chemical dependence of Northwestern Memorial Hospital. *Obstetrics and Gynecology, 73,* 715–720.

Kelley, S. J., Walsh, J. H., & Thompson, K. (1991). Birth outcomes, health problems, and neglect with prenatal exposure to cocaine. *Pediatric Nursing, 17*(2), 130–136.

Lasky, R. E., Tyson, J. E., Rosenfeld, C. R., Krasinski, D., Dowling, S., & Grant, N. F. (1987). Disappointing follow-up for indigent high-risk newborns. *American Journal of Diseases of Children, 141,* 101–105.

Lawson, M. S., & Wilson, G. S. (1980). Parenting among women addicted to narcotics. *Child Welfare, 59*(2), 67–79.

Lester, B. M., Corwin, M. J., Sepkoski, C., Seifer, R., Peucker, M., McLaughlin, S., & Golub, H. (1991). Neurobehavioral syndromes in cocaine-exposed newborn infants. *Child Development, 62,* 694–705.

Lewin, K. (1931). Environmental forces in child behavior and development. In C. Murchison (Ed.), *A handbook of child psychology.* Worcester, MA: Clark University Press.

Lief, N. (1976). Some measure of parenting behavior for addicted and nonaddicted mothers. In *Symposium on Comprehensive Health Care for Addicted Families and Their Children* (NIDA Monograph, U.S. Public Health Service). Washington, DC: US Government Printing Office.

Lief, N. R. (1985). The drug user as a parent. *International Journal of the Addictions, 20*(1), 63–97.

Little, B. B., Snell, L. M., Palmore, M. K., & Gilstrap, L. C. (1988). Cocaine use in pregnant women in a large public hospital. *American Journal of Perinatology, 5,* 206–207.

MacGregor, S. N., Keith, L. G., Chasnoff, I. J., Rosner, M. A., Chisum, G. M., Shaw, P., Minogue, J. P., & Min, D. (1987). Cocaine use during pregnancy: Adverse perinatal outcome. *American Journal of Obstetrics and Gynecology, 157,* 686–689.

Marshall, A. B. (1991, September). State-by-state legislative review. *Perinatal addiction research and education update.* Chicago: NAPARE.

Maslow, A. (1954). *Motivation and personality.* New York: Harper & Row.

Mayer, J., & Black, R. (1977). Child abuse and neglect in families with an alcohol or opiate addicted parent. *Child Abuse and Neglect, 1,* 85–91.

McLloyd, V. C. (1990). Minority children: Introduction to the special issue. *Child Development, 61*, 263–266.

Moore, K. G. (Ed.). (1992). State laws on pregnant women and substance abuse, 1991. *State Legislative.* (Available from the American College of Obstetricians and Gynecologists, 409 12th Street SW, Washington, DC 20024-2188).

Murray, H. J. (1938). *Explorations in personality.* New York: Oxford University Press.

Myers, B. J., Olson, H. C., & Kaltenbach, K. (1992). Cocaine-exposed infants: Myths and misunderstandings. *Zero to Three, 13*(1), 1–5.

Nichtern, S. (1973). The children of drug abusers. *Journal of the American Academy of Child Psychiatry, 12*(1), 24–31.

Ogbu, J. (1987). Cultural influences on plasticity in human development. In J. J. Gallagher & C. T. Ramey (Eds.), *The malleability of children* (pp. 155–170). Baltimore: Brookes.

Oro, A. S., & Dixon, S. D. (1987). Perinatal cocaine and methamphetamine exposure: Maternal and neonatal correlates. *Journal of Pediatrics, 111*, 571–578.

Pollin, W. (1985). The danger of cocaine. *Journal of the American Medical Association, 254*, 98.

Punishing women for their behavior during pregnancy: A public health disaster. (1993). *Reproductive Freedom in Focus.* (Available from The Center for Reproductive Law and Policy, 120 Wall Street, New York, 10005.)

Riley, J. G., & Porat, R. (1987). Abnormal pneumograms in infants with in utero cocaine exposure [Abstract]. *Pediatric Research, 21*, 262A.

Rist, M. C. (1991). The shadow children. *Illinois Council For Exceptional Children, 40*, 5–11.

Rodning, C., Beckwith, L., & Howard, J. (1989). Prenatal exposure to drugs and its influence on attachment. *Annals of the New York Academy of Sciences, 562*, 353–354.

Rodning, C., Beckwith, L., & Howard, J. (1991). Quality of attachment and home environments in children prenatally exposed to PCP and cocaine. *Development and Psychopathology, 3*(4), 351–366.

Rutter, M. (1982). Prevention of children's psychosocial disorders: Myths and substance. *Pediatrics, 70*, 883–894.

Ryan, L., Ehrlich, S., & Finnegan, L. (1987). Cocaine abuse in pregnancy: Effects on the fetus. *Neurotoxicology and Teratology, 9*, 295–299.

Sameroff, A. J. (1975). Early influences of development: Fact or fancy? *Merrill-Palmer Quarterly, 21*(4), 267–294.

Sameroff, A. J. (1986). Environmental context of child development. *Journal of Pediatrics, 109*(1), 192–200.

Sameroff, A. J., & Chandler, M. J. (1975). Reproductive risk and the continuum of caretaking casualty. In F. D. Horowitz, M. Hetherington, S. Scarr-Sameroff, & G. Siegel (Eds.), *Review of child development research* (Vol. 4, pp. 187–244). Chicago: University of Chicago Press.

Sameroff, A. J., & Fiese, B. H. (1990). Transactional regulation and EI. In S. J. Meisels & J. P. Shonkoff (Eds.), *Handbook of early childhood intervention* (pp. 119–149). Cambridge: Cambridge University Press.

Sameroff, A. J., & Seifer, R. (1983). Familial risk and child competence. *Child Development, 54*, 1254–1268.

Schneider, J. W., Griffith, D. R., & Chasnoff, I. J. (1989). Infants exposed to cocaine in utero: Implications for development assessment and intervention. *Infants and Young Children, 2*, 25–36.

Schutter, L. S., & Brinker, R. P. (1992). Conjuring a new category of disability from prenatal cocaine exposure: Are the infants unique biological or caretaking casualties? *Topics in Early Childhood Special Education, 11*(4), 84–111.

Segal, E. A. (1991). Social policy and intervention with chemically dependent women and their children. *Child and Adolescent Social Work, 8*(4), 285–295.

Shonkoff, J. P., Hauser-Cram, P., Krauss, M. W., & Upshur, C. C. (1992). Development of infants with disabilities and their families. *Monographs of the Society for Research in Child Development, 57*(6, Serial No. 230).

Silber, S. (1989). Family influences on early development. *Topics in Early Childhood Special Education, 8*(4), 1–23.

Simeonsson, R. J., Cooper, D. H., & Scheiner, A. P. (1982). A review and analysis of early intervention programs. *Pediatrics, 69,* 635–641.

Smith, I. E. (1992). An ecological perspective: The impact of culture and social environment on drug-exposed children. *OSAP Prevention Monograph 11: Identifying the needs of drug-affected children: Public policy issues* (pp. 93–108).

Solnit, A. (1984). Keynote address: Theoretical and practical aspects of risks and vulnerabilities in infancy. *Child Abuse and Neglect, 8,* 133–144.

Steele, B. (1987). Psychodynamic factors in child abuse. In R. E. Helfer & R. S. Kempe (Eds.), *The battered child* (4th ed., pp. 81–114). Chicago: University of Chicago Press.

Seifer, R. (1983). Familial risk and child competence. *Child Development, 54,* 1254–1268.

Stokols, D. (1992). Environmental quality, human development, and health: An ecological view. *Journal of Applied Developmental Psychology, 13,* 121–124.

Struthers, J. M., & Hansen, R. L. (1992). Visual recognition memory in drug-exposed infants. *Journal of Developmental and Behavioral Pediatrics, 13,* 108–111.

Stump, J. (1992). *Our best hope: Early intervention with prenatally drug-exposed infants and their families.* Washington, DC: Child Welfare League of America.

Toufexis, A. (1991, May 13). Innocent victims. *Time,* pp. 56–60.

Vega, W. A., Kolody, B., Hwang, J., & Noble, A. (1993). Prevalence and magnitude of perinatal substance exposures in California. *New England Journal of Medicine, 329,* 850–854.

Viadero, D. (1989, October, 25). Drug-exposed children pose special problems. *Education Week,* pp. 1, 10–11.

Viadero, D. (1992, January 29). New research finds little lasting harm for 'crack' children. *New York Times,* pp. A1, A10.

Waller, M. B. (1992–1993). Helping crack-affected children succeed. *Educational Leadership, 50*(4), 57–60.

Young, S. L., Vosper, H. J., & Phillips, S. A. (1992). Cocaine: Its effects on maternal and child health. *Pharmacotherapy, 12*(1), 2–17.

Zeanah, C. H., & McDonough, S. (1989). Clinical approaches to families in early intervention. *Seminars in Perinatology, 13*(6), 35–38.

Zuckerman, B., Frank, D. A., Hingson, R., Amaro, H., Levenson, S. M., Kayne, H., Parker, S., Aboagye, K., Fried, L. E., Cabral, H., Timperi, R., & Bauchner, H. (1989). Effects of maternal marijuana and cocaine use on fetal growth. *New England Journal of Medicine, 320,* 762–768.

18

▼▼▼▼▼▼▼

Cocaine Exposure and Intervention in Early Development

Tiffany Field
University of Miami School of Medicine

Cocaine use is reported to be as high as 10% to 15% in pregnant women (Singer, Garber, & Kliegman, 1991). Cocaine exposure has been associated with a greater rate of perinatal complications including spontaneous abortion, placenta previa, intrauterine growth retardation, intraventricular hemorrhage, cardiac anomalies, low birth weight, low head circumference, and prematurity (Burkett, Yasin, & Palow, 1990; Chasnoff, 1987; Coles, Platzman, Smith, James, & Falek, 1991; Hadeed & Siegel, 1989; Porat & Brodsky, 1991; Richards, Kulkarni, & Bremner, 1990; Rosenak, Diamont, Yaffe, & Hornstein, 1990). In addition, behavioral studies have noted a tendency for cocaine-exposed newborns to show more stress behaviors than nonexposed infants including restlessness, irritability, hypertonia, tremors/clonus, and abnormal reflexes (Dixon, Bresnahan, & Zuckerman, 1990). These, together with signs of fetal stress including increased heart rate, lower vagal tone, and lower APGAR scores, suggest more subtle central nervous system involvement (Richards et al., 1990).

In this chapter, data from our cocaine-exposure studies are reviewed including a study on the neonatal behavior of cocaine-exposed full-term infants, a study on differences between cocaine-exposed and nonexposed preterm infants, a study in which cocaine-exposed preterm infants were provided extra stimulation, and a study on grade school children exposed to cocaine in utero. These questions were addressed for the following reasons: (a) the data on cocaine-exposed full-term infants' performance on the Brazelton Neonatal Assessment Scale are mixed, with some investigators reporting very minimal effects and others reporting more pronounced effects; (b) in the case of the preterm, cocaine-exposed infant, the contribution of prematurity itself or the effects of cocaine exposure on top of prematurity have not been studied; (c) because supplemental stimulation has positive effects on preterm infants, the same may apply to cocaine-exposed preterm infants if they are provided extra stimulation; and (d) the cocaine-exposed children's behavior problems highlight the importance of early interventions.

NEONATAL BEHAVIOR OF FULL-TERM, COCAINE-EXPOSED INFANTS

Until recently little was known about the behavior of newborns exposed to cocaine in utero. A study by Chasnoff and his associates (Chasnoff, Burns, Schnoll, & Burns, 1985) reported inferior performance on only one of the Brazelton Neonatal Behavioral Assessment Scale (NBAS) scores, namely state organization. However, these limited findings may have related to the small sample size as well as the use of a global scoring system. Lester, Als, and Brazelton (1982) developed a more sensitive scoring system to detect more specific behavior differences. This system was used in our study on newborn behavior of cocaine-exposed full-term infants (Eisen, Field, Bandstra, Roberts, Morrow, & Larson, 1991). A Neonatal Stress Scale was also used to record stress behaviors during the NBAS. The stress scale was developed to describe stress behaviors of cocaine-exposed newborns during the Brazelton Assessment, including tremors, restlessness, irritability, excessive high-pitched crying, hypertonia, abnormal reflex behavior, abnormal Moro reflex, excessive mouthing, tachypnea, autonomic stability, gastrointestinal signs (e.g., vomiting and diarrhea).

In this study 26 full-term neonates with a positive urine screen for cocaine were compared to 26 neonates with negative urine screens for cocaine and marijuana. These neonates averaged 38 weeks gestational age, 2,400 grams birth weight and 4 days chronological age. The two groups of primarily inner-city, African-American, low socioeconomic status (SES) mothers did not differ on demographic factors. However, more cocaine-using mothers were single (23 vs. 14), cigarette smokers (18 vs. 3), and alcohol drinkers (17 vs. 2). Marijuana use was reported by 39% of the cocaine-using mothers, cigarettes and alcohol combined by 27%, and only 15% of the mothers used cocaine alone, suggesting that 85% of the cocaine-using sample were polydrug users.

The cocaine-exposed newborn group did not differ from the nonexposed group on gender distribution, gestational age, chronological age, birth weight, birth length, or postnatal complications (see Table 18.1). However, the cocaine-exposed neonates had smaller head circumferences and more obstetric complications. The cocaine-exposed neonates also tended to show more stress behaviors, particularly abnormal reflex behavior and autonomic instability. It is interesting that on this scale maternal alcohol use contributed more to the variance than cocaine use. The only variables that entered a stepwise regression were obstetric complications

TABLE 18.1
Perinatal Data

Measures	Cocaine	Control	p
Gestational age (weeks)	38.5	38.2	ns
Chronological age (days)	4.5	4.0	ns
Birth weight (g)	2,472.5	2,411.3	ns
Head circumference (cm)	31.8	32.3	.05
Birth length (cm)	46.3	46.5	ns
Obstetric complications[a]	82.8	87.0	.03
Postnatal complications[a]	127.8	120.7	ns

[a]Higher score is optimal.

and maternal alcohol use, which together contributed to 24% of the variance. On the NBAS the cocaine-exposed neonates received inferior scores on the habituation cluster, suggesting that they required more trials to habituate the stimuli than the nonexposed neonates (see Table 18.2).

Cocaine use was the only significant variable in the stepwise regression accounting for a significant amount of the variance in the habituation score. Another group has also reported inferior performance on the habituation items of the NBAS by cocaine-exposed neonates (Coles, Platzman, Smith, & James, 1990). This finding is perhaps not surprising inasmuch as habituation is related to dopaminergic function, and cocaine has been implicated in dopamine dysfunction (Cole & Robbins, 1989). Given that habituation has been related to central nervous system dysfunction and inferior intellectual development in other drug-exposed infants (Streissguth, Barr, & Martin, 1983), these findings highlight the need for intervention.

DIFFERENTIATING COCAINE-EXPOSED FROM NONEXPOSED PRETERM NEONATES ON NEONATAL BEHAVIOR AND HORMONES

One of the most frequent perinatal complications associated with cocaine exposure is prematurity. Many of the medical and behavior complications attributed to intrauterine cocaine exposure are the same as those associated with prematurity (Young, Vosper, & Phillips, 1992). Despite the association between cocaine exposure and prematurity, most studies on cocaine-exposed infants have been conducted with full-term infants. It is conceivable that cocaine exposure effects may be more pronounced for less mature, more vulnerable premature infants versus full-term infants.

The purpose of the next study was to compare cocaine-exposed preterm infants with nonexposed preterm infants to determine the combined effects of cocaine exposure and prematurity (Scafidi, Field, Wheeden, Schanberg, Kuhn, Symanski,

TABLE 18.2
Means for the Neonatal Stress Scale and Brazelton Cluster Scores

Measures	Cocaine	Control	p
Neonatal Stress Scale score	3.2	2.2	.07
Brazelton cluster scores			
Habituation	5.7	6.3	.03
Orientation	5.5	4.9	ns
Motor maturity	5.2	5.1	ns
Range of state	3.9	4.2	ns
Regulation of state	6.1	5.8	ns
Autonomic stability	6.0	5.9	ns
No. of abnormal reflexes	4.3	3.7	ns

Zimmerman & Bandstra, in press). For this study 30 preterm newborns (15 females) with a positive urine toxicology for cocaine (mean gestational age = 30 weeks, mean birth weight = 1,239 grams) and 30 preterm neonates (18 females) with a negative toxicology (mean gestational age = 30 weeks, mean birth weight = 1,212 grams) were recruited following random stratification on demographic variables. The groups did not differ on SES or ethnic composition (68% African-American, 18% Caucasian, 7% Hispanic). Obstetric and postnatal complications were summarized by the scales designed by Littman and Parmelee (1978). The infants' behavior was observed on the NBAS (Brazelton, 1984), and sleep–wake behavior was recorded for a 45-min period and scored using an adaptation of Thoman's sleep state criteria (Scafidi, Field, Schanberg, Bauer, Tucci, Roberts, Morrow, & Kuhn, 1990; Thoman, 1975). Finally, urine was collected over an 8-hr period and was assayed for norepinephrine, epinephrine, dopamine, and cortisol. In addition, blood samples taken from heelsticks were assayed for glucose and insulin.

The results suggested that the cocaine-exposed preterm infants were significantly more compromised than the preterm infants who had not been exposed on virtually all measures including demographic factors, medical complications, NBAS scores, sleep–wake behavior, and catecholamine and hormone levels. First, the cocaine-using mothers were more often single and averaged a higher parity (4 vs. 2), although the groups did not differ on maternal age or ethnicity. Although the cocaine-exposed infants did not differ from nonexposed infants on the traditional birth measures—including gestational age, birth weight, birth length, Apgar scores, or postnatal complications—the cocaine-exposed infants had more obstetric complications (lower scores), smaller head circumference, and they were in the neonatal intensive care unit (NICU) for longer periods of time (see Table 18.3). Although they also averaged a greater daily weight gain in the NICU, perhaps because they were there longer and achieved a higher weight gain trajectory in their extra days in the NICU, they were also on more medications (typically caffeine) and had a greater incidence of intraventricular hemorrhage.

TABLE 18.3
Means of Demographic Variables for Cocaine-Exposed
and Nonexposed Preemies

	Nonexposed M	Cocaine-Exposed M	p
Gestational age (weeks)	30.0	30.2	ns
Birth weight (g)	1231.8	1211.9	ns
Birth length (cm)	38.3	37.5	ns
Ponderal Index	2.19	2.23	ns
Head circumference (cm)	27.2	26.2	.02
Apgar 1 min	5.3	5.6	ns
Apgar 5 min	7.2	7.3	ns
OCS[a]	78.1	66.1	.006
Intraventricular hemorrhage	26.0%	73.0%	.001
PNF[a]	70.5	69.9	ns
Medications	32.2%	70.0%	.003
Days in NICU	12.1	18.3	.03
Average daily weight gain in NICU	−5.4	1.0	.003
Parental visits (% of sample)	80.6%	43.3%	.003
Parental visits with touch	77.4%	40.0%	.002
Parental visits with holding	67.7%	40.0%	.03
Parental visits with feeding	51.6%	23.3%	.02

[a]Higher score is optimal.

The intraventricular hemorrhage rating for the cocaine-exposed group was most frequently a Grade 1. The fact that the cocaine-using mothers visited their infants less frequently and touched, held, and fed them less frequently when they visited them could relate to the mothers' drug-using behavior and lifestyle and/or the more fragile condition of their immature infants.

On the NBAS, the cocaine-exposed infants did surprisingly better on the habituation cluster than the nonexposed infants, possibly due to accelerated development related to intrauterine stress or possibly because they were "shutting down" sooner because of their stress condition (see Table 18.4). In contrast, their performance was inferior on the range of state and regulation of state factors, and they received more depressed scores on the Lester depression cluster. On the supplemental items, they received lower scores on cost of attention, regulatory capacity, and regulation of state.

During the 45-min sleep–wake behavior recordings (scored second by second on a laptop computer from time lapse videotapes), the cocaine-exposed infants showed different sleep patterns (see Table 18.5). First, they spent less time in quiet sleep (40% vs. 63% time), and more time in indeterminate sleep (31% vs. 14%). In addition, they showed significantly more multiple limb movements (30% vs. 13% of the time), more mouthing behaviors (9% vs. 5%) and more tremulousness (11% vs. less than 1%). These sleep behavior differences suggested not only that the cocaine-exposed preterm infants were showing less mature sleep

TABLE 18.4
Means for the Brazelton Cluster Scores and the Kansas Supplements

	Nonexposed M	Cocaine-Exposed M	p
Habituation	5.1	5.9	.02
Orientation	3.2	3.6	ns
Motor	3.3	3.4	ns
Range of state	4.2	3.4	.01
Regulation of state	5.4	4.0	.01
Autonomic response	6.4	5.8	ns
Reflexes	6.6	8.3	ns
Depression	5.4	7.4	.04
Excitability	1.5	1.6	ns
Quality of alertness	5.0	4.3	ns
Cost of attention	6.4	5.4	.01
Examiner persistence	5.7	4.9	ns
General irritability	7.5	7.3	ns
Robustness and endurance	5.6	5.0	ns
Regulatory capacity	6.1	4.8	.04
Regulation of state	6.6	5.1	.03
Motor tone	4.7	4.2	ns

behavior than the nonexposed preterms (i.e., they were spending less time in quiet sleep), but also that their sleep was more disorganized as suggested by the high levels of indeterminate sleep. The latter finding is disturbing given that indeterminate sleep was the one neonatal variable that was inversely related to 12-year-old IQ scores in the Sigman and Parmelee (1989) longitudinal follow-up study.

Finally, the cocaine-exposed preterm infants had higher levels of urinary norepinephrine, dopamine, and cortisol (see Table 18.6). These results were surprising given that the infants' urine was sampled long after acute drug effects would be apparent (at 1 month postpartum). An earlier study (Hertzel, Christensen, Pedersen, & Kuhl, 1982) reported elevated catecholamines that could have

TABLE 18.5
Means for Percentage of Time of States and Behaviors for
Cocaine-Exposed and Nonexposed Preemies

	Nonexposed M	Cocaine-Exposed M	p
Quiet sleep	63.3	39.8	.01
Indeterminate sleep	14.0	31.2	.002
Multiple limb movements	12.8	29.9	.006
Mouthing	4.5	8.6	.05
Tremulousness	0.2	11.0	.001
No movement	64.0	45.4	.001

TABLE 18.6
Medians for Catecholamine, Glucose, and Hormone Levels

	Nonexposed Median	Cocaine-Exposed Median	p
24-Hour Urine			
Norepinephrine (ng/mg/creatine)	47.50	72.00	.02
Epinephrine (ng/mg/creatinine)	4.00	3.40	ns
Dopamine (ng/mg/creatinine)	1420.00	1554.00	.05
Cortisol (ng/mg/creatinine)	214.00	430.00	.002
Creatinine (mg/dL)	12.58	11.97	ns
Plasma			
Glucose (mg/dL)	70.00	71.00	ns
Insulin (μ units/mL)	17.15	13.50	.05

simply related to the residual effects of cocaine. However, the elevated catecholamines and cortisol in this study may have derived from chronic sympathetic and adrenal-cortical activity. Enhanced norepinephrine levels could relate to enhanced maturity of the sympathetic nervous system, as reported earlier for preterm infants receiving supplemental stimulation (Kuhn, Schanberg, Field, Symanski, Zimmerman, Scafidi, & Roberts, 1991). This enhanced development may relate to excessive stress in the perinatal period. The elevated urinary cortisol levels (a tonic measure of stress) may also explain the decreased salivary cortisol response to stressors noted earlier by Gardner, Karmel, and their colleagues (Magnano, Gardner, & Karmel, 1992). The chronic level of stress may lead to a less rigorous response to stress because of differences in threshold secretion. The lower levels of plasma insulin in the cocaine-exposed preterm newborns could also result from enhanced sympathetic and adrenergic activity (Hertzel et al., 1982). As Scafidi et al. (in press) concluded, there is reason to be concerned; that is, many of the findings (e.g., inferior state regulation, indeterminate sleep, intraventricular hemorrhage) are known to contribute to developmental delay, suggesting the need for early intervention for cocaine-exposed preterm neonates.

AN EARLY INTERVENTION FOR COCAINE-EXPOSED PRETERM INFANTS

Massage therapy is noted to facilitate growth and development in healthy, preterm newborns. Following a 10-day period of 45 min of massage per day, preterm infants showed greater weight gain, more active and alert behavior, and greater motor maturity (Field, Schanberg, Scafidi, Bauer, Vega-Lahr, Garcia, Nystrom, & Kuhn, 1986; Scafidi, Field, Schanberg, Bauer, Vega-Lahr, & Garcia, 1986; Scafidi et al., 1990). In addition, these infants were discharged from the hospital 6 days earlier for a hospital cost savings of approximately $3,000 per infant. Further, the massaged preterm infants showed a later advantage at 8 months of age. Their weight percentiles were higher and their Bayley Mental and Motor Scale scores were superior (Field, Scafidi, & Schanberg, 1987). Because massage therapy was noted to facilitate weight gain and more mature behaviors in preterm infants, and because those effects appeared to persist in the form of growth and development advantages later in infancy (8 months), these effects were predicted to extend to infants who were cocaine-exposed in addition to being born prematurely.

The sample for the cocaine intervention study was comprised of 30 preterm cocaine-exposed neonates who were approximately 30 weeks gestational age and 1,200 grams birth weight and who had a moderate number of obstetric and postnatal complications. Only cocaine-exposed infants with a positive urine or meconium toxicology screen or a positive maternal self-report for cocaine use were recruited for the study. These infants could be more accurately described as polydrug-exposed neonates because approximately 85% of them were also exposed to alcohol, tobacco, and/or marijuana. Only newborns who were considered medically stable and were free from ventilatory assistance and receiving no intravenous medications or feedings were admitted to the study. The cocaine-exposed newborns were then randomly assigned based on a random stratification procedure to the treatment or control groups. Fortunately this procedure yielded equivalence between the groups on the important variables such as gestational age, birth weight, duration of time in the NICU, and weight at the beginning of the study (Wheeden, Scafidi, Field, Ironson, Valdeon, & Bandstra, 1993).

The massage therapy was provided for three 15-min periods during 3 consecutive hours for a 10-day period. The 15-min stimulation session consisted of three standardized 5-min phases. In the first and third phases stroking with moderate pressure was provided to different body parts and during the middle phase the upper and lower limbs were also moved into flexion and extension, as in bicycling movements. For the first and third phases, which were stroking with pressure, the infant's head, the back of the neck and shoulders, the upper back down to the waist, the thigh to the foot, and the shoulder to the wrist were stroked for six 10-sec strokes for each body part. The movements were slow and moved from the top to the bottom and back to the top, as for example, from the top of the infant's head down the side of the face to the neck and back up to the top of the head. In the middle phase the infant was placed in a supine position and passive flexion and extension movements were done on each arm, then each leg, and then both legs simultaneously.

The data suggested that the massaged infants were helped in several ways. First, for the postnatal complications data an interaction effect suggested that by the 10th day the massaged infants were showing fewer postnatal complications on the Littman and Parmelee Scale (Littman & Parmelee, 1978) and on a more comprehensive severity index called the Newfoundland Scale (Schreiner & Sexton, in press; see Table 18.7). The massaged infants also averaged a 28% greater weight gain ($M = 33$ grams vs. 26 grams) over the treatment period despite the

TABLE 18.7
Means for Perinatal Data

	Massage	Control	p
Maternal age	25.5	25.1	ns
Parity	4.1	3.7	ns
Gestational age (weeks)	29.7	30.8	ns
Birth weight (g)	1,158.3	1,265.4	ns
Birth length (cm)	36.8	38.8	ns
Head circumference (cm)	25.8	26.6	ns
Ponderal Index[a]	2.4	2.2	ns
Apgar			
1 min	5.9	5.3	ns
5 min	7.5	6.9	ns
10 min	8.4	7.8	ns
Obstetric complications[b]	69.0	63.1	ns
Postnatal complications[b]	70.9	71.3	ns
Newfoundland Scale[c]	7.1	7.2	ns
Number of ICU days	20.3	16.2	ns
Weight at study onset	1,458.0	1,488.0	ns

Note. All comparisons were nonsignificant.
[a]Ponderal Index = birth weight/length^3 × 100. [b]Higher score is optimal. [c]Lower score is optimal.

fact that they consumed similar amounts of formula and calories. In addition, another group by repeated measures analysis interaction effect suggested that the massaged infants had better motor scores at the end of the 10-day study period, whereas the motor scores of the control infants remained the same. The massaged infants also tended to show improved orientation behaviors by the last day of the study. In addition, fewer stress behaviors were noted by Day 10 in the massaged infants versus the control infants on a scale that taps stress behaviors of drug-exposed infants (Eisen et al., 1991; see Table 18.8).

TABLE 18.8
Means for Brazelton Clusters and Performance

	Massage		Control		
	Day 1	Day 10	Day 1	Day 10	p[a]
Habituation	5.7	6.0	6.6	6.4	ns
Orientation	3.9	4.9	3.2	3.2	.06
Motor maturity	3.8	5.0	3.7	3.4	.02
Range of state	3.6	4.1	2.7	3.5	ns
Regulation of state	4.6	5.9	3.0	4.8	ns
Autonomic	5.8	5.7	5.2	5.4	ns
Reflexes[b]	11.9	7.9	8.6	6.4	ns
Stress behaviors[b]	2.7	1.6	2.2	2.3	.05

Note. [a]Significance for interaction effects. [b]Lower score is optimal.

These findings are consistent with those from studies on the use of massage therapy with preterm infants. The weight gain was predictable even though the mediating mechanism for the weight gain is not yet known. Some preliminary data suggest that the massage therapy may be increasing vagal activity, which in turn is stimulating the production of food absorption hormones such as glucose and insulin. Hopefully, like the preterm infants who received massage therapy, these infants will continue to show a weight advantage. The growth and development advantage noted for the preterm infants at 8 months could derive from better parent–infant interactions, which could be stimulated by the better motor and orientation scores of these infants during the neonatal period. It appears, then, that this is another high-risk infant group that benefits from this cost-effective early intervention.

CLASSROOM BEHAVIOR OF GRADE-SCHOOL CHILDREN EXPOSED TO COCAINE

The benefits of the early intervention just described are highlighted by the behavior problems noted for older, grade-school-age children who had been exposed to cocaine and were not provided with any early intervention. In the early 1990s large numbers of the so-called "crack babies" started entering grade-school (Chira, 1990). Currently, cocaine-exposed children represent large proportions of special education classes for behaviorally disordered children. Anecdotal reports from teachers of these classes suggest that the children exhibit many of the same behaviors as attention deficit hyperactivity disorder (ADHD) and conduct disorder (CD) children (Chira, 1990). However, they also tend to be mean (engage in unprovoked physical aggression) and have little empathy, remorse, or awareness of the repercussions of their aggressive behavior. In one of the only follow-up studies of prenatal cocaine exposure (Rodning, Beckwith, & Howard, 1989) there is the suggestion of the cocaine toddlers' apparent inability to modulate arousal and the toddlers' abnormal emotional responses. For example, cocaine-exposed toddlers did not show typical distress responses when separated from attachment figures.

According to teachers' anecdotal reports (Chira, 1990) cocaine-exposed children demonstrate behaviors common to both ADHD and CD diagnoses. They are hyperactive, overwhelmed by too much stimuli, show poor attention span and are aggressive and violent. They apparently require even more attention from teachers than ADHD and CD children, often needing one-on-one supervision. What seems to distinguish cocaine-exposed children from ADHD and CD children are teachers' descriptions that they are particularly mean, nasty, and frequently lacking signs of emotion. These descriptions suggest antisocial, psychopathic behavior.

Appreciating the problems of retrospective studies, particularly when in utero drug exposure is confounded by poor postnatal environments and childrearing, we attempted to document in a more systematic way the classroom behavior that has been inadequately reported by these children's grade-school teachers. For these observations we attended the special education classes in two different schools and conducted interviews and classroom observations of a group of 18 cocaine-exposed children and 16 ADHD children. The cocaine exposure had been made known to the school authorities by the children's grandparents.

The children's principal teacher was asked to complete the Teacher's Report Form (Achenbach & Edelbrock, 1986). This scale provides a profile of problem behavior syndromes (plus scales indicating adaptive behavior in school perform-ance) for children 4 to 16 years old. This scale is summarized by the internalizer and externalizer factors.

The children were given the Center for Epidemiology Studies Depression Scale (CES–D; Radloff, 1977) and the Empathy Scale (Bryant, 1982), which is adapted from the Mehrabian and Epstein (1972) Adult Empathy Scale. It contains questions such as "It's hard for me to see why someone else gets upset." The children were also given the Social Anxiety Scale for Children, Revised (LaGreca & Stone, 1993). This is a self-report measure of social anxiety, with statements such as "I worry about being teased." It yields three factors: fear of negative evaluation, social avoidance and distress with new or unfamiliar peers, and social avoidance and distress, generalized.

Finally, each child was observed for four different 10-min periods using a 10-sec time-sample unit observation system in the classroom. The behaviors of the teacher were also coded if and when he or she was interacting with the child being observed. Running behavior observations were first conducted to select behaviors for the coding system. The behaviors coded include out of seat, fidgeting, staring into space, off-task, disorganized behavior, positive and negative verbal and physical behavior toward the teacher and toward the peers (for a total of 8 behaviors), attention seeking, and noncompliant behavior.

When the cocaine-exposed grade-school children were compared to the ADHD children, their teacher-rated Achenbach and Conners scores were more problematic than those of the ADHD children and in the clinical range for externalizing problems. In addition, they scored higher on the CES–D Scale, and they showed more disturbed classroom behaviors, including more fidgeting, staring into space, off-task behavior, and attention-seeking, noncompliant behavior vis-à-vis their teachers, and aggressive behavior with their peers (see Table 18.9). Surprisingly, no differences were noted on the Children's Empathy and Social Anxiety Scale scores.

It would seem that instead of showing different types of behaviors than the ADHD children, the cocaine-exposed children simply displayed more of the same kinds of behaviors. It is possible that the mean, nonempathic behavior that is typically noted by teachers to distinguish the cocaine-exposed children from the ADHD children was not observed in this study because the special education classrooms were particularly well organized and the teachers exercised behavior management techniques that seemed to effectively control these children's be-havior. In addition, the use of study carrels and interactive television within those

TABLE 18.9
Cocaine-Exposed Children's Data

Scales	Cocaine-Exposed	ADHD	p
CES-D	16.9	11.1	.03
Teacher CBCL			
Internalizer	71.7	58.1	.05
Externalizer	66.0	53.6	.05
Classroom behaviors (% time)			
Fidgeting	13.0	8.5	.05
Staring in space	5.3	3.9	.05
Off-task behavior	28.0	20.5	.02
Attention seeking	4.0	1.8	.005
Noncompliant behavior	10.0	3.7	.001
Aggressive behavior	2.6	1.7	.05

carrels may have enabled the children to be less impulsive because of lower arousal levels. Nonetheless, the higher levels of aggressive, externalizing behavior on top of attention difficulty highlights the need for further longitudinal follow-up studies and early intervention programs for children exposed to cocaine.

In summary, these studies combined suggest minimal effects of cocaine exposure on the neonatal behavior of full-term infants in contrast to several negative effects of cocaine exposure on less mature preterm infants. The preterm infants who were exposed to cocaine showed more perinatal complications, less optimal neonatal behavioral assessment scores, more disorganized sleep patterns and stress behaviors during sleep, and increased sympathetic activity, as suggested by elevated norepinephrine and cortisol levels and decreased insulin levels. These conditions may have been compounded by fewer visits from their mothers and less physical contact when they did visit. Fortunately, many of these negative effects could be reversed by the massage therapy intervention used with the cocaine-exposed preterm infants. The behaviors noted—namely fewer postnatal complications, greater weight gain, and better motor and orienting behavior—in the massaged infants certainly would contribute to better parent–infant interactions, which in turn would facilitate growth and development. Because parents can be taught to massage their own infants, this is a potentially cost-effective intervention. The study on cocaine-exposed grade-school children suggested that they have attention problems, and they are more noncompliant with their teachers and aggressive with their peers. These data highlight the importance of finding effective early intervention programs.

ACKNOWLEDGMENTS

This research was supported by an NIMH Research Scientist Award (#MH00331), an NIMH Research Grant (#MH46586) and an NIDA Research Grant (#DA06900) to Tiffany Field.

REFERENCES

Achenbach, T. M., & Edelbrock, C. S. (1988). *Teacher's Report Form.* Burlington, VT: Authors.

Brazelton, T. B. (1984). *Neonatal Behavioral Assessment Scale.* Philadelphia: Lippincott.

Bryant, B. K. (1982). An index of empathy for children and adolescents. *Child Development, 53,* 413–425.

Burkett, G., Yasin, S., & Palow, D. (1990). Perinatal implications of cocaine exposure. *Journal of Reproductive Medicine, 35,* 35–42.

Chasnoff, I. J. (1987). Perinatal effects of cocaine. *Contemporary Obstetrics and Gynecology, 14,* 163–179.

Chasnoff, I., Burns, W. J., Schnoll, S. H., & Burns, K. (1985). Cocaine use in pregnancy. *New England Journal of Medicine, 313,* 666–669.

Chira, S. (1990, May 25). Crack babies turn five, and schools brace. *New York Times,* pp. A1, A11.

Cole, B. J., & Robbins, T. W. (1989). Effects of 6-hydroxydopamine lesions of the nucleus accumbens septi on performance of a 5-choice serial reaction time task in rats: Implications for theories of selective attention and arousal. *Behavioral Brain Research, 33,* 165–179.

Coles, C. D., Platzman, K. A., Smith, I. E., & James, M. (1990, April). *Effects of maternal use of cocaine and alcohol on neonatal behavior.* Paper presented at the International Conference on Infant Studies. Montreal, Canada.

Coles, C., Platzman, K., Smith, I., James, M., & Falek, A. (1991). Effects of cocaine, alcohol, and other drugs used in pregnancy in neonatal growth and neurobehavioral status. *Neurotoxicology and Teratology, 13*(4), 1–11.

Dixon, S., Bresnahan, K., & Zuckerman, B. (1990). Cocaine babies: Meeting the challenge of management. *Contemporary Pediatrics, 22,* 70–92.

Eisen, L., Field, T., Bandstra, E., Roberts, J., Morrow, C., & Larson, S. (1991). Perinatal cocaine effects on neonatal stress behavior and performance on the Brazelton scale. *Pediatrics, 88,* 477–480.

Field, T., Scafidi, F., & Schanberg, S. (1987). Massage of preterm newborns to improve growth and development. *Pediatric Nursing, 13*(6), 385–387.

Field, T., Schanberg, S. M., Scafidi, F., Bauer, C. R., Vega-Lahr, N., Garcia, R., Nystrom, J., & Kuhn, C. M. (1986). Tactile/kinesthetic stimulation effects on preterm neonates. *Pediatrics, 77*(5), 654–658.

Hadeed, A. J., & Siegel, S. R. (1989). Maternal cocaine use during pregnancy: Effect on the newborn infant. *Pediatrics, 84,* 205–210.

Hertzel, J., Christensen, N. J., Pedersen, D. A., & Kuhl, C. (1982). Plasma noradrenaline and adrenaline in infants of diabetic mothers at birth and at two hours of age. *Acta Paediatrica Scandinavia, 71,* 941–945.

Kuhn, C., Schanberg, S., Field, T., Symanski, R., Zimmerman, E., Scafidi, F., & Roberts, J. (1991). Tactile/kinesthetic stimulation effects on sympathetic and adrenocortical function in preterm infants. *Journal of Pediatrics, 119,* 434–440.

LaGreca, A. M., & Stone, W. L. (1993). The Social Anxiety Scale for Children—Revised: Factor structure and concurrent validity. *Journal of Clinical Child Psychology, 22,* 17–27.

Lester, B. M., Als, H., & Brazelton, T. B. (1982). Regional obstetric anesthesia and newborn behavior: A reanalysis toward synergistic effects. *Child Development, 53,* 687–692.

Littman, D., & Parmelee, A. (1978). Medical correlates of infant development. *Pediatrics, 61,* 470–474.

Magnano, C. L., Gardner, J. M., & Karmel, B. Z. (1992). Differences in salivary cortisol levels in cocaine-exposed and noncocaine-exposed NICU infants. *Developmental Psychobiology, 25,* 93–103.

Mehrabian, A., & Epstein, N. (1972). A measure of emotional empathy. *Journal of Personality, 40,* 525–543.

Porat, R., & Brodsky, N. (1991). Cocaine: A risk factor for necrotizing enterocolitis. *Journal of Perinatology, 11,* 30–32.

Radloff, L. S. (1977). A CES-D Scale: A self-report depression scale for research in the general population. *Applied Psychological Measurement, 1,* 385–401.

Richards, I. S., Kulkarni, A. P., & Bremner, W. F. (1990). Cocaine-induced arrhythmia in human fetal myocardium in vitro: Possible mechanism for fetal death. *Pharmacology and Toxicology, 66,* 150–154.

Rodning, C., Beckwith, L., & Howard, J. (1989). Characteristics of attachment organization and play organization in prenatally drug-exposed toddlers. *Developmental Psychopathology, 1,* 277–289.

Rosenak, D., Diamont, Z., Yaffe, H., & Hornstein, D. (1990). Cocaine: Maternal use during pregnancy and its effect on the mother, fetus, and the infant. *Obstetrical and Gynecological Survey, 45,* 348–359.

Scafidi, F., Field, T., Schanberg, S., Bauer, C., Tucci, K., Roberts, J., Morrow, C., & Kuhn, C. M. (1990). Massage stimulates growth in preterm infants: A replication. *Infant Behavior and Development, 13,* 167–188.

Scafidi, F., Field, T., Schanberg, S., Bauer, C., Vega-Lahr, N., & Garcia, R. (1986). Effects of tactile/kinesthetic stimulation on the clinical course and sleep/wake behavior of preterm neonates. *Infant Behavior and Development, 9,* 91–105.

Scafidi, F. A., Field, T., Wheeden, A., Schanberg, S., Kuhn, C., Symanski, R., Zimmerman, E., & Bandstra, E. (in press). Cocaine-exposed preterm neonates show behavioral and hormonal differences.

Schreiner, A. P., & Sexton, M. E. (in press). The ability of a perinatal risk inventory to predict developmental outcome. *Pediatrics.*

Sigman, M., & Parmelee, A. (1989, January). *Longitudinal predictors of cognitive development.* Paper presented at the AAAS Meeting, San Francisco, CA.

Singer, L. T., Garber, R., & Kliegman, R. (1991). Neurobehavioral sequelae of fetal cocaine exposure. *Journal of Pediatrics, 119,* 667–672.

Streissguth, A. P., Barr, H. M., & Martin, D. C. (1983). Maternal alcohol use and neonatal habituation assessed with the Brazelton scale. *Child Development, 54,* 1109–1118.

Thoman, E. B. (1975). Early development of sleeping behaviors in infants. In N. R. Ellis (Ed.), *Aberrant development in infancy: Human and animal studies* (pp. 28–39). New York: Wiley.

Wheeden, A., Scafidi, F., Field, T., Ironson, G., Valdeon, C., & Bandstra, E. (1993). Massage effects on cocaine-exposed preterm neonates. *Journal of Developmental and Behavioral Pediatrics, 14,* 318–322.

Young, S. L., Vosper, H. J., Phillips, S. A. (1992). Cocaine: Its effects on maternal and child health. *Pharmacotherapy, 12,* 2–17.

Author Index

The letter *f* following a page number indicates a figure; *n* denotes a footnote; and *t* indicates tabular material.

A

Aase, J., 155, *160*
Abel, E. L., 336, *349*
Abercrombie, E. D., 44, 44*f*, *55*
Aboagye, K., 71, *94*, 111, 118, 123, *127*, 143, *159*, 179, 202, 230–232, *250*, 252, 255, *269*, 287, *303*, 305, 306, 307, 309, 310, 311, 312, 313, *328*, *332*, 335, 336, 338, *350*, *353*
Abrams, R. M., 236, *245*
Achenback, T. M., 365, *367*
Acker, D., 336, *349*
Acredolo, C., 281, *283*
Adamse, M., 265, *271*
Ager, J. W., 113, 114, 120, 121*f*, 122, *125*, *127*, 144, 155, *160*, *162*
Ahdieh, H., 179, *201*
Ahmad, G., 8, *14*
Ainsworth, M. D. S., 291, *302*
Akbari, H. M., 11, 13, *14*, 81*t*, *90*, *91*, 211, 224, 235, *245*, 247, 254, 267
Akimoto, K., 234, *246*
Akiyama, H., 43, 45, *54*
Akunne, H. C., 10, *16*
Alessandri, S. M., 123, *124*, 172, 174, 175, 176, *177*, *178*, 258, *267*, 275, 279, 280, *282*, 320, 323, *326*, 337, *349*
Alfonso, D., 11, *14*

Ali, S. F., 8, 9, 10, 12, 13, *14*, *16*, *17*, 80*t*, *94*, 211, 220, *226*, 235, *249*
Allanson, J. E., 255, *269*
Allred, E. N., 47, *54*
Alpern, L., 289, *303*
Al-Rawi, N. J., 49, *53*
Als, H., 241, *248*, 356, *367*
Al-Tikriti, S., 49, *54*
Alvaro, I., 81*t*, *94*
Amaro, H., 71, *94*, 111, 118, 123, *127*, 143, *159*, *162*, 179, 202, 230–232, *250*, 252, 255, 259, 262, *267*, *269*, 272, 287, *303*, 305, 306, 307, 309, 310, 311, 312, 313, 320, *328*, *332*, 335, 336, 338, *350*, *353*
Amin-Zaki, L., 49, *53*, *54*
Amuroso, L. P., 199, *201*
Anastasiow, N. J., 325, *326*
Anday, E. K., 71, *91*, 236, *246*, 257, *267*, 336, *350*
Anders, T. F., 275, *285*
Anderson, C., 325, *332*
Anderson, D. R., 76, 78*t*, 82*t*, 83, 87*t*, *93*, 242, 244, *247*
Anderson, D. W., 46, *55*
Anderson, G. M., 233, *248*
Anderson, J., 22, *38*, 236, *249*
Anderson, P. H., 10, *14*
Anderson-Brown, T., 9, *14*
Andrzejczak, A. L., 79*t*, *91*

369

Aneshensel, C. S., 320, *328*
Anisfeld, E., 257, *267*
Anton, S. F., 264, *270*
Archer, T., 8, *17*
Ardila, A., 265, *267*
Arendt, R., 111, *127*, 257, *267*
Arevalo, R., 11, *14*
Arilla, E., 81*t*, *94*
Arnold, H. M., 76, 78*t*, 81*t*, 86, 87*t*, 88*t*, *92*,
    131, *159*, 210, 212, 214*f*, 215, 219,
    225, 244, *247*
Aronson, M., 115, *124*
Asarnow, R., 115, *126*
Asensio, D. C., 144, *161*, 182, 188, *202*
Ashby, C. R., Jr., 10, *16*, 82*t*, *93*, 211, 220,
    226, 235, *248*
Ashby, S., 102*t*, 103, *108*, 243, *247*
Ashe, W. K., 77*t*, 80*t*, 87*t*, *94*, 242, *249*
Athalie, F., 221, 222*f*, *225*
Axelrod, J., 12, *14*
Azmitia, E. C., 11, 13, *14*, 81*t*, *90*, *91*, 211,
    224, 235, *245*, 247, 254, *267*
Azuma, S. D., 34, *37*, 102*t*, 103, 104, *107*,
    108, 153, *158*, 242, *246*, 288, *302*

B

Babb, S., 234, *249*
Bachicha, J. A., 306, 309, 310, 311, 312, *330*
Bachman, J. G., 307, *330*
Badger, E., 342, *349*
Bailey, D. N., 180, *200*
Bakeman, R., 281, *283*
Bakir, F., 49, *53*
Baldwin, J., 224, *226*
Bales, W. R., 307, *331*
Baley, J., 102*t*, 104, *109*
Ball, G. C., 60, *65*
Bancalari, E., 237, *246*
Bandstra, E. S., 164, *177*, 183, 186, 200, *200*,
    237, 241*t*, *246*, 247, 257, *269*, 306,
    328, 335, *349*, 356, 357–358, 361,
    362, 363, *367*, *368*
Banerjee, S. P., 235, *249*
Bannoura, M. D., 211, *227*
Barker, D. J. P., 45, *54*
Barker, J. L., 9, *15*
Barkov, B. A., 237, *249*
Barkow, H., 275, *285*
Barnard, K. E., 118, *124*
Barnett, D., 261, *268*

Barnette, D. M., 307, 309, 310, *328*
Barocas, R., 34, *37*
Barr, H. M., 52, *55*, 111, 112, 113, 113*n*, 114,
    115, 116, 120, *126*, *127*, 131, 142,
    143, 149, 153, 155, *159*, *160*, *162*,
    207, 224, *227*, 307, 311, 312, *332*,
    357, *368*
Barratt, M. S., 165, *178*
Barrett, K. C., 274, *283*
Barrett, M. E., 106, *108*, 147, *159*, 252, *268*,
    307, 312, *326*
Barrett, P., 46, *54*, 111, *126*
Barron, S., 80*t*, *91*, 216, 223–224, *224*
Baselt, R., 146, *158*
Bass, E. W., 211, *225*
Bateman, D., 146, *158*
Bateman, D. A., 311, *332*
Bates, J. E., 274, 279, *283*
Batra, K. K., 307, 309, 310, 311, 312, *328*
Bauchner, H., 71, *94*, 111, 118, 123, *127*,
    143, *159*, 179, *202*, 230–232, *250*,
    252, 255, 259, *269*, 272, 287, *303*,
    306, 307, 309, 310, 311, 312, 313,
    320, *332*, 335, 336, 338, *350*, *353*
Bauer, C. R., 358, 361, *367*, *368*
Bauman, P. S., 260, 265, *267*, 325, *326*, 344,
    349
Baumgartner, W. A., 144, 145, *158*
Bautista, D. B., 154, *162*, 237, 239, *246*
Baxter, A., 346, *349*
Baxter, J., 180, *202*
Bayley, N., 113, *124*, 256, *267*
Bean, X., 154, *162*, 237, 239, *246*
Beardslee, W. R., 319, *332*
Beck, A. T., 117*t*, *124*, 319, *326*
Beckman, L. J., 321, *326*
Beckwith, L., 34, *37*, 102*t*, 103, *109*, 115,
    123, *126*, *127*, 151, *161*, 260, 261,
    271, 278, *285*, 288, 291, *302*, *303*,
    337, 344, 345, *351*, *352*, 364, *368*
Bee, H. L., 118, *124*
Beeghly, M., 155, *162*
Behar, L. B., 294, *302*
Behnke, M., 99, 100*t*, 101, *109*, 263, *272*,
    306, 307, 308*t*, 309, 310, 311, 312,
    313, 316, 319, 325, *326*, *328*, *332*
Bejar, R., 71, *92*, 338, *350*
Belenky, Y., 235, *249*
Bell, C. A., 348, *350*
Bell, J., 77*t*, 79*t*, 87*t*, 88*t*, *94*, 167, *178*, 212, *226*
Bellinger, D. C., 47, 52, *53*, *54*, 113, *124*
Bellucci, P. A., 325, *328*

Bendell, D., 306, *328*
Bendersky, M., 166, *177, 178*
Benzon, H. T., 9, *14*
Berendes, H. W., 312, *329*
Bergeman, C. S., 253, *267*
Berger, O., 47, *54,* 113, *125*
Berger, T. W., 44, 44*f, 55*
Bernardi, E., 260, *267*
Berner, J., 265, *270*
Bernheimer, H., 44–45, *53*
Bernstein, V. J., 261, 262, *267, 269*
Berry, J., 265, *267*
Berry, P., 277, *284*
Berzins, J., 319, *331*
Besharov, D. J., 252, *267,* 336, *349*
Bickerstaff, J., 342, *349*
Biegon, A., 13, *14*
Bier, M., 47, *54,* 113, *125*
Bierman, J. M., 32, *39*
Bihun, J. T., 116, 121, *125*
Bilitzke, P. J., 78*t,* 81*t,* 87*t, 91,* 211, *225,* 242, *246*
Billings, R. L., 116, *125*
Billman, D., 257, *268*
Bingol, N., 24, *37,* 71, *91,* 255, *268,* 309, 310, 312, 336, *349*
Birkmayer, W., 44–45, *53*
Black, R., 260, *268,* 344, *351*
Blackhurst, D. W., 307, *332*
Blahd, W. H., 144, 145, *158*
Blehar, M. C., 291, *302*
Bloom, F. E., 9, 13, *16*
Blume, S. B., 325, *326*
Boehrer, J. D., 232, *248*
Bondy, S. C., 8, *14*
Bookstein, F. L., 111, 113*n, 126, 127,* 143, 153, 155, *162*
Bookstein, G., 149, *159*
Bornschein, R. L., 47, *54,* 113, *125*
Bornstein, M. H., 19, *38,* 72, *93,* 99, 100*t,* 101, 107, *108,* 111, 112, *126,* 164, *177, 178,* 230, 241*t,* 242, 245, *248,* 253, 255, 257, 258, 262, 265, *268,* 270, 272, 274, 276, *283*
Bottoms, S., 114, *125*
Boukydis, C. F. Z., 25, *38*
Bowman, R. S., 113, *124*
Boyd, C. J., 265, *268,* 322, *326*
Boyd, T., 120, *125*
Brackbill, Y., 168, *177*
Brackfield, S., 277, *284*
Bradley, R. H., 117*t,* 118, 118*n, 124*

Brady, M., 144, *161,* 179, 180, 182, 183, 188, 189, 190, *201, 202,* 232, *248,* 307, 309, 310, 312, *331*
Brake, S. C., 62, *66*
Branch, D. G., 144, *161*
Brandt, C., 155, *162*
Braun, S. B., 74–75, 79*t, 92*
Braunwald, K., 261, *268*
Brazelton, T. B., 25, *38,* 164, 176, *177,* 241, *246, 248,* 257, *268,* 276, *283,* 305, *326,* 356, 358, *367*
Breau, A. M., 294, *302*
Brem, F. S., 34, *38*
Bremner, W. F., 355, *368*
Breslow, N. E., 97, 99, *107*
Bresnahan, K., 207, *227,* 230, 242, *250,* 305, *332,* 355, *367*
Bridger, W., 294, *302*
Bridger, W. H., 116, *125*
Bridges, F. A., 277, *283*
Brill, N. J., 113, *126,* 261, *271*
Brinker, R. P., 337, 345, 346, *349, 352*
Britt, G. C., 129, *161*
Brodsky, N. L., 111, *125,* 335, *349,* 355, *368*
Bromet, E., 319, *326*
Bromwich, R. M., 342, 343, *349*
Bronfenbrenner, U., 339, 340, *349*
Brooks-Gunn, J., 169, 170, *178,* 257, *270*
Brown, B. R., 321, *326*
Brown, J. V., 281, *283*
Brown, R. T., 111, 115, 116, *124*
Brown, Z. A., 131, 142, *160, 162,* 207, *227,* 307, 311, 312, *332*
Brown-Woodman, P. D. C., 8, *17,* 75, 81*t, 94*
Brumitt, G. A., 116, *125*
Bryant, B. K., 365, *367*
Buckley, S., 154, *162,* 239, *246*
Bugental, D. B., 321, *326*
Buhfiend, C. M., 235, *249*
Bull, D., 22, *38,* 236, *249*
Bunsey, M., 223, *227*
Burbacher, T. M., 51, *53,* 116, *125*
Burchfield, D. J., 236, *245*
Buring, J. E., 96, 99, *108*
Burke, M. E., 307, 309, 310, *329*
Burkett, G. T., 335, *349,* 355, *367*
Burns, K. A., 71, *91,* 99, 100*t,* 101, 102, *108,* 131, *159,* 164, *177,* 179, *200,* 256, 257, 261, *268,* 278, *283,* 287, *302,* 305, 306, 309, 311, 312, 312–313, 313, *319, 326,* 336, *349,* 356, *367*

Burns, R. B., 322, *326*
Burns, W. J., 71, *91,* 99, 100*t,* 101, *108,* 131, *159,* 164, *177,* 179, 180, *200, 201,* 261, *268,* 278, *283,* 287, *302,* 305, 306, 309, 311, 312, 312–313, 313, 319, *326,* 336, *349,* 356, *367*
Burton, L. E., 77*t,* 80*t,* 87*t, 94,* 242, *249*
Buss, A. H., 274, 275, *283, 284*
Bussey, M. E., 179, *201,* 232, *246*
Butler, N. R., 312, *328*
Byck, R., 251, *268*
Byers, R. K., 46, *53*
Byrd, L. D., 10, *14*
Byrd, S. E., 232, *248*

C

Cabral, H., 26, *39,* 71, *94,* 111, 118, 123, *127,* 143, *159, 162,* 179, *202,* 230–232, 233, 242, *247, 250,* 252, 255, 259, *267, 269,* 272, 287, *303,* 305, 306, 307, 309, 310, 311, 312, 313, 320, *328, 332,* 335, 336, 338, *350, 353*
Cairns, D., 102*t,* 104, *109*
Caldwell, B. M., 117*t,* 118, 118*n, 124*
Caldwell, J., 294, *303*
Callahan, C. M., 142, 144, *158, 160,* 183, 186, 199, *200*
Calne, D. B., 42, *53*
Calsyn, D. A., 143, *161*
Camacho, T., 319, *329*
Campbell, D., 71, *93,* 99, 100*t,* 101, 102, 102*t,* 104, *109,* 241*t, 248,* 306, 309, 310, *330*
Campbell, H., 257, *270*
Campbell, S., 294, *302*
Campbell, S. B., 294, *302*
Campos, J. J., 274, 276, 279, *283, 284*
Carboni, S., 234, *248*
Carey, W. B., 274, 275, *283, 285*
Carlson, V., 261, *268*
Carlsson, A., 45, *54*
Carmichael, F. J., 12, *14*
Carmichael Olson, H., 149, 152, 153, 155, *158, 159, 160, 162*
Carpenter, R. W., 59, 64, *66*
Carr, J. N., 344, *349*
Cartwright, P. S., 307, 308*t,* 309, 310, *326*
Carvey, P. M., 235, *249*
Carzoli, R. P., 236, *246*

Casanova, O. Q., 307, 309, 310, 311, 312, *326*
Casella, G. A., 317, *330*
Cassidy, J., 289, 290, *302*
Castor, D., 321, *326*
Castro, R., 11, *14*
Celada, T., 265, *270*
Cha, C. M., 25, *39*
Chambers, C. D., 264, *268*
Chan, K., 236, 240, *246*
Chan, M. K., 233, *249*
Chandler, M. J., 32, *39,* 124, *126,* 306, *331,* 340, *352*
Chang, J., 146, *158*
Chang, M., 237, *246*
Chasnoff, I. J., 28, 34, *37,* 71, 72, *91, 93,* 99, 100*t,* 101, 102, 102*t,* 103, 104, 106, *107, 108, 109,* 111, 123, *124,* 131, 138, 147, 152, 153, 154, *158, 159, 161,* 164, *177,* 179, 180, *200, 201,* 230, 241*t,* 242, 243, *246,* 252, 255, 256, 257, *268, 270,* 278, *283, 285,* 287, 288, *302, 303,* 305, 306, 307, 309, 310, 311, 312, 312–313, 313, 314*t,* 319, 324, *326, 330,* 335, 336, 337, 338, *349, 351, 352,* 355, 356, *367*
Chasnoff, M. D., 232, *246*
Chavez, C. J., 59, *66,* 179, 180, *201, 202*
Chawarska, K., 258, *270*
Checola, R. T., 24, *39*
Chen, C., 237, *246*
Chen, W.-J., 77*t,* 80*t,* 87*t,* 88*t, 92,* 167, *177,* 212, 215, 215*f,* 216, 217*f,* 224, *225*
Cherukuri, R., 311, 312, *326,* 338, *350*
Chess, S., 274, 275, *284, 286*
Chethik, L., 261, *268*
Children's Defense Fund, 343, 344, *350*
Chintalapally, S., 311, *330*
Chira, S., 364, *367*
Chisum, G. M., 131, *161,* 179, *201,* 287, *303,* 306, 309, 310, 311, 312, *330,* 336, 338, *349, 351*
Chisum, R. N., 71, *93,* 255, *270*
Chitwood, D., 183, 186, 200, *200*
Christensen, N. J., 360, 361, *367*
Church, M. W., 76, 77*t,* 78*t,* 79*t,* 80*t,* 81*t,* 87*t, 91, 94,* 132, 153, *159,* 211, *225,* 242, *246*
Church, S., 62, 65, *66,* 242, *249*
Church, W. H., 10, *14*
Cicchetti, D., 131, *159,* 260, 261, *268, 271,* 277, *283,* 339, *350*

Clancy, R. R., 235, *247*
Clark, C. R., 254, *268*
Clark, G. D., 144, *158,* 183, 186, 199, *200,*
  201
Clark, K. E., 6, *17,* 22, *38,* 255, 272
Clark, R., 261, *268*
Clark, V. A., 320, *328*
Clarke, C., 274, *284*
Clarkson, T. W., 49, *53, 54*
Clarren, S. K., 336, *350*
Clatterbaugh, H. E., 307, *331*
Clayton, R. R., 335, *350*
Clement, C., 264, *271*
Clow, D. W., 80*t, 91,* 211, *225*
Cobb, S., 322, *326*
Coen, R. W., 278, *283,* 336, *350*
Cohen, D. J., 115, 116, *126,* 233, *248*
Cohen, M. E., 71, *91,* 236, *246,* 257, *267,*
  336, *350*
Cohen, S., 322, *326*
Cohen, S. E., 115, *126, 127*
Cohn, J. F., 306, 319, *327*
Coldren, J. R., 115, *124*
Cole, B. J., 357, *367*
Cole, J., 22, *38,* 238, *248*
Coleman, M., 8, *16*
Coleman-Hardee, M., 10, *16*
Coles, B. J., 258, *268*
Coles, C. D., 71, *91,* 99, 100*t,* 101, 102, *108,*
  111, 112, 114, 115, 116, 122, *124,*
  127, 129, 152, 157, *159,* 164, *177,*
  241*t, 246,* 257, *268,* 305–306, 307,
  309, 311, 312, 313, 324, 325, *327,*
  329, 344, *350,* 355, 357, *367*
Collins, A., 8, *16*
Colombo, J., 115, *124,* 257, *268*
Comfort, M., 322, *327*
Commissiong, J. W., 234, *246*
Comstock, G., 320, *327*
Condry, J. C., 325, *327*
Condry, S., 325, *327*
Cone-Wesson, B., 235, *249,* 278, *285*
Conlon, M., 99, 100*t,* 101, *109,* 263, 272,
  306, 307, 309, 310, 311, 312, 313,
  316, 319, 325, *326, 328, 332*
Connell, D., 306, 319, *327*
Cook, C., 151, *162*
Cooper, D. H., 339, *353*
Cooper, R., 179, *201*
Cooper, S., 322, *327*
Cooper, T. B., 8, *16*
Coppolillo, H. P., 344, *350*

Cornelius, M., 112, *124,* 336, *350*
Corrigall, W., 234, *249*
Corwin, M. J., 24, *38,* 71, *93,* 153, *160,* 237,
  238, *248,* 278, *285,* 287, *302,* 337, *351*
Costin, L. B., 348, *350*
Courtwright, D. T., 252, *269*
Coustan, D. R., 307, 309, 310, *329*
Covino, B. G., 9, *14*
Cox, C., 49, *54*
Coyle, J. T., 12, *14*
Coyne, J., 319, *329*
Craig, T. J., 319, *327*
Crandall, M. E., 6, *14*
Crandall, R., 322, *327*
Crane, M. M., 307, *332*
Cregler, L. L., 24, *37*
Crnic, K. A., 323, *327*
Crockenberg, S., 281, *283*
Cross, A., 322, *327*
Cross, C. K., 318, *329*
Crutchfield, S., 278, *283,* 336, *350*
Cruz, A. D., 179, *201*
Cunningham, N., 257, *267*
Curley, F. J., 24, *37*
Curro, F. A., 8, *16*
Cutler, S., 155, *160*

D

Dabiri, C., 275, *284*
Daley, S., 336, *350*
Damlugi, S. F., 49, *53*
Danzger, B., 176, *178*
Darby, B. L., 115, *127,* 143, *162*
Dark, K., 236, *249*
Darmani, N. A., 61, *65*
Darr, C., 146, *159*
Datta, S., 9, *14*
Davidson, C. E., 341, *350*
Davidson-Ward, S. L., 237, 239, *246*
Davis, C. M., 74, 79*t, 94*
Davis, F., 309, 310, 311, 312, *329*
Davis, M., 236, *246*
Day, L., 236, 240, *246*
Day, N., 112, *124*
Day, N. E., 97, 99, *107*
Day, N. L., 71, *93,* 99, 100*t,* 102, *109,* 111,
  114, *126,* 129, 152, 157, *159, 161,*
  241*t, 248,* 255, *269,* 306, 309, 310,
  311, 312, 313, 317, 324, *327, 331,*
  336, *350*

Debanne, S., 122, *127*
Deck, J. H. N., 234, *249*
deCosta, B., 10, *16*
Dekio, S., 147, *159*
Delaney, C. J., 143, *161*
Delke, I., 306, 307, 309, 310, 311, 312, 313, *330*
Dempsey, J., 275, 277, *284*
Deposito, F., 179, *201*
Derryberry, D., 274, 275, *283, 285*
Des Rosiers, M. H., 11, *17*
Desmond, M. M., 59, *65,* 288, *303*
DeVane, C. L., 74–75, 79*t, 92*
Dhahir, H. I., 49, *53*
Di Paolo, T., 240, *246*
di Porzio, U., 9, *15*
Diamont, Z., 355, *368*
Diaz, V., 24, *37,* 71, *91,* 255, *268,* 308*t,* 309, 310, 312, 314*t,* 336, *349*
Dietrich, K. N., 47, *54,* 113, *125*
Dincheff, B. A., 79*t, 91*
Ding, X. Y., 240, *248*
Dinnies, J., 146, *159*
Dirkes, D., 71, *91*
Dirkes, K., 99, 100*t,* 102, *108,* 256, 257, *268,* 305, *326*
Disney, E. R., 257, *269,* 287, 288, 289, *302*
DiStabile, P., 107, *109*
DiVitto, B., 277, *284*
Dixon, S. D., 71, *92,* 179, *201,* 232, *246,* 255, *269, 271,* 278, *283, 285,* 336, 338, *350, 352,* 355, *367*
Dobbing, J., 73, *92*
Doberczak, T. M., 22, *37,* 235, *246,* 278, *283*
Dodd, P. A., 236, 240, *246*
Dodge, K., 300, *302*
Doherty, R. A., 49, *53*
Dohrenwend, B. P., 323, *327*
Dohrenwend, B. S., 323, *327*
Dolan, A. B., 275, *285*
Dombrowski, M. P., 307, 310, 312, *327*
Don, A., 155, *159*
Dougherty, F. E., 260, 265, *267,* 325, *326,* 344, *349*
Dougherty, L. M., 274, *284*
Dow-Edwards, D. L., 5, 7, 8, 10, 11, 12, 14, *15, 65, 66,* 73–74, 77*t,* 79*t,* 80*t,* 81*t,* 82*t,* 87*t,* 89, 90, *92, 93,* 131, 132, *159,* 235, 242, 244, *246, 247, 249,* 254, *269*
Dowler, J. K., 116, *125*
Dowling, S., 346, *351*

Downs, S. W., 348, *350*
Doyle, A., 176, *177*
Dreshfield, L., 80*t, 92*
Driscoll, C. D., 209, *225*
Drucker, E., 60, *66,* 102, 105, 107, *109*
Duara, S., 237, *246*
Dufford, M. T. W., 60, *66*
Duhart, H. M., 9, 10, 12, 13, *17*
Dunn, L., 319, *326*
Dunn, L. M., 117*t,* 118, *125*
Dunst, C. J., 275, *283,* 318, 322, *327,* 346, *350*
Durand, D. J., 24, *37,* 179, *201,* 255, *269,* 278, *284*

E

Eaton, W., 319, 320, *327*
Ebrahimi, M., 239, *249*
Edelbrock, C. S., 365, *367*
Edwards, J. E., 321, *327*
Egeland, B., 291, *303,* 319, *327*
Ehrlich, S. M., 179, *202,* 255, *272,* 287, *303,* 325, *331,* 336, 338, *352*
Eichhorn, D. H., 165, *178*
Einarson, T., 95, 102*t,* 103, *108,* 157, *160,* 207, *225,* 243, *247*
Einarson, T. R., 27, 28, *38,* 71, *93,* 129, *160*
Eisen, A., 42, *53*
Eisen, L. N., 99, 100*t,* 101, *108,* 164, *177,* 241*t, 247,* 257, *269,* 306, *328,* 356, 363, *367*
Ekman, P., 168, *177,* 276, *283*
El-Bizri, H., 75, 80*t, 92*
Eldredge, L., 22, *38,* 236, *249*
Elkind, L., 336, *351*
Ellinwood, F. H., 253, *269*
Enright, M., 165, *178*
Enters, E. K., 61, *65*
Epstein, N., 365, *367*
Erbaugh, J., 117*t, 124,* 319, *326*
Erickson, M. F., 319, *327*
Erickson, S., 111, 115, 116, *124*
Erlich, S., 131, *161*
Ernhart, C., 112, 122, *127*
Ernhart, C. B., 119, 120, *125*
Erting, C., 281, *285*
Ervin, F., 264, *271*
Ervin, M. G., 236, 240, *246*
Escamilla-Mondanaro, J., 344, *350*
Estes, N. A. M., 336, *350*

Evans, A. S., 97, 99, *108*
Evans, A. T., 307, 309, 310, 311, 312, *328*
Evans, M. I., 307, 310, 312, *327*
Evans, R. I., 339, *350*
Ewing, L. J., 294, *302*
Eyler, F. D., 99, 100*t*, 101, *109*, 263, 272, 306, 307, 309, 310, 311, 312, 313, 316, 319, 325, *326, 328, 332*

F

Factor, E. M., 82*t, 92*
Fagan, J. F., III, 116, *125*
Fagen, J. W., 275, 276, *283*
Falek, A., 71, *91*, 99, 100*t*, 101, 102, *108*, 111, 112, 114, 115, 116, 122, *124, 127*, 164, *177*, 241*t, 246*, 257, *268*, 305–306, 307, 309, 311, 312, 313, *327*, 355, *367*
Fanshel, D., 343, 344, *350*
Fantel, A. G., 75, 79*t, 92*, 131, 132, *159*
Farel, A. M., 320, *329*
Farran, A. C., 277, *286*
Farrar, H. C., 254, *269*, 307, *328*
Fechter, L. D., 6, *16*
Feigenbaum, A., 102*t*, 103, *108*, 243, *247*
Feil, L. A., 318, *331*
Fein, G. G., 116, *125*
Feldman, J., 155, *158, 162*, 306, 307, 309, 310, 311, 312, 313, *326, 330*, 338, *350*
Feraru, E., 62, 63, *66*
Ferrari, L., 257, *267*
Ferré, C., 309, 310, 311, 312, *329*
Fetters, L., 155, *162*
Fick, C. M., 321, *329*
Fico, T. A., 10, 14, *15*, 63, 65, *66*, 74, 77*t*, 79*t*, 80*t*, 87*t*, 89, *92, 93*, 235, *246*
Fidell, L. S., 119, *127*
Field, T. F., 254, *269*
Field, T. M., 99, 100*t*, 101, *108*, 164, *177*, 241*t, 247*, 254, 257, 264, *269*, 275, 277, 281, *283, 284*, 306, 319, *327*, *328*, 356, 357–358, 358, 361, 362, 363, *367, 368*
Fiese, B. H., 340, 341, *352*
Fiks, K. B., 288, *302*
Fink, D. J., 307, 309, 310, 311, 312, *330*
Finnegan, L. P., 58, *66*, 131, *161*, 179, *202*, 235, *247*, 255, 272, 287, *303*, 305, 325, *328, 331*, 336, 338, *352*

Finnell, R. H., 75, 80*t, 92*
Fiszman, M. L., 9, *15*
Fleckenstein, L. K., 276, *283*
Foley, S., 264, *272*
Foote, S. I., 254, *271*
Forman, R., 144, 148, *159, 160*
Foss, J. A., 80*t*, 81*t, 91, 92, 94*, 131, *159, 161*, 224, *226*, 237, *247*
Fox, H. E., 307, 309, 310, 311, 312, *330*
Foy, B., 11, *15*
Fraiberg, S., 281, *284*
Frambes, N. A., 10, *16*, 74, 79*t*, 80*t*, 87*t*, 89, 94, 167, *178*, 210, 211, 212, 213*f*, 220, *226, 227*, 235, 242, 243, *249*
Francis, E. Z., 208, 209, *225, 226*
Frank, D. A., 26, *39*, 71, 72, *94*, 111, 118, 123, *127*, 143, 154, *157, 159*, 179, *202*, 230–232, 233, 240, 242, *247, 248, 250*, 252, 255, 256, 262, *269, 272*, 287, *303*, 305, 306, 307, *309*, 310, 311, 312, 313, 324, *328, 332*, 335, 336, 338, *350, 353*
Frank, M. A., 72, *93*, 99, 100*t*, 101, *108*, 111, *126*, 164, *178*, 255, 257, *270*
Frankenfield-Chernicoff, M., 307, *331*
Frankowski, J. J., 116, 121, *125*
Frazier, W. A., 346, *349*
Freed, L. A., 10, 11, 14, *15*, 74, 79*t*, 80*t*, 90, 92, 131, *159*, 235, *246, 247*, 254, *269*
Freed-Malen, L. A., 8, 14, *15*, 74, 82*t*, 90, 92
Freeman, R. C., 322, *330*
Freeseman, L. J., 115, *124*
Freier, C., 28, *37*, 71, 72, *91*, 102*t*, 103, *108*, 111, 123, *124*, 154, *159*, 230, 243, *246*, 256, 262, *268, 269*, 278, *283*, 288, *302*, 337, *349*
French, F. E., 32, *39*
Frentzen, B., 306, 307, 309, 310, 311, 312, 313, 316, *328*
Frerichs, R. R., 320, *328*
Freud, A., 348, *351*
Frick, G. S., 10, 11, 14, *15*
Fried, L., 143, *159*, 230–232, *250*, 252, 255, *269*, 305, 309, 310, 311, 312, *328*, 335, 338, *350*
Fried, L. E., 71, *94*, 111, 118, 123, *127*, 179, *202*, 252, *267*, 287, *303*, 306, 307, 309, 310, 311, 312, 313, *332*, 336, *353*
Fried, P. A., 111, 112, *125*, 192, *201*

Friesen, W., 276, *283*
Frye, K. F., 118, *125*
Fuchs, M., 24, *37*, 71, *91*, 255, 268, 308*t*, 309, 310, 312, 336, *349*
Fujinaga, M., 8, *15*
Fulroth, R. F., 24, *37*, 179, *201*, 255, *269*, 278, *284*
Fung, Y. K., 79*t*, *92*, 235, *247*

G

Gaensbauer, T., 277, *284*
Gagnon, W. A., 216, 223–224, *224*
Galanter, M., 322, *328*
Gamagaris, Z., 63, 65, *66*, 74, 79*t*, 89, *92*
Gansau, C., 89, *93*
Garbarino, J., 176, *177*, 346, *350*
Garber, R., 129, *161*, 355, *368*
Garcia, D., 196, *201*
Garcia, G., 196, 198, *201*
Garcia, R., 319, *328*, 361, *367*, *368*
Garcia-Coll, C. T., 25, 34, *38*, 274, *284*
Gardner, J. M., 154, *161*, 240, *248*, 361, *367*
Garmezy, N., 34, *37*
Garruto, R. M., 45, *54*
Gartner, L. M., 180, *201*
Gaughran, J., 274, *283*
Gause, S., 144, *161*, 179, 180, 189, 190, *201*, 307, 309, 310, 312, *331*
Gautieri, R. F., 24, *38*
Gawin, F. H., 21, *37*, 253, 265, *269*, 271, 319, *328*
Gay, J. W., 307, *331*
Geffen, G. M., 254, *268*
Geffen, L. B., 254, *268*
Geggel, R. L., 336, *350*
George, S. K., 307, 309, 310, *328*
Gerber, M. M., 336, *350*
Gerhardt, K. J., 236, *245*
Gerhardt, T., 237, *246*
Gervasio, C., 184, 185, *201*
Gessa, G. L., 234, *248*
Gessner, P. K., 79*t*, *91*
Gfroerer, J., 179, *201*
Ghodsian, M., 319, *328*
Giannetta, J., 111, *125*
Gilbaud-Wallston, J., 318, *328*
Gilliam, G., 176, *177*
Gillogley, K. M., 307, 309, 310, 311, 312, *328*
Gilstrap, L. C., 307, 309, 311, 312, *329*, 335, *351*

Gingras, J. L., 233, 237, *249*, 312, *329*
Giordano, M., 80*t*, *92*
Gissen, A. J., 9, *14*
Giunta, C. T., 141, *162*
Gladen, B. C., 113, *125*, *126*
Gladstone, D., 107, *108*, 132, *160*
Glamann, D. B., 232, *248*
Glasdonte, D., 72, *93*
Glass, L., 306, 307, 309, 310, 311, 312, 313, *326*, *330*, 338, *350*
Glassman, M. B., 288, *302*
Glezer, I., 235, *249*
Glotzer, D., 263, *270*
Gluck, D. S., 294, *302*
Godolphin, W., 180, *201*
Goeders, N. E., 253, *269*
Gold, M. S., 335, *350*
Goldberg, D., 336, *351*
Goldberg, M., 311, *331*
Goldberg, S., 102*t*, 103, *108*, 176, *178*, 243, *247*, 257, *270*, 277, *284*
Goldberg, S. R., 9, *16*
Golden, M., 294, *302*
Golden, N. L., 114, *125*
Golden, R., 62, 63, *66*
Golding, J., 312, *328*
Goldman, P. S., 51, *54*
Goldman-Rakic, P. S., 263, *269*
Goldsmith, H. H., 274, 276, 279, *283*, *284*
Goldstein, J., 348, *351*
Goldstein, P. J., 325, *328*
Goldstein, S., 306, 319, *328*
Golub, H. L., 24, *38*, 71, *93*, 153, *160*, 237, 238, *248*, 278, *285*, 287, *302*, 337, *351*
Gomby, D. S., 252, *269*
Gonzalez, R., 155, *158*
Goodlett, C., 155, *162*
Goodman, G. S., 115, 116, *125*
Goodwin, G. A., 76, 78*t*, 81*t*, 86, 87*t*, 88*t*, *92*, 131, *159*, 210, 211, 212, 214*f*, 215, 219, *225*, 244, *247*, 259, *269*
Gordon, M., 32, *38*
Gorinson, H. S., 62, 63, *66*
Gorski, R. A., 77*t*, 80*t*, 87*t*, *93*, 211, *226*
Goshko, M., 325, *330*
Gospe, S. M., 236, 243, *247*
Gottesman, N., 319, *327*
Gottfried, A. W., 116, *125*
Grace, A. A., 44, 44*f*, *55*
Graham, K., 27, 28, *38*, 71, *93*, 95, 102*t*, 103, *108*, 129, 144, 148, 157, *159*, *160*, 180, *201*, 207, *225*, 243, *247*

Granger, R. H., 19, *38,* 72, *93,* 99, 100*t,* 101,
  107, *108,* 111, 112, *126,* 164, *178,*
  230, 241*t,* 242, 245, *248,* 255, 257,
  258, *270*
Granick, S., 321, *326*
Grant, K. S., 116, *125*
Grant, N. F., 346, *351*
Grant, T. M., 131, 142, 144, *158, 160, 162,*
  183, 186, 199, *200,* 207, *227,* 307,
  311, 312, *332*
Greenbaum, R., 77*t,* 79*t,* 87*t,* 88*t, 94,* 167,
  178, 212, *226*
Greenberg, M., 281, *285*
Greenberg, M. T., 323, *327*
Greenberg, R., 277, *284*
Greene, J., 71, *93,* 99, 100*t,* 101, 102, 102*t,*
  104, *109,* 241*t, 248,* 306, 309, 310,*330*
Greene, N. M., 22, 24, *38,* 253, *271*
Greene, T., 120, *125*
Greenspan, S., 34, *37,* 132, 154, *160*
Greenwald, M., 144, *159, 160,* 180, *201*
Greer, S., 305, *331*
Greig, N., 10, *16*
Griffin, J. F., 307, 309, 310, *329*
Griffin, M. L., 264, *271,* 319, *328, 332*
Griffith, D., 262, *269*
Griffith, D. R., 28, *37,* 71, 72, *91,* 99, 100*t,*
  102, 102*t,* 103, 104, *108,* 111, 123,
  124, 154, *159,* 230, 243, *246,* 256,
  257, *268,* 278, *283,* 288, *302,* 305,
  326, 336, 337, *349; 352*
Griffith, E. M., 322, *327*
Grilli, M., 9, *15*
Gromisch, D. S., 24, *37,* 71, *91,* 255, *268,*
  308*t,* 309, 310, 312, 314*t,* 336, *349*
Grose, E. A., 8, 10, 11, 12, 14, *15*
Grossmann, K., 277, *284*
Grossmann, K. E., 277, *284*
Guerrero, I., 179, *201*
Guest, I., 75, 80*t, 92*
Guinan, J. F., 322, *328*
Gunderson, V. M., 116, *125*
Gunn, P., 277, *284*
Gunnoe, C., 46, *54,* 111, *126*
Guo, H., 61, *65*
Guy, L., 319, *328*

H

Hadeed, A. J., 24, *37,* 255, *269,* 309, 310,
  312, *328,* 336, *351,* 355, *367*
Hadfield, M. G., 253, *269*

Haertzen, C. A., 59, 64, *66*
Haith, M. M., 115, 116, *125*
Hall, L. A., 319, 320, *329*
Hallock, N., 275, 277, *284*
Halstead, A. C., 180, *201*
Hamamura, T., 234, *246*
Hamberger, K., 223, *227*
Hamel, C., 241*t, 248*
Hamel, S. C., 5, *16,* 71, *93,* 95, 99, 100*t,* 101,
  102, 102*t,* 104, *109,* 129, 132, 153,
  161, 164, *178,* 207, *226,* 305, 306,
  309, 310, 319, *330*
Hammer, R. P., Jr., 80*t, 91,* 211, *225*
Hammer-Knisely, J., 236, *246*
Hammond, M. A., 118, *124*
Hammond, P. B., 47, *54,* 113, *125*
Hanbauer, I., 9, *15*
Handler, A., 308*t,* 309, 310, 311, 312, 314*t,*
  329
Handmaker, N., 155, *160*
Handmaker, S., 155, *160*
Hans, S. L., 58, *65,* 111, 113, 124, *125,* 261,
  262, *267, 269, 270,* 305, *329*
Hansen, R. L., 236, 243, *247,* 258, 272, 307,
  309, 310, 311, 312, *328,* 337, 338,
  339, 341, *351, 353*
Hanson, J. W., 255, *269*
Hanson, M. J., 277, *285*
Hara, T., 8, *16*
Hardy, P., 113, *125*
Harel, S., 325, *326*
Hargreaves, W. A., 59, *65*
Hart, R. P., 82*t, 92*
Hartel, D., 60, *66*
Hasen, T. N., 237, *249*
Hatcher, R., 180, *201,* 319, *326*
Hauser, W. A., 311, *332*
Hauser-Cram, P., 340, 344, *352*
Hauth, J. C., 307, 309, 310, *328*
Haver, V. M., 143, *161*
Haviland, J. M., 276, *285*
Hawkins, S., 102*t,* 104, *109*
Hawley, T. L., 257, *269,* 287, 288, 289, *302*
Hazan, C., 115, 116, *125*
Heagarty, M., 146, *158*
Healy, B., 306, *328*
Heaton, R. K., 265, *271*
Heimler, R., 257, *268*
Heinicke, C. M., 344, 345, *351*
Helsing, K., 320, *327*
Hembree, E. A., 274, *284*

Henderson, M. G., 10, 13, *15, 77t,* 80*t,* 87*t,*
    92, 235, 242, *247*
Hennekens, C. H., 96, 99, *108*
Henriquez, R., 336, *349*
Henson, L. G., 111, 113, 124, *125,* 262, *269*
Hepner, A., 11, *15*
Herman, C. S., 113, 114, 120, 122, *127*
Hermans, R. H. M., 6, 8, *16*
Herren, T., 22, *38,* 238, *248*
Hertzel, J., 360, 361, *367*
Herzberg, D. S., 265, *267*
Heyser, C. J., 10, *16,* 76, 77*t,* 78*t,* 80*t,* 81*t,*
    82*t,* 85, 86, 87*t,* 88*t,* 92, 93, 131, *159,*
    161, 167, *177,* 210, 211, 212, 214*f,*
    215, 215*f,* 216, 217*f,* 218, 219*f,* 220,
    221, 222*f,* 224, 225, 226, 235, 244,
    247, 248, 259, *269*
Hickok, J. M., 11, *17*
Hill, V. A., 144, 145, *158*
Hillis, L. D., 232, *248*
Hiltunen, A. J., 8, *17*
Hinde, R. A., 274, *284*
Hinesby, R. K., 264, *268*
Hingson, R., 71, *94,* 111, 118, 123, *127,* 143,
    159, 179, *202,* 230–232, *250,* 252,
    255, 262, *269, 272,* 287, *303,* 305,
    306, 307, 309, 310, 311, 312, 313,
    328, 332, 335, 336, 338, *350, 353*
Hinkin, C. E., 265, *267*
Hirschfeld, R. M. A., 318, *329*
Hochberg, E., 71, *93,* 99, 100*t,* 101, 102,
    102*t,* 104, *109,* 241*t, 248,* 306, 309,
    310, *330*
Hoffman, J., 25, *38*
Hoffmann, H., 77*t,* 79*t,* 87*t,* 88*t, 94,* 167, *178,*
    212, *226*
Hogarty, P. S., 114, *126,* 164, 165, *178*
Hogue, C. J. R., 312, *329*
Hohmann, M., 6, *15*
Holipas, N., 336, *349*
Hollenbeck, A. R., 8, *17*
Hollingshead, A. B., 317, *329*
Hollinshead, W. H., 307, 309, 310, *329*
Holmes, P. A., 78*t,* 80*t,* 87*t, 91*
Holson, R. R., 9, 10, 12, 13, *17*
Homel, P., 274, *283*
Hopkins, E., 336, *351*
Horn, P. T., 239, *247*
Hornstein, D., 355, *368*
Hornykiewicz, O., 44–45, *53*
Horowitz, F., 281, *285*
Houy, J., 236, *246*

Howard, J., 34, *37,* 102*t,* 103, *109,* 123, *126,*
    151, *161,* 260, 261, *271,* 278, *285,*
    288, 291, *302, 303,* 337, 343, *351,*
    352, 364, *368*
Howes, C., 289, 298, *302, 303*
Howze, K., 336, *351*
Howze, W. M., 336, *351*
Hoyme, H. E., 255, *269*
Hrdina, P. D., 11, *15*
Hughes, H. E., 8, 10, 11, 12, 14, *15,* 74, 81*t,*
    82*t,* 90, *92, 93*
Hull, C. L., 346, *351*
Hume, R. F., 312, *329*
Humphrey, H. E. B., 111, 120, *125*
Hunt, C. E., 71, *91,* 179, *201,* 241*t, 246*
Hunt, H. F., 62, *66*
Hunter, D., 46, *54*
Hurlburt, N., 114, *126,* 164, *178*
Hurt, H., 111, *125,* 335, *349*
Hutchings, D. E., 5, *15,* 62, 63, 65, *66,* 74,
    77*t,* 79*t,* 87*t,* 89, *92, 93,* 99, *108,* 129,
    132, 149, 157, *160,* 207, 225, 242,
    249, 324, *329*
Hwang, J., 307, 309, 310, *332,* 335, *353*

I

Ignar, D., 240, *247*
Imaizumi, S., 123, *124,* 174, *177,* 258, *267,*
    279, 280, *282,* 320, 323, *326,* 337,
    349
Ingersoll, E. W., 257, *272*
Ingham, J. G., 321, *329*
Inglass, T. H., 24, *37*
Inkelis, S. H., 336, *351*
Ironson, G., 362, *368*
Irukayama, K., 49, *55*
Isaacson, R. L., 51, *54*
Isenberg, S. J., 336, *351*
Israel, Y., 12, *14*
Itagaki, S., 43, 45, *54*
Izard, C. E., 168, 170, *178,* 274, 276, *284*

J

Jackson, G. H., 211, *226*
Jacobs, B. L., 22, *37*
Jacobson, J. L., 111, 113, 114, 116, 118, 120,
    121*f,* 121, 123, *125, 126,* 149, 153,
    160, 207, 225

Jacobson, L., 325, *331*
Jacobson, S. W., 111, 113, 114, 116, 118,
    118*n*, 120, 121*f*, 121, 123, *125, 126,*
    149, 155, *160,* 207, *225*
Jaffe, J. H., 58, *66*
James, H., 77*t*, 80*t*, 87*t*, *94,* 242, *249*
James, M. E., 71, *91,* 99, 100*t*, 101, 102, *108,*
    111, *124,* 164, *177,* 241*t*, *246,* 257,
    268, 305–306, 307, 309, 311, 312, 313,
    325, *327, 329,* 355, 357, *367*
James, S., 320, *331*
Jarbe, T. U. C., 8, *17*
Jasinski, D. R., 59, 64, *66*
Jaskir, J., 165, *178*
Jasperse, D., 112, *124,* 336, *350*
Javitch, J. A., 10, *15*
Jellinek, M., 325, *330*
Jellinger, K., 44–45, *53*
Jenkins, V., 318, 322, *327*
Jenner, P., 45, *54*
Jeremy, R. J., 111, 113, 124, *125,* 261, *267*
Jewett, T., 255, *269*
Jidoi, J., 147, *159*
Joe, J. C., 234, *249*
Johanson, I. B., 211, *227*
Johns, J. M., 76, 78*t*, 82*t*, 83, 87*t*, *93,* 211,
    225, 242, 244, *247*
Johnson, H., 318, *331*
Johnson, H. L., 262, *269,* 288, *302*
Johnson, J. H., 321, 323, *329, 331*
Johnston, L. D., 307, *330*
Jonakait, G. M., 82*t*, *92*
Jones, B. E., 59, 64, *66*
Jones, C. L., 24, *38*
Jones, K. L., 112, *126,* 255, *269,* 336, *351*
Jones, M., 260, *267*
Jones, M. T., 240, 240–241, *248*
Joshi, V., 179, *201*
Justice, J. B., 10, *14*

K

Kagan, J., 274, *284,* 289, *303*
Kale, W. L., 323, *329*
Kaliva, P. W., 75, 80*t*, *92*
Kalkoske, M., 319, *327*
Kaltenbach, K., 58, *66,* 337, *352*
Kandall, S. R., 22, *37,* 180, *201,* 235, *246,*
    278, *283*
Kaplan, D., 71, *91,* 179, *201,* 241*t*, *246*
Kaplan, G., 319, *329*

Kaplan-Estrin, M. G., 113, 114, 121*f*, *125*
Karmel, B. Z., 154, *161,* 240, *248,* 361, *367*
Kasari, C., 262
Kaufman, A. S., 295, *303*
Kaufman, N. L., 295, *303*
Kay, D. C., 59, 64, *66*
Kaye, K., 336, *351*
Kayne, H., 71, *94,* 111, 118, 123, *127,* 143,
    149, 179, *202,* 230–232, *250,* 252, 255,
    269, 287, *302, 303,* 305, 306, 307,
    309, 310, 311, 312, 313, *328, 332,*
    335, 336, 338, *350, 353*
Kean, J., 180, *202*
Kearns, G. L., 254, *269,* 307, *328*
Keeler, M. H., 319, *329*
Keith, L. G., 71, *93,* 131, *161,* 179, *201,* 255,
    270, 287, *303,* 306, 307, 309, 310,
    311, 312, *326, 330,* 336, *351*
Kelley, N. E., 71, *91,* 236, *246,* 257, *267*
Kelley, S. J., 336, *351*
Kelsey, J. L., 97, 99, *108*
Kemp, V. H., 321, *329*
Kendall, K. A., 129, *161*
Kendjelic, E. M., 211, *227*
Kennard, M. A., 51, *54*
Kennedy, C., 11, *17*
Keogh, B. K., 275, *285,* 294, *303*
Kerns, K., 155, *159*
Kessel, S. S., 312, *329*
Kessler, L., 319, 320, *327*
Keve, T. M., 6, *14, 15*
Key, T. C., 6, *16,* 22, *38,* 240, *248,* 255, *271*
Khalidi, A., 49, *53*
Khalsa, J. H., 179, *201*
Khandabi, P., 34, *37,* 291, *302*
Khantzian, E. J., 263, *270*
Khantzian, N. J., 263, *270*
Kidwell, D. A., 147, *160*
Kikert, R., 234, *249*
Killam, A. P., 312, *329*
Kim, T., 24, *39*
Kimmel, C. A., 208, 209, *225, 226*
Kirchner, G. L., 52, *55,* 115, *127*
Kirstein, C. L., 74, 77*t*, 79*t*, 80*t*, 87*t*, 88*t*, 89,
    91, 94, 167, *178,* 210, 211, 212, 213*f*,
    225, 226, 227, 242, 243, *249*
Kish, S. J., 234, *249*
Kistin, N., 309, 310, 311, 312, *329*
Kjarasch, S. J., 263, *270*
Klaassen, C. D., 122, *126*
Klebanoff, M. A., 312, *331*
Kleber, H. D., 21, *37,* 264, *272*

Klein, J., 144, 148, *159, 160,* 180, *201*
Klein, V. R., 309, 310, 311, 312, *329*
Kleinbaum, D. G., 97, *108,* 119, *126*
Kleinman, J. C., 312, *329*
Klemka-Walden, L. M., 233, 237, *249*
Klerman, G., 318, *332*
Kletter, R., 71, *91,* 179, *201,* 241*t, 246*
Kleven, M. S., 234, *247*
Kliegman, R., 102*t,* 104, *109,* 129, *161,* 355, 368
Knapp, D. K., 179, 184, 185, 190, 194, 195, 198, *201, 202*
Knapp, S., 11, *15*
Knobloch, H., 32, *38*
Ko, D., 61, *65*
Kodituwakku, P., 155, *160*
Koegler, S. M., 9, *15*
Kolody, B., 307, 309, 310, *332, 335, 353*
Koob, G. F., 9, *16*
Koontz, A. M., 312, *329*
Kopera-Frye, K., 155, *160*
Koren, G., 27, 28, *38,* 71, 72, *93,* 95, 102*t,* 103, 107, *108,* 129, 132, 144, 148, 153, 157, *159, 160,* 180, *201,* 207, 225, 243, *247,* 324, *329*
Koslowski, B., 176, *177,* 276, *283*
Kosofsky, B. E., 132, 152, 153, *160*
Kosten, T. R., 264, *272,* 319, *332*
Kotch, L. E., 216, 223–224, *224*
Krafchuk, E., 275, *285*
Krafft, K. M., 113, *125*
Kraft, K. M., 47, *54*
Kramer, H. K., 11, *14,* 81*t, 91,* 211, *224,* 235, 245, *247,* 254, *267*
Krasinski, D., 346, *351*
Krauss, M. W., 340, 344, *352*
Kreitman, N. B., 321, *329*
Kresbach, P., 179, *202*
Kropenske, V., 343, *351*
Kuhar, M. J., 9, *16*
Kuhl, C., 360, 361, *367*
Kuhn, C. M., 240, *247,* 306, *328,* 357–358, 361, *367, 368*
Kuhn, T. S., 19, *38*
Kuhnert, B. R., 114, *125*
Kulkarni, A. P., 355, *368*
Kullama, L., 236, 240, *246*
Kupper, L. L., 97, *108,* 119, *126*
Kurkjian, M. F., 77*t,* 79*t,* 87*t, 94*
Kurtz, S. L., 8, *17,* 77*t,* 79*t,* 87*t, 94*
Kuzma, J., 122, *127*
Kwon, C., 240

Kyllerman, M., 115, *124*

L

La Greca, A. M., 321, *332,* 365, *367*
Lamb, M. E., 262, *268,* 274, *283*
Lamb, R. J., 9, *16*
Lambert, G., 311, *332*
Lancaster, J. S., 122, *124*
Landau, C., 232, *248*
Landress, H. J., 106, *108,* 147, *159,* 252, *268,* 307, 312, *326*
Lange, R. A., 232, *248*
Lange, U., 319, *328*
Lange, W. R. R., 60, *65*
Langston, J. W., 43, *54*
Lariviere, N. A., 216, *225*
Larson, S. K., 99, 100*t,* 101, *108,* 164, *177,* 241*t, 247,* 257, *269,* 306, *328,* 356, 363, *367*
Lasky, R. E., 346, *351*
Lau, Y.-S., 79*t,* 92, 235, *247*
Lauder, J. M., 11, *16,* 22, *38,* 254, *270*
Laughery, J., 265, *270*
Lavee, Y., 318, *330*
Lavine, L., 46, *55*
Lawson, M. S., 260, 265, *270,* 343, 344, *351*
Le Moal, M., 220, *225, 226*
Lee, B. L., 252, *271*
Lee, H., 165, *178*
Lefcourt, H. M., 321, *329*
Legido, A., 235, *247*
Leitner, D. S., 71, *91,* 236, *246,* 257, *267,* 336, *350*
Leonard, M. F., 277, *285*
Leskawa, K. C., 211, *226*
Lester, B. M., 22, 24, 25, 26, 30, 31, 34, *38,* 71, *93,* 101, *108,* 153, *160,* 237, 238, 241, *248,* 278, *285,* 287, *302,* 337, *351,* 356, *367*
Levandoski, N., 335, *349*
Levenson, H., 318, *329*
Levenson, S. M., 71, *94,* 111, 118, 123, *127,* 143, *159,* 179, *202,* 230–232, 233, 242, *247, 250,* 252, 255, *269,* 287, *303,* 305, 306, 307, 309, 310, 311, 312, 313, *328, 332,* 335, 336, 338, *350, 353*
Leventhal, J. M., 260, *272*
Levesque, D., 240, *246*
Levine, T. E., 122, *126*

Leviton, A., 46, 47, 52, *53, 54,* 111, 113, *124, 126*
Levitsky, D. A., 223, 227
Levitt, P., 12, *16*
Lewin, K., 346, *351*
Lewis, D. E., 336, *349*
Lewis, K., 237, *248*
Lewis, M., 123, *124,* 164, 165, 166, 169, 170, 171, 172, 174, 175, 176, *177, 178,* 257, 258, 262, *267, 270,* 275, 276, 279, 280, *282, 285,* 320, 323, *326,* 337, *349*
Lidsky, T. J., 235, *249*
Lief, N., 344, *351*
Lief, N. R., 344, *351*
Lifschitz, M. H., 288, *303*
Lilienfeld, A. M., 32, *38*
Lin, D., 235, *249*
Lingerfelt, B., 275, *283*
Link, E. A., 232, *248*
Linn, P., 281, *285*
Lipson, A. H., 8, *17,* 75, 81*t, 94*
Lipton, D. S., 322, *330*
Little, B. B., 307, 309, 310, 311, 312, *329,* 335, *351*
Littman, D., 358, 362, *367*
Lizardo, E., 196, *202*
Lo, E. S., 235, *249*
Lochry, E. A., 224, *226*
Locke, B. Z., 320, *332*
Lockitch, G., 180, *201*
Lodder, D. E., 129, *161*
Loevinger, J., 117*t, 126*
Longo, L. D., 6, 8, *16*
Lopez, R., 24, *38*
Lord, E. E., 46, *53*
Low, J., 277, *285*
Lucena, J., 182, *201, 202*
Lund, C. A., 151, *161*
Luthar, S., 264, *270*
Lutiger, B., 27, 28, *38,* 71, *93,* 129, *160*
Lynn, S. N., 180–181, *202*
Lyons-Ruth, K., 289, *303,* 306, 319, *327*

M

Maag, L., 325, *332*
Mac, E., 184, 185, 198, *201, 202*
Mac Hee, K., 24, *39*
MacDonald, N. R., 10, *16,* 78*t,* 82*t,* 87*t, 93*

MacGregor, S. N., 71, 91, *93,* 99, 100*t,* 131, *161,* 179, *201,* 207, *226,* 255, *270,* 287, *303,* 306, 307, 309, 310, 311, 312, *326, 330,* 336, *351*
Macklin, M., 24, *39*
MacPhail, B. J., 75, 79*t, 92*
Mactutus, C. F., 6, *16*
Magnano, C. L., 154, *161,* 240, *248,* 361, *367*
Magura, S., 322, *330*
Mahalik, M. P., 24, *38*
Maher, C., 46, *54,* 111, *126*
Main, M., 176, *177,* 260, *270,* 276, *283*
Malatesta, C. A., 276, *285*
Malatesta, C. Z., 274, *284*
Malmud, E., 111, *125*
Malowany, D., 62, 65, *66,* 242, *249*
Mandell, A. J., 11, *15*
Manly, J. T., 339, *350*
Mann, D. E., 24, *38*
Manschreck, T., 265, *270*
Mansky, P. A., 59, 64, *66*
Mantel, N., 46, *55*
Marcus, J., 261, 262, *267, 270*
Mark, H., 24, *37*
Markowitz, M., 102, 105, *109*
Marques, P. R., 145, *161*
Marsden, C. D., 43, *54*
Marsh, D. O., 49, *54*
Marshall, A. B., 337, *351*
Martens, J. M., 11, *16*
Martier, S., 112, 113, 114, 120, 121*f,* 122, *125, 127,* 144, 155, *160, 162*
Martin, B. R., 61, *65*
Martin, D. C., 52, *55,* 112, 113, 114, 115, 120, *127,* 151, *161,* 357, *368*
Martin, J. C., 112, *127,* 131, 151, *161, 162,* 207, 227, 307, 311, 312, *332*
Martin, R. A., 321, *329*
Martin, W. R., 59, 64, *66*
Martyn, C. N., 45, *54*
Marwah, J., 6, *16,* 240, *248*
Masana, M. I., 9, *15*
Maslow, A., 346, *351*
Massman, A., 240–241, *248*
Masten, A., 34, *37*
Mateer, C., 155, *159*
Matera, C., 307, 309, 310, 311, 312, *330*
Matheny, A. P., 275, *285*
Matheson, C. C., 289, *302*
Mathews, S. V., 75, 82*t, 94*
Matis, R., 306, 319, *327*
Matthews, J. C., 8, *16*

Mattis, S. B., 34, *38*
Mattran, K. M., 8, *17*, 77*t*, 79*t*, 87*t*, *94*
Mattson, M. P., 254, *270*
Mattson, S. N., 216, 223–224, *224*
Maycock, D. E., 207, *227*
Mayer, J., 260, *268*, 344, *351*
Mayes, L. C., 19, 22, *38*, 72, *93*, 99, 100*t*,
    101, 107, *108*, 111, 112, *126*, 164,
    178, 230, 241*t*, 242, 245, *248*, 253,
    255, 256, 257, 258, 259, 265, *268*, *270*
Maynard, E. C., 199, *201*
Mayock, D. E., 131, *162*, 307, 311, 312, *332*
Mayrent, S. L., 96, 99, *108*
Mazze, R. I., 8, *15*
McCall, R. B., 102, *108*, 114, *126*, 164, 165,
    178, 274, *284*
McCalla, S., 306, 307, 309, 310, 311, 312,
    313, *330*
McCann, E. M., 237, *248*
McCarten, K., 233, 242, *247*
McConnaughey, M. M., 10, 13, *15*, 235, *247*
McCreary, R., 180, *202*
McDevitt, S. C., 274, 275, *283*, *285*
McDonough, S., 339, *353*
McGaughey, P. J., 129, *161*
McGeer, E. G., 42, 43, 45, *53*, *54*
McGeer, P. L., 43, 45, *54*
McGivern, R. F., 77*t*, 80*t*, 87*t*, *93*, 211, *226*
McGrath, M. M., 34, *38*
McGuiness, D., 258, *271*
McGurk, H., 164, 165, *178*
McInerny, J., 336, *350*
McKinzie, D. L., 76, 78*t*, 81*t*, 86, 87*t*, 88*t*, *92*,
    131, *159*, 210, 212, 214*f*, 215, 219,
    221, 222*f*, *225*, 244, *247*
McLaughlin, F. J., 307, 309, 310, *326*
McLaughlin, M. K., 6, *14*, *15*
McLaughlin, S., 24, *38*, 71, *93*, 153, *160*, 237,
    238, *248*, 278, *285*, 287, *302*, 337, *351*
McLloyd, V. C., 345, *352*
McMillen, B. A., 10, 13, *15*, 76, 77*t*, 78*t*, 80*t*,
    82*t*, 83, 87*t*, *92*, *93*, 211, *225*, 235,
    242, 244, *247*
Meadow, K. P., 281, *285*
Means, L. W., 76, 78*t*, 82*t*, 83, 87*t*, *93*, 211,
    225, 242, 244, *247*
Means, M. J., 76, 78*t*, 82*t*, 83, 87*t*, *93*, 211,
    225, 242, 244, *247*
Medoff-Cooper, B., 277, *285*
Mehrabian, A., 365, *367*
Meisels, S. J., 325, *330*
Meisenhelder, J. B., 321, *330*

Melamed, J., 319, *326*
Mele, A., 10, *16*
Melendez, M., 257, *267*
Melis, F., 234, *248*
Mendelson, M., 117*t*, *124*
Mendolson, M., 319, *326*
Merikangas, K. R., 264, *270*, *271*, *272*
Meyer, J., 22, *38*, 238, *248*
Meyer, J. S., 10, *16*, 78*t*, 82*t*, 87*t*, *93*
Meyer, L. S., 216, 223–224, *224*
Meyers, C. P., 60, *65*
Michael, J. L., 264, *271*, 319, *330*, *332*
Mieczkowski, T., 148, *161*, 265, *268*, 322, *326*
Miettinen, O. S., 98, *108*
Milhorat, T. H., 14, *15*, 74, 79*t*, 90, *92*, 131,
    159, 235, *247*, 254, *269*
Millard, W. J., 10, *16*
Miller, E. D., 8, *16*
Miller, J. C., 235, *248*
Miller, J. S., 77*t*, 78*t*, 80*t*, 82*t*, 87*t*, 88*t*, *92*,
    167, *177*, 211, 212, 215, 215*f*, 216,
    217*f*, 224, *225*
Miller, L., 6, *16*, 22, *38*, 240, *248*, 255, *271*
Miller, M., 151, *162*
Miller, N., 63, 65, *66*
Miller, P. M., 321, *329*
Miller, R. K., 6, 7, *17*
Miller, R. L., 74–75, 79*t*, *92*
Miller, S. I., 122, *127*
Miller, T., 325, *328*
Miller, W. C., 319, *329*
Mills, J. L., 129, 141, 148, 152, *161*
Min, D., 336, *351*
Minabe, Y., 10, *16*, 82*t*, *93*, 211, 220, *226*,
    235, *248*
Minkoff, H. L., 306, 307, 309, 310, 311, 312,
    313, *326*, *330*, 338, *350*
Minnefor, A., 179, *201*
Minnes, S., 257, *267*
Minogue, J. P., 71, *93*, 131, *161*, 179, *201*,
    255, *270*, 287, *303*, 306, 309, 310,
    311, 312, *330*, 336, *351*
Minor, B. G., 8, *17*
Mirin, M., 319, *332*
Mirin, S. M., 264, *271*, 319, *328*, *330*, *332*
Mirochnick, M., 22, *38*, 233, 238, 240, *248*
Mirsky, A., 155, *162*
Mitchell, D. W., 115, *124*, 257, *268*
Mock, F., 117*t*, *124*
Mock, J., 319, *326*
Mohammed, A. K., 8, *17*
Moldestad, M., 264, *268*

Molina, V. A., 76, 78*t*, 81*t*, 82*t*, 85, 86, 87*t*, 88*t*, 92, *93*, 131, *159*, 210, 211, 212, 214*f*, 215, 219, *225*, *226*, *227*, 244, 247, 259, *269*
Moliterno, D. J., 232, *248*
Montare, A., 294, *302*
Montes, M., 195, *202*
Montes, N., 183, 186, *201*
Moody, C. A., 76, 78*t*, 80*t*, 81*t*, 86, 87*t*, 88*t*, 92, 131, *159*, 210, 211, 212, 214*f*, 215, 219, 220, *225*, *226*, *227*, 244, *247*, 259, *269*
Moomjy, M., 307, 309, 310, 311, 312, *330*
Moore, K. G., 335, 337, *352*
Moore, L., 131, *162*, 207, *227*, 307, 311, 312, *332*
Moore, R. Y., 12, 13, *16*
Moore, T. R., 6, *16*, 22, *38*, 240, *248*, 255, *271*
Morales, V., 198, *201*
Morgenstern, H., 97, *108*
Morishima, H. O., 8, *16*
Morissette, M., 240, *246*
Morris, A. J., 262, *270*
Morrison, J. H., 254, *271*
Morrow, C., 99, 100*t*, 101, *108*, 164, *177*, 241*t*, *247*, 257, *269*, 306, *328*, 356, 358, 361, 363, *367*, *368*
Mottet, N. K., 116, *125*
Msall, M. E., 255, *269*
Mule, S. J., 317, *330*
Mullen, M. K., 25, *38*
Muller, K. E., 119, *126*
Murphy, J. M., 325, *330*
Murphy, S. P., 236, *246*
Murray, H. J., 346, *352*
Murray, J., 28, *37*, 71, 72, *91*, 102*t*, 103, *108*, 111, 123, *124*, 154, *159*, 256, *268*, 278, *283*, 288, *302*, 337, *349*
Murtadha, M., 49, *53*
Musto, D., 251, *271*
Myers, B. A., 129, *161*
Myers, B. J., 337, *352*
Myers, G. J., 49, *54*
Myers, J. K., 319, 320, *330*, *332*
Myers, T., 240–241, *248*

N

Nakla, M., 8, *14*
Naluz, A., 144, *161*, 182, 188, *202*
Nanda, D., 311, *330*

Nathan, M. A., 235, *249*
Nathanielsz, P. W., 240, 240–241, *248*
National Institute of Medicine, 312, *330*
National Institute on Drug Abuse (NIDA), 60, *66*
National Research Council, 42, *54*
Nau, H., 89, 90, *93*
Needleman, H. L., 46, 47, 52, *53*, *54*, 111, 113, *124*, *126*
Needlman, R., 233, 240, *248*
Neerhof, M. G., 207, *226*, 307, 309, 310, 312, *330*
Negus, B. H., 232, *248*
Nemeth, P., 257, *268*
Nero, T. J., 62, *66*
Neto, G. S., 237, *246*
Neubert, D., 89, *93*
Neuspiel, D. R., 5, *16*, 71, *93*, 95, 99, 100*t*, 101, 102, 102*t*, 104, 105, 107, *108*, *109*, 129, 132, 152, 153, *161*, 164, *178*, 207, *226*, 241*t*, *248*, 305, 306, 309, 310, 319, 324, *330*
Newton, J. R., 113, *124*
Nichols, M. L., 113, *124*
Nichtern, S., 343, 344, *352*
Nicklas, N., 319, *326*
NIDA. *See* National Institute on Drug Abuse (NIDA)
Niswander, K. R., 32, *38*
Noble, A., 307, 309, 310, *332*, 335, *353*
Noble, L. M., 24, *39*
Nobrega, J. N., 234, *249*
Nomura, Y., 9, *17*
Norman, A. B., 80*t*, *92*
Norris, D., 34, *37*, 291, *302*
Novack, A. H., 144, *158*, 183, 186, 199, *200*
Nugent, E. A., 253, *269*
Nulman, I., 102*t*, 103, *108*, 243, *247*
Nystrom, J., 361, *367*

O

O'Brien, E. J., 322, *330*
Ochs, H. D., 60, *66*
O'Connor, M. J., 113, *126*, 261, 262, *271*
O'Donnell, K. J., 312, *329*
Oehlberg, S. M., 305, 325, *328*
Ogbu, J., 342, *352*
Oh, W., 25, *38*, *39*, 199, *201*
Ohr, P. S., 275, 276, *283*
Olegard, R., 115, *124*

Oleske, J., 179, *201*
Olson, D. H., 318, *330*
Olson, H. C., 337, *352*
O'Malley, P. M., 307, *330*
O'Malley, S., 265, *271*
O'Neill, J. M., 116, 121, *125*
Oro, A. S., 179, *201,* 255, *271,* 278, *285,* 338, *352*
Orr, S., 320, *331*
O'Shea, J., 77*t,* 79*t,* 87*t,* 88*t, 94,* 167, *178,* 212, *226*
Osman, M., 74, 79*t,* 89, *92*
Osmond, C., 45, *54*
Osofsky, J. D., 176, *178*
Osol, G., 6, *15*
Oster, H., 168, *177*
Osterloh, J. D., 252, *271*
Ostrea, A. R., 183, 186, 190, 194, 195, *201, 202*
Ostrea, E. M., Jr., 59, *66,* 144, *161, 162,* 179, 180, 180–181, 182, 183, 184, 185, 186, 188, 189, 190, 194, 195, 196, 197, 198, *201, 202,* 232, *248,* 307, 309, 310, 312, *331*
Otsuki, S., 234, *246*
Overbeck, G. W., 76, 77*t,* 78*t,* 79*t,* 80*t,* 87*t, 91*
Owiny, J. R., 240, 240–241, *248*

P

Pacis, M., 198, *201*
Padbury, J., 236, 240, *246*
Padgett, R. J., 116, 121, *125*
Pagan, M., 336, *349*
Page, C., 321, *329*
Palmore, M. K., 307, 310, *329,* 335, *351*
Palow, D. C., 335, *349,* 355, *367*
Pandey, U., 61, *65*
Parekh, A., 311, 312, *326,* 338, *350*
Parker, S., 71, *94,* 111, 118, 123, *127,* 179, *202,* 230–232, *250,* 287, *303,* 305, 306, 307, 309, 310, 311, 312, 313, 320, *328, 331, 332,* 335, 336, 338, *350, 353*
Parkhurst, E., 32, *38*
Parks, P. M., 144, *161,* 182, 183, 188, *202,* 232, *248*
Parmelee, A. H., 115, *126, 127,* 358, 360, 362, *367, 368*
Parrish-Johnson, J. C., 52, *55,* 115, *127*
Parsons, O., 321, *326*

Pasamanick, B., 32, *38*
Pastuszak, A., 102*t,* 103, *108,* 243, *247*
Pasulka, P., 61, *66*
Patch, V. D., 264, *271*
Paterson, J. A., 8, *16*
Patlak, C. S., 11, *17*
Patterson, C. B., 262, *270*
Pauls, D., 264, *271, 272*
Pedersen, D. A., 360, 361, *367*
Peeke, H. V., 236, *249*
Peresie, H., 46, *54,* 111, *126*
Peris, J., 10, *16*
Perry, B., 61, *66*
Perry, S., 306, *328*
Pert, A., 10, *16*
Peters, A. J., 236, *245*
Peters-Martin, P., 274, *285*
Peterson, M. A., 77*t,* 80*t,* 87*t, 93,* 211, *226*
Peterson, S. E., 254, *271*
Pettigrew, K. D., 11, *17*
Peucker, M., 24, *38,* 71, *93,* 153, *160,* 237, 238, *248,* 278, *285,* 337, *351*
Phillips, B., 24, *37,* 179, *201,* 255, *269,* 278, *284*
Phillips, S. A., 336, *353, 357, 368*
Phillipsen, L., 34, *37,* 291, *302*
Phipps, B. S., 183, 186, 199, *200*
Phipps, P., 144, *158*
Piaget, J., 176, *178*
Pippenger, C. E., 64, *66*
Pittman, R. K., 266, *271*
Pitts, D. K., 6, *16,* 240, *248*
Pizzi, W. J., 61, *66*
Platzman, K. A., 71, *91,* 99, 100*t,* 101, 102, *108,* 111, 115, 116, *124,* 129, 152, *159,* 164, *177,* 241*t, 246,* 257, *268,* 305–306, 307, 309, 311, 312, 313, *327,* 344, *350,* 355, *357, 367*
Plessinger, M. A., 6, 7, *17,* 255, *272*
Plomin, R., 253, *267,* 274, 275, *283, 284*
Poitrast, F. G., 325, *330*
Pollin, W., 335, *352*
Pollitt, K., 106, *109*
Porat, R., 336, *352,* 355, *368*
Portner, J., 318, *330*
Posner, M. I., 254, *271*
Pottenger, M., 320, *332*
Powell, G. F., 277, *285*
Pranzatelli, M. R., 11, *16*
Preston, P., 307, 309, 310, *328*
Pribram, K. H., 258, *271*
Price, J., 307, 309, 310, *328*

Prindle, R. A., 24, *37*
Pringle, G. F., 74, 81*t*, 90, *93*
Prusoff, B. A., 264, *271*, *272*, 320, *332*
Pullis, M. E., 294, *303*
Pyun, K. H., 60, *66*

Q

Quinn, D., 325, *330*

R

Rabinowitz, M. B., 47, 52, *53*, 113, *124*
Radloff, L. S., 318, 319, 320, *331*, 365, *368*
Rae, D. S., 319, *331*
Raese, J., 234, *249*
Ragozin, A. A., 323, *327*
Rainbow, T. C., 13, *14*
Raisys, V. A., 144, *158*, 183, 186, 199, *200*, *201*
Rajachandran, L., 76, 78*t*, 81*t*, 86, 87*t*, 88*t*, 92, 131, *159*, 210, 211, 212, 214*f*, 215, 219, *225*, 244, *247*, 259, *269*
Ramazzotto, L. J., 8, *16*
Ramey, S. L., 131, *162*, 207, *227*, 307, 311, 312, *332*
Rao, G. S., 75, 82*t*, *94*
Rauch, H. C., 81*t*, *91*
Raum, W. J., 77*t*, 80*t*, 87*t*, *93*, 211, *226*
Raymundo, A. L., 144, *161*, 179, 180, 182, 189, 190, *201*, *202*, 307, 309, 310, 312, *331*
Rayner, R., 168, *178*
Raynes, A. E., 264, *271*
Reddix, B., 235, *249*, 278, *285*
Reece, H., 305, 309, 310, 311, 312, *328*, 335, 338, *350*
Reed, J. A., 79*t*, *92*, 235, *247*
Reed, M., 46, *54*
Reed, R., 111, *126*
Rees, D. C., 208, 209, *225*, *226*
Regan, D. O., 305, 325, *328*, *331*
Reid, A. A., 10, *16*
Reivich, M., 11, *17*
Renyi, A. L., 11, *16*
Repacholi, B., 289, *303*
Reppert, S. M., 75, 82*t*, *94*
Resnik, R., 6, *16*, 240, *248*, *255*, *271*
Retzky, S. S., 207, *226*, 307, 309, 310, 312, *330*

Reznick, J. S., 274, *284*
Rhoads, D. L., 323, *331*
Rhymes, J. P., 277, *285*
Rice, D. C., 51, *54*
Rice, K. C., 10, *16*
Richards, I. S., 355, *368*
Richardson, G. A., 71, *93*, 99, 100*t*, 102, *109*, 111, 112, 114, *124*, *126*, 129, 152, 157, *159*, *161*, 241*t*, *248*, 306, 308*t*, 309, 310, 311, 312, 313, 314*t*, 324, *327*, *331*, 336, *350*
Richie, J. M., 22, 24, *38*, 253, *271*
Riley, E. P., 80*t*, 81*t*, *91*, 92, *94*, 123, *126*, 131, *159*, *161*, 209, 216, 223, 223–224, 224, *224*, *225*, *226*, 237, *247*
Riley, J. G., 336, *352*
Rist, M. C., 336, *352*
Ritchie, H. E., 8, *17*, 75, 81*t*, *94*
Ritz, M. C., 9, *16*
Rivkees, S. A., 75, 82*t*, *94*
Robbins, T. W., 258, *268*
Roberts, C. S., 319, *332*
Roberts, D. E., 107, *109*
Roberts, J. P., 99, 100*t*, 101, *108*, 164, *177*, 257, *269*, 306, *328*, 356, 358, 361, 363, *367*, *368*
Roberts, R., 319, *329*
Robeson, C., 72, *93*
Robeson, D., 132, *160*
Robeson, N., 107, *108*
Robies, N., 336, *350*
Robieux, I., 72, *93*, 107, *108*, 132, *160*
Robins, L. N., 129, 141, 148, 152, *161*
Robinson, L. K., 255, *269*
Robinson, N. L., 77*t*, 80*t*, 87*t*, *94*, 242, *249*
Robinson, N. M., 323, *327*
Robinson, S. E., 61, *65*
Robles, N., 112, *124*
Robson, P.J., 321, *331*
Rodier, P. M., 51, *53*
Rodning, C., 34, *37*, 102*t*, 103, *109*, 123, *126*, 151, *161*, 260, 261, *271*, 278, *285*, 288, 291, *302*, *303*, 337, *352*, 364, *368*
Rodriguez, M., 11, *14*
Rodriguez, V., 335, *349*
Rodriguez-Sanchez, M. N., 81*t*, *94*
Rogan, W. J., 113, *125*, *126*
Rogosch, F. A., 260, *271*
Rolfs, R. T., 311, *331*
Rolsten, C., 74, 79*t*, *94*
Romero, A., 183, 184, 185, 186, 188, 189, 194, 195, 196, *201*, *202*

Rose, S. A., 116, *125*
Rosecan, J. S., 22, *39*
Rosen, T. S., 62, 64, *66*, 262, *269*, 288, *302*
Rosenak, D., 355, *368*
Rosenberg, M., 318, 321, 322, *331*
Rosenblum, L. A., 262, *270*
Rosenfeld, C. R., 346, *351*
Rosenthal, J., 265, *270*
Rosenthal, R., 325, *331*
Rosenweig, B., 183, 186, 199, *201*
Rosner, M. A., 71, *93*, 131, *161*, 179, *201*,
    255, *270*, 287, *303*, 306, 309, 310,
    311, 312, *329*, *330*, 336, *351*
Ross, D. F., 325, *327*
Ross, F., 319, *331*
Ross, M. G., 236, 240, *246*
Ross, S. B., 11, *16*
Rosselli, M., 265, *267*
Rossen, J. D., 232, *248*
Rossetti, Z. L., 234, *248*
Rothbart, M. K., 254, *271*, 274, 275, 276,
    277, 279, *283*, *284*, *285*
Rothman, K. J., 96, 98, 99, *109*
Rothman, R. B., 10, *16*
Rotter, J. B., 321, *331*
Rouillard, C., 240, *246*
Rounsaville, B. J., 264, *270*, *271*, *272*
Roxas, R., Jr., 182, *201*
Rubenstein, J., 289, *303*
Rubio, E., 179, *202*
Rudraveff, M. E., 305, 325, *328*
Ruesch, N., 257, *267*
Ruff, H. A., 258, *272*
Ruiz, B., 74, *79t*, *94*
Rush, D., 101, 106, *109*
Rutter, M., 124, *126*, 319, *331*, 339, *352*
Ryan, L., 131, *161*, 179, *202*, 255, *272*, 287,
    303, 336, 338, *352*

S

Saady, J. J., 61, *65*
Saarni, C., 276, *285*
Sabel, K.-G., 115, *124*
Sachs, B. P., 336, *349*
Sadowsky, D., 240, 240–241, *248*
Saitoh, M., 145, *161*
Sakamoto, M., 145, *161*
Sakurada, O., 11, *17*
Salamy, A., 22, *38*, 236, *249*
Saleh, W. E., 321, *329*

Saleri, V., 190, 197, *202*
Salfi, M., 236, *249*
Salwen, M., 311, *330*
Salwin, M., 306, 307, 309, 310, 311, 312,
    313, *330*
Sambamoorthi, U., 112, *124*, 336, *350*
Sameroff, A. J., 32, 34, *39*, 124, *126*, 275,
    285, 306, 318, *331*, 340, 341, *352*
Sampson, P. D., 52, *55*, 111, 113n, 115, 116,
    126, *127*, 143, 149, 153, 155, *159*,
    162, 224, 227
Samuels, S. J., 307, 309, 310, 311, 312, *328*
Sanberg, P. R., 80t, *92*
Sandberg, D., 319, *328*
Sandin, B., 115, *124*
Sandman, B. M., 115, *127*
Sands, J., 73, *92*
Sarason, B. R., 322, *331*
Sarason, I. G., 318, 321, 322, 323, *329*, *331*
Sargent, T., 263, *270*
Sashidharan, S. P., 321, *329*
Sasidharan, P., 257, *268*
Saulys, A., 146, *159*
Sauvain, K. J., 307, *332*
Savich, R. W., 179, *201*, 232, *246*
Saxon, A. J., 143, *161*
Scafidi, F. A., 357–358, 361, *362*, *367*, *368*
Scalzo, F. M., 9, 10, 12, 13, *16*, *17*, 80t, *94*,
    211, 220, *226*, 235, *249*
Schallert, T., 45, *54*
Schanberg, S. M., 306, *328*, 357–358, 358,
    361, 362, *367*, *368*
Scheiner, A. P., 339, *353*
Schell, A., 47, *54*
Scher, M., 112, *124*, 336, *350*
Scherling, D., 252, 255, 256, *272*
Schlesselman, J. J., 97, 99, *109*, 119, *126*
Schneider, J. W., 102t, 103, *109*, 278, *285*,
    337, *352*
Schneiderman, J., 144, *159*, 160, 180, *201*
Schneyer, M., 265, *270*
Schnoll, S. H., 61, *65*, *66*, 71, *91*, 99, 100t,
    101, *108*, 131, *159*, 164, *177*, 179,
    200, 278, *283*, 305, 306, 307, 309,
    311, 312, 312–313, 313, *326*, 336,
    349, 356, *367*
Schorge, J. O., 307, 309, 310, *326*
Schottenfeld, R., 99, 100t, 101, *108*, 111, *126*,
    164, *178*, 255, 257, *270*
Schottenfield, R., 72, *93*
Schraeder, B., 277, *285*
Schreiner, A. P., 362, *368*

Schuetz, S., 154, *162*, 237, 239, *246*
Schuster, C. R., 59, *66*
Schutter, L. S., 337, 345, *352*
Schutzman, D. L., 307, *331*
Schwartz, P. M., 116, *125*
Sciarra, J. J., 310, 311, 312, *329*, 336, *351*
Scott, H. D., 307, 309, 310, *329*
Scott, K., 6, 7, *17*
Scott, M., 155, *162*
Scribani, L. A., 74, 81*t*, 90, *93*
Segal, E. A., 335, 343, *352*
Segal, S., 180, *201*
Sehgal, S., 154, *162*, 237, 239, *246*
Seiden, L. S., 234, *247*
Seidler, F. J., 8, 9, 13, *14, 15, 16*, 82*t*, *94*, 233, 235, *249*
Seifer, R., 24, 34, *37, 38*, 71, *93*, 153, *160*, 237, 238, *248*, 278, *285*, 337, 340, *351, 352, 353*
Seifert, M. F., 81*t*, *94*
Seltzer, M. L., 115, *126*
Selwyn, P. A., 60, *66*
Senie, R. T., 22, *37*, 235, *246*, 278, *283*
Sepkoski, C., 24, *38*, 71, *93*, 153, *160*, 237, 238, *248*, 278, *285*, 287, *302*, 337, *351*
Sette, W. F., 122, *126*
Sexton, M. E., 362, *368*
Shah, S., 236, *249*
Shanks, C. A., 9, *14*
Shannak, K., 234, *249*
Shanzer, S., 22, *37*, 235, *246*, 278, *283*
Shapiro, N. R., 224, *226*
Sharrar, R. G., 311, *331*
Shaul, P. W., 25, *39*
Shaw, P., 71, *93*, 131, *161*, 179, *201*, 255, 270, 287, *303*, 306, 309, 310, 311, 312, *330*, 336, *351*
Shaywitz, B. A., 115, 116, *126*
Shaywitz, S. E., 115, 116, *126*
Shear, H., 95, *108*, 157, *160*, 207, *225*
Shennum, W. A., 321, *326*
Shepherd, G. M., 253, *272*
Sherlock, J. D., 10, *16*, 78*t*, 82*t*, 87*t*, *93*
Shields, A., 260, *271*
Shih, L., 235, *249*, 278, *285*
Shinohara, M., 11, *17*
Shiono, P. H., 252, *269*, 312, *331*
Shipley, T. E., 322, *327*
Sholomskas, D., 320, *332*
Shonkoff, J. P., 325, *330*, 340, 344, *352*
Shryne, J. H., 211, *226*
Shulman, H. H., 275, 277, *284*

Siddiqi, Q., 322, *330*
Siegal, M., 318, *331*
Siegel, J. M., 323, *331*
Siegel, L. S., 118, *126*
Siegel, S. R., 24, *37*, 255, *269*, 309, 310, 312, 328, 336, *351*, 355, *367*
Sierer, R., 89, *93*
Sigman, M. D., 113, 115, *126, 127*, 164, *177*, 262, 360, *368*
Sigman, N., 261, *271*
Sikich, L., 11, *17*
Silber, E., 322, *331*
Silber, S., 340, 344, *353*
Silverstein, J., 115, *124*
Silvestre, M. A., 182, *201, 202*
Silvestri, J. M., 235, *249*
Simeonsson, R. J., 339, *353*
Simkowski, K., 179, *202*
Simon, H., 220, *225, 226*
Simpkins, J. W., 74–75, 79*t*, *92*
Singer, J., 307, *331*
Singer, J. M., 276, *283*
Singer, L., 111, *127*, 257, *267*
Singer, L. T., 102*t*, 104, *109*, 116, *125*, 129, *161*, 355, *368*
Sison, C., 197, *202*
Slikker, W., 9, 10, 12, 13, *17*
Sloan, L. B., 307, *331*
Slotkin, T. A., 8, 9, 13, *14, 15, 16*, 82*t*, *94*, 233, 235, *249*
Smialek, T., 180, *201*
Smith, D. W., 112, 122, *126, 127*, 336, *350*, *351*
Smith, E., 288, *303*
Smith, G., 325, *330*
Smith, I. E., 71, *91*, 99, 100*t*, 101, 102, *108*, 111, 112, 114, 115, 116, 122, *124*, *127*, 164, *177*, 241*t*, *246*, 257, *268*, 305–306, 307, 309, 311, 312, 313, *327*, 344, *353*, 355, 357, *367*
Smith, J., 49, *53*
Smith, J. E., 253, *269*
Smith, R. F., 8, *17*, 77*t*, 79*t*, 87*t*, *94*
Snell, L. M., 307, 309, 310, 311, 312, *329*, 335, *351*
Snidman, N., 274, *284*
Snyder, S. H., 10, *15*
Snyder, S. W., 307, *331*
Sobrian, S. K., 77*t*, 80*t*, 87*t*, *94*, 242, *249*
Sokol, R. J., 112, 113, 114, 116, 120, 121*f*, 122, *125, 126, 127*, 144, 155, *160, 162*
Sokoloff, L., 11, *17*

Sollogub, A. C., 319, *332*
Solloguls, A. C., 319, *330*
Solnit, A., 340, 344, *353*
Solnit, A. J., 277, *285*, 348, *351*
Solomon, J., 260, *270*
Solomon, Z., 319, *326*
Sorg, J., 6, *16*, 22, *38*, 240, *248*, 255, *271*
Sostek, A. M., 275, 277, *284*, *285*
Soto, L., 257, *267*
Spangler, G., 277, *284*
Sparber, S. B., 60, 61, 63, *66*
Spear, L. P., 10, 11, *14*, *16*, 74, 76, 77*t*, 78*t*,
    79*t*, 80*t*, 81*t*, 82*t*, 85, 86, 87*t*, 88*t*, 88*t*,
    89, *91*, *92*, *93*, *94*, 131, 132, 149, 154,
    159, *161*, 167, *177*, *178*, 208, 209,
    210, 211, 212, 213*f*, 214*f*, 215, 215*f*,
    216, 217*f*, 218, 219*f*, 220, 221, 222*f*,
    224, *224*, *225*, *226*, *227*, 235, 242,
    243, 244, 245, *247*, *248*, *249*, 254,
    259, *267*, *269*
Spear, N. E., 76, 77*t*, 78*t*, 79*t*, 80*t*, 81*t*, 82*t*,
    86, 87*t*, 88*t*, *92*, *94*, 131, *159*, 167,
    177, *178*, 210, 211, 212, 214*f*, 215,
    215*f*, 216, 217*f*, 218, 219*f*, 220, 221,
    222*f*, 224, *225*, *226*, 244, *247*
Spencer, J. R., 9, *15*
Spencer, P., 42, *53*
Spencer, P. S., 45, 46, *54*
Spielmann, H., 89, *93*
Spierer, A., 336, *351*
Spitz, H. L., 22, *39*
Spitzer, A. R., 235, *247*
Spizzirri, C. L., 274, *284*
Spunger, L. B., 277, *286*
Spunt, B. J., 325, *328*
Spyker, J. M., 50, 50*f*, *55*
Sryne, J. H., 77*t*, 80*t*, 87*t*, *93*
Stack, C. M., 179, *201*, 232, *246*
Stanger, C. L., 312, *329*
Stanton, M. E., 208, 209, *227*, 243, 245, *249*
Steele, B., 164, *177*, 183, 186, 200, *200*, 344,
    353
Steele, B. M., 99, 100*t*, 101, *108*, 241*t*, *247*,
    257, *269*, 306, *328*
Steele, B. W., 335, *349*
Steele, R. E., 318, 319, *332*
Stein, L. I., 113, *124*
Steinberg, M. R., 260, *272*
Steitelberger, F., 44, *53*
Stenberg, C., 274, *283*
Stenmark, D. E., 323, *329*
Stern, D. N., 176, *178*

Stevens, M., 144, *161*, 179, 180, 189, 190,
    201, 307, 309, 310, 312, *331*
Stevens, R., 311, *330*
Stewart, C. W., 9, 10, 12, 13, *17*
Stiles, K. M., 47, *53*
Stoffer, D., 112, *124*, 336, *350*
Stokes, D. L., 77*t*, 80*t*, 87*t*, *94*, 242, *249*
Stokols, D., 339, *353*
Stone, R. K., 24, *37*, 71, *91*, 255, *268*, 309,
    310, 312, 336, *349*
Stone, W. L., 365, *367*
Strauss, M. E., 59, *66*, 179, 180, *201*, 202
Streissguth, A. P., 52, *55*, 111, 112, 113,
    113*n*, 114, 115, 116, 120, 122, *126*,
    127, 131, 141, 142, 143, 144, 149,
    151, 153, 155, *158*, *159*, *160*, *161*,
    162, 183, 186, 199, *200*, 207, 209,
    224, *225*, 227, 255, 272, 307, 311,
    312, *332*, 336, *351*, 357, *368*
Strichartz, G. R., 9, *14*
Stricker, E. M., 44, 44*f*, *55*
Stringer, S. A., 321, *332*
Strittmatter, S. M., 10, *15*
Stromland, K., 151, *162*
Stroufe, L. A., 289, *303*
Strumwasser, S., 265, *267*
Strupp, B. J., 223, *227*
Struthers, J. M., 236, 243, *247*, 258, 272, 337,
    353
Stryker, J. C., 180, 180–181, *201*, *202*
Stump, J., 343, *353*
Succop, P. A., 47, *54*, 113, *125*
Suess, G., 277, *284*
Sullivan, M. C., 34, *38*
Sullivan, M. W., 123, *124*, 169, 170, 171, 172,
    174, 175, 176, *177*, *178*, 258, *267*, 275,
    279, 280, 282, 320, 323, *326*, 337, *349*
Sullivan, T. P., 207, *226*, 307, 309, 310, 312,
    330
Summers, R. J., 11, *15*
Surtees, P. G., 321, *329*
Swann, A. C., 253, *272*
Symanski, R., 357–358, 361, *367*, *368*
Syme, S. L., 322, *326*
SYSTAT, 104, *109*
Szumowski, E. K., 294, *302*

T

Tabachnick, B. G., 119, *127*
Tamis-LeMonda, C. S., 262, *268*, *272*
Tan, S., 237, *246*

Tanafranca, M., 196, 202
Tannenbaum, L., 190, 202
Tanner, P., 8, 16
Tarr, J. E., 24, 39
Taylor, C. I., 319, 329
Taylor, P., 112, 124, 336, 350
Taylor, P. M., 317, 327
Teiling, A. K. Y., 8, 17
Tellegen, A., 34, 37
Templeton, V. H., 107, 109
Tennant, C., 260, 267
Thoman, E. B., 257, 272, 358, 368
Thomas, A., 274, 275, 284, 286
Thomas, K., 179, 201
Thompson, A., 344, 345, 351
Thompson, K., 336, 351
Thompson, W. D., 97, 99, 108
Thrasher, S., 183, 186, 196, 202
Thullen, J., 113, 125
Thurkauf, A., 10, 16
Tikriti, S., 49, 53
Tilak, J. P., 78t, 80t, 87t, 91
Tilden, V. P., 323, 332
Timperi, R., 71, 94, 111, 118, 123, 127, 179, 202, 230–232, 250, 287, 303, 306, 307, 309, 310, 311, 312, 313, 332, 336, 353
Ting, G., 275, 284
Tingelstad, J., 113, 125
Tippett, J., 322, 331
Tippetts, A. S., 145, 161
Todd, R. D., 11, 17
Toloyan, S., 75, 80t, 92
Toth, S. L., 260, 271
Toufexis, A., 336, 353
Towey, J. P., 62, 66
Tracey, K. J., 336, 349
Trivette, C. M., 318, 322, 327
Tronick, E. Z., 22, 23, 26, 30, 31, 34, 38, 39, 155, 162, 306, 319, 327
Trulson, M. E., 234, 249
Tsubaki, F., 49, 55
Tucci, K., 358, 361, 368
Tully, M., 113, 125
Turner, L. M., 77t, 80t, 87t, 94, 242, 249
Tyrala, E. E., 75, 82t, 94
Tyson, J. E., 346, 351
Tytun, A., 336, 351

U

Udom, C. E., 6, 16
Ulissey, M. J., 234, 249

Ulleland, C. N., 336, 351
Ulrey, G. L., 337, 338, 339, 341, 351
Unzner, L., 277, 284
Upshur, C. C., 340, 344, 352
Utarnachitt, D., 198, 201
Utarnachitt, R., 198, 201
Uzuka, M., 145, 161

V

Valcarcel, M., 25, 38
Valdeon, C., 362, 368
Valencia, G., 306, 307, 309, 310, 311, 312, 313, 330
Valentine, J., 9, 10, 12, 13, 17
Van, G. W. G., 265, 267
van der Loos, H., 8, 17
Van Natta, P. A., 319, 327
Vance, S. D., 322, 327
van-de-Bor, M., 239, 249
VanWaes, M., 75, 80t, 92
Varma, D. R., 75, 80t, 92
Vaughn, B., 291, 303
Vega, W. A., 307, 309, 310, 332, 335, 353
Vega-Lahr, N., 319, 328, 361, 367, 368
Vest, T. A., 307, 309, 310, 329
Viadero, D., 336, 353
Vinci, R., 71, 94, 111, 118, 123, 127, 179, 202, 230–232, 250, 263, 270, 287, 303, 305, 306, 307, 309, 310, 311, 312, 313, 328, 332, 335, 338, 350
Vohr, B. R., 25, 38
Volpe, J. J., 22, 26, 39, 130, 132, 153, 162
Vorhees, C. V., 85, 94, 122, 122f, 127, 131, 162
Vosper, H. J., 336, 353, 357, 368

W

Wachs, T. D., 274, 285
Wachsman, L., 154, 162, 237, 239, 246
Waddington, C. H., 32, 39
Waddington, J. L., 53, 55
Wagener, D. K., 317, 327
Wagner, D., 257, 267
Wagner, J. M., 211, 226, 227
Wall, S., 291, 302
Waller, M. B., 336, 353
Walsh, J. H., 336, 351
Walther, F. J., 239, 249

Wandersman, L. P., 318, *328*
Wang, C., 61, *66*
Wang, R. Y., 10, *16*, 82*t*, *93*, 211, 220, *226*, 235, *248*
Warburton, D., 154, *162*, 239, *246*
Ward, C. H., 117*t*, *124*, 319, *326*
Ward, S., 154, *162*
Warren, W. B., 307, 309, 310, 311, 312, *330*
Wasiewski, W. W., 237, *249*
Wasserman, D. R., 260, *272*
Wasserman, E., 179, *202*
Wasserman, W., 60, *66*
Watermaux, C., 113, *124*
Waternaux, C., 47, 52, *53*
Waters, E., 289, 291, *302, 303*
Waters, L. K., 321, *327*
Watkinson, A., 111, 112, *125*
Watkinson, B., 192, *201*
Watson, J. B., 168, *178*
Watson, T., 176, *178*
Wayne, R. H., 180–181, *202*
Weathers, W. T., 307, *332*
Weathersby, E., 155, *160*
Weaver, D. R., 75, 82*t*, *94*
Webb, D., 335, *349*
Webber, M. P., 311, *332*
Webster, W. L., 81*t*, *94*
Webster, W. S., 8, *17*, 75, 81*t*, *94*
Wedgewood, R. J., 60, *66*
Weese-Mayer, D. E., 233, 235, 237, *249*
Weese-Mayer, D. W., 232, *248*
Weinberg, M. K., 155, *162*
Weiss, B., 43, 48, 48*f*, 51, 52, *53, 55*
Weiss, R. D., 264, *271*, 319, *328, 330, 332*
Weissman, M. M., 264, *272*, 318, 319, 320, *330, 332*
Weisstein, C., 265, *270*
Weksberg, R., 102*t*, 103, *108*, 243, *247*
Welch, R., 144, *162*
Welch, R. A., 307, 310, 312, *327*
Wellisch, D. K., 260, *272*
Werner, E. E., 32, *39*
Wessler, R., 117*t*, *126*
West, J., 155, *162*
Westerink, B., 234, *249*
Wharton, G. G., 8, *17*
Wheeden, A., 357–358, 361, 362, *368*
Whitaker-Azmitia, P. M., 11, *14*, 81*t*, *91*, 211, *224*, 254, *267*
White, K., 322, *327*
White, R. W., 176, *178*
Wiesel, T. N., 8, *17*

Wietzman, M., 263, *270*
Wiggins, R. C., 74, 79*t*, *94*
Wilber, C. H., 264, *272*
Willard, J. E., 232, *248*
Willey, S., 336, *349*
Williams, M. T., 319, *332*
Williams-Petersen, M. G., 129, *161*
Wilson, G. S., 58, 59, *65, 66*, 180, *202*, 260, 265, *270*, 288, *303*, 343, 344, *351*
Wilson, J. M., 234, *249*
Wilson, R. S., 275, *285*
Winblad, B., 45, *54*
Windh, R., 240, *247*
Winniford, M. W., 232, *248*
Wippman, J., 289, *303*
Wise, R. A., 25, *39*, 253, *272*
Wise, W. E., 336, *349*
Wobie, K., 325, *332*
Wolfe, H. M., 307, 310, 312, *327*
Wolkind, S., 319, *328*
Woo, M. S., 237, *246*
Wood, R. D., 211, *227*
Woods, J. R., 6, 7, *17*, 255, *272*, 314*t*
Woods, N. S., 99, 100*t*, 101, *109*, 263, *272*, 306, 307, 309, 310, 311, 312, 313, 316, 319, 325, *326, 328, 332*
Woolsey, T. A., 8, *17*
Woolverton, W. L., 234, *247*
World Health Organization, 58, *66*
Wu, P. Y. K., 278, *285*
Wyzga, R. E., 52, *55*

Y

Yablonsky-Alter, E., 235, *249*
Yaffe, H., 355, *368*
Yamashita, T. S., 102*t*, 104, *109*, 111, *127*
Yase, Y., 45, *54*
Yasin, S., 355, *367*
Yee, H., 183, 185, 186, 188, 196, *202*
Yoon, J. J., 24, *39*
Yoottanasumpun, V., 77*t*, 79*t*, 87*t*, 88*t*, *94*, 167, *178*, 212, *226*
Yoshikawa, D., 146, *158*
Yotsumoto, I., 9, *17*
Young, S. L., 336, *353*, 357, *368*

Z

Zajac, C. S., 78*t*, 80*t*, 87*t*, *91*
Zajicek, E., 319, *328*

Zax, M., 34, *37*
Zeanah, C. H., 339, *353*
Zelson, C., 179, *202*
Zeskind, P. S., 25, *38*
Zhang, Z., 46, *55*
Ziedonis, D. M., 319, *332*
Zigmond, M. J., 44, 44*f, 55*
Zimmerman, E., 357–358, 361, *367, 368*
Zimmerman, E. A., 306, *328*
Zimmerman, L. T., 211, *225*
Zingman, T. M., 107, *109*
Zmitrovich, A. C., 62, 65, *66,* 242, *249*

Zubrycki, E. M., 80*t, 92*
Zuckerman, B. S., 19, 22, 26, *38, 39,* 71, 72, *93, 94,* 107, *108,* 111, 112, 118, 123, *126, 127,* 129, 130, 132, 143, 152, 153, 154, 155, 157, *159, 162,* 179, *202,* 207, *227,* 230–232, 233, 238, 240, 241*t,* 242, 245, *247, 248,* 250, 252, 255, 256, 258, 259, 262, *267, 269, 270, 272,* 287, *303,* 305, 306, 307, 309, 310, 311, 312, 313, 319, 320, 324, *328, 331, 332,* 335, 336, 338, *350, 353,* 355, *367*
Zuddas, A., 9, *15*

Subject Index

A

Absolute alcohol per day, 113
Acquired immunodeficiency syndrome, 60–61
Alzheimer's disease, 46
Amyotrophic lateral sclerosis, 45
Amyotrophic lateral sclerosis–Parkinsonism
    dementia, 45–46
Anesthesia, cocaine, 8–9
Animal models, 208–210
    cross-species comparability, 208–209

B

Bayley scales of infant development, 113–115
    apical test, 115
Beck depression inventory, 319
Bingeing, 113
Birth to Three Project, 157
Bonferroni correction, 117
Boston City Hospital, 232
Brazelton neonatal behavioral assessment
    scale, 36–37

C

Cancer, 42–43
Caregiver–infant interaction, 276–277, 306
    compensatory mechanisms, 281
    infant temperament, 280–282

Center for Epidemiologic Studies Depression
    Scale, 320
Central nervous system
    developmental exposure models, 71–90
    hyperexcitability, 64
Children
    prenatal alcohol exposure
        sustained attention deficit, 115
Chronicity, 113
Clarkson, Thomas, 49
CNS, see Central nervous system
Cocaine
    abuse
        history, 251
        mother–infant interaction, 306
        parents, 251–266
        pregnant women, 305–325
        psychosocial, 305–325
    addiction, 252
    anesthetic effects, 8–9
    brain development, 253–256
    CNS stimulant, 71–90, 253
    depression, 318–320
    developmental toxicity, 5–14
    distractibility, 254
    environment issues, 30
    hypoxia, 255
    incipient hazards, 41–53
    infant development effects
        attention and arousal, 252, 257

Cocaine *(Cont.)*
  infant development effects *(Cont.)*
    central nervous system, 252–256
    parental functioning, 252
    parenting impairment, 264
    passive absorption of crack smoke, 263
    pathways, 263–266
    psychiatric disorders, 263–264
    psychopathology, 264
  life stress, 323–324
  locus of control, 321
  maternal drug abuse, 35
  monoaminergic neurotransmitters, 254–255
  poverty, 30, 34–35
  prenatal exposure, *see* Prenatal cocaine
    exposure
  reuptake inhibitor, 5–6
    dopamine, 5–6, 9–11, 253
    norepinephrine, 6, 12–13, 253–255
    serotonin, 5–6, 11–12, 253
  risk assesssment, 41–42
    dose–response assessment, 42, 51
    exposure assessment, 42
    hazard identification, 42, 51
    risk characterization, 42
    risk confirmation, 52
  self-esteem, 321–322
  social support, 321–322
  systemic blood pressure, 8
  teenage mothers, 35
Codeine, 57
Committee on the Aquirement of the Drug
  Habit, 251
Confounder
  definition, 96–98
    main interest association, 97–98
    not an intermediate variable, 98
    outcome condition risk factor, 97
  misclassification, 98–99
  prenatal cocaine exposure research, 95–107
  simulated data set, 104–106
Cross-modal transfer test, 116

D

Depression
  child abuse, 320
  cocaine, 318–320
Dopamine
  homovanillic acid, 234–235
  reuptake inhibition, 5–6, 9–11, 253

F

Family Support Scale, 322
FAS, *see* Fetal alcohol syndrome
Fetal alcohol syndrome, 111–124
Fetal cocaine syndrome, 337
Fluoxetine, 11–12
Fostering-crossfostering design, 84–85

G

General Cognitive Index, 295

H

Heroin, 57
Homovanillic acid, 233–234
Howes Peer Play Scale, 298
Human behavioral teratology, 111
Human immunodeficiency virus, 60
Hypoxia, 6–8, 13, 255

I

Infant
  cocaine effect, 99–104
    confounding, 99
    polydrug exposure, 103
    tobacco smoke exposure, 101–102
  detecting teratogenic effects, 113–117
    Bayley Scales of Infant Development,
      113–115
    fixation duration, 115–116
    processing speed, 116
    reaction time, 115–116
  facial expression, 171–173
  information processing
    arm retraction, 168–169
    emotional responsivity, 172
    learning procedures, 167–174
  prematurity effects, 31–33
    cocaine-exposed, 361–364
    cocaine-exposed vs. nonexposed, 357–361
  temperament, 274–277
    assessment, 274
    caregiver–infant interaction, 276–277,
      280–282
    emotional behavior, 276–277
    learning, 275–276
    pre- and postnatal risk factors, 277–278
    prematurity, 277
    psychological preparedness, 275

Infant, cocaine-exposed, 355–366
emotional responsivity, 175–176
learning, 174
neonatal behavior, 356–357
temperament, 273–282
emotional responsivity, 273
learning, 273
positive vs. negative reactivity, 279
social functioning, 273
Infant Behavior Questionnaire, 279

L

Lead poisoning, 46–48
Levenson Locus of Control Scale, 321
Life experiences survey, 323

M

McCarthy Scales of Children's Abilities, 294–295
Meconium, 232
assay development, 183–187
drug interference, 184–185
gas chromatography/mass spectroscopy, 186–187
intra-assay precision, 184
radioimmunoassay, 183–186
sensitivity/specificity, 184, 191–193
clinical studies, 187–190
drug analysis, 179–200
acute drug exposure, 198
animal studies, 180–183
chronic drug exposure, 198
fatty acid ethyl esters, 198
infant studies, 195–198
maternal hair correlation, 193–194
monkey, 181
nicotine, 195
rat, 181–182
serial, 190–191
Medical complications score, 166
Mental Development Index, 113
Mercury poisoning, see Methylmercury poisoning
Methadone, 57–65
acquired immunodeficiency syndrome, 60–61
animal studies, 60–64
cognitive development, 58
heroin addiction treatment, 57, 59–60
human immunodeficiency virus, 60
pregnancy, 59–60

Methylmercury poisoning, 48–51
cerebral palsy, 49
Michigan alcoholism screening test, 115
MOMS project, 156
Monkey, 181
Morphine, 57
Movement assessment of infants, 103
Mythology of severe risk, 95

N

Naloxone, 62
National Institute on Drug Abuse Household Survey, 20
Neonatal Stress Scale, 356
Norepinephrine
reuptake inhibition, 6, 12–13, 253–255

O

Opioid, 57
withdrawal, 58–59

P

Parental attitudes research instrument, 260
Parkinson's disease, 43–45
PCP, see Phencyclidine
Peabody Picture Vocabulary Test-Revised, 118
Phencyclidine, 287–301
Polydrug use, 30
Postpolio syndrome, 45
Prenatal alcohol exposure, 21, 111–124
dose–response analysis, 120–123
differential susceptibility, 122
thresholds, 121–122
research
confounding influence control, 117–120
exposure assessment, 112–113
maternal self-report, 118–119
multivariate analysis, 119–120
quality of parenting, 118
sample selection, 112–113
Prenatal cocaine exposure
autonomic nervous system activity, 238–240
blood pressure, 239–240
circulating catecholamines, 238–239
brain
electrical activity, 235–236
growth, 230–233
injury, 232–233

Prenatal cocaine exposure *(Cont.)*
  brainstem
    cry analysis, 237–238
    respiratory control, 237
    startle response, 236–237
  child outcome, 19–37
  cognition and behavior, 242–244
    classical conditioning, 243
    conditioned discrimination task, 244
    methodological problems, 242–243
  cognitive function, 207–224
    rat classical conditioning, 212–223
  cohort study, 129–157
  early intervention, 335–348
    ecological framework, 338–339, 344–345
    foster care families, 347–348
    individualized family service plan, 341–344
    inner city, 345–348
    redefinition, 341–343
    re-education, 341, 343–344
    remediation, 341–342
    social support, 346–347
    systems theory, 339–340
    transactional model of development, 340
  emotional behavior, 278–279
  endocrine changes, 240–241
  epidemiology, 20, 307
  fetal effects, 22–26
    action, 23
    affect, 23
    arousal, 23, 25–26
    attention, 23
    brain development, 22
    cry characteristics, 24–25
    direct, 24–26
    Four A's of Infancy, 23
    growth retardation, 24–25
    indirect, 24–26
    neuroregulatory mechanism, 22–23
  human *versus* animal outcome measures,
      231
  infant outcome, 256–259
    arousal regulation, 257–258, 263
    attention, 257
    developmental functioning, 256
    habituation, 257–258
    recognition memory tasks, 258
  infant temperament, 278–279
  neonatal neurobehavioral organization, 241–242
  neurobehavioral outcome survey, 27–30
  neurochemistry, 233–235
    homovanillic acid, 233–234

  neurodevelopmental assessment, 26–27
  neurophysiological effects, 229–245
    levels, 229–230
  parenting environment, 259–263
    aggression, 259
    alcohol abuse, 262
    attachment behavior, 260–261
    consistency, 265
    family discord, 265
    maternal responsiveness, 261–262, 265
    neglect, 260
    physical abuse, 260
  perinatal problems, 311–313
    matched sample outcome, 313–316
    socioeceonomic status, 312
  pharmacology, 21–22
  preschool-age children, 287–301
    attachment quality, 290–293, 299–300
    attention, 288
    cognition, 288
    compliance, 295, 298
    follow-up assessment, 293–297
    insensitivity, 298
    IQ scores, 288
    maternal addiction, 289
    parent frustration threshold, 296
    peer relations, 289–290, 298–299
    social skill problems, 300
    spontaneous play, 290–294
    structured delay task, 294
  research, 72–73
    animal models, 73
    behavior teratologic experiments, 75–83
    confounding problem, 95–107
    cross-sectional *versus* longitudinal, 338
    dose rate, 88–90
    exposure periods, 73–74
    exposure routes, 74–76
    fostering-crossfostering design, 84–85
    maternal factors, 85–86
    nutrition, 83–84
    rat, 83–90
  rural population
    longitudinal study, 316–318
    psychosocial assessments, 318
  sociodemographic and lifestyle differences,
      307–311
    age, 307–309
    education, 309
    elective abortions, 310
    gravidity/parity, 310
    marital status, 309

polydrug use, 309–310
prenatal care, 310
race, 309
sexually transmitted disease, 311
socioeconomic status, 309
weight gain, 310
studies, 163–176
confounding variables, 164, 337
drug use identification, 163
intraventricular hemorrhage, 165–166
IQ, 164–165
measures, 164–167
methodological problems, 28, 129–157
toxicology assays, 20–21
hair analysis, 20
meconium, 20
self-report, 20–21, 29
urine analysis, 20, 29
Prenatal PCP exposure, 287–301
Psychomotor Development Index, 113

Q

Quinpirole, 10

R

Radioimmunoassay of postpartum maternal
hair, *see* RIAH
Rall, David, 41
Rat
behavioral teratologic research, 83–90
hypoxia, 6–8
meconium, 181–182
prenatal cocaine exposure, 210–224
behavioral alterations, 211
classical conditioning task, 212–223
cognitive alterations, 212–223
conditional discrimination task, 218
gender-specific, 219–221
heart-rate orienting response, 221–223
neural alterations, 211
reversal performance deficit, 218–220
sensory pre-conditioning, 216–218
RIAH, 144–148
self-reporting correlation, 145–147
Rosenberg Self-Esteem Scale, 321–322

S

Seattle cocaine and pregnancy study, 130–157

follow-up cohort, 138–141
demographics, 139–140
hypotheses, 131–132
prenatal substance exposure, 142–148
confounding, 152–153
data analysis, 152
data collection, 149–151
development over time, 148–155
individual differences, 153–154
long-term consequences, 154–155
measurement methods, 143–145
meconium, 144
RIAH, 144–148
self-reporting, 143
urine analysis, 143
public health policy, 155–157
birth to three project, 157
MOMS project, 156
sample maintenance, 141–142
sample selection, 131–132, 133
demographic subgroups, 135
hospital screening questionnaire,
133–137, 143
postpartum maternal interview, 137, 143
recruiting subjects, 133
self-reporting, 135
sample stratification, 137–138
Serotonin
reuptake inhibition, 5–6, 11–12, 253
Synaptogenesis, 254

T

Thalidomide, 42
Toddler
cocaine effect, 99–104
confounding, 99
polydrug exposure, 103
tobacco smoke exposure, 101–102

V

Visual recognition memory test, 116

W

Women
cocaine use, 305–325
low socioeconomic status, 305